The Future of Pharma Across All Sectors in the Artificial Intelligence Era

Next Generation Technology Driven Personalized Medicine and Smart Healthcare Series

The Future of Pharma Across All Sectors in the Artificial Intelligence Era

Edited by

Miltiadis Lytras
Computer Science Department, College of Engineering, Effat University, Jeddah, Saudi Arabia

Ahmed M. Shaman
Research and Innovation Institute, Ministry of Defense Health Services, Riyadh, Saudi Arabia

Patricia Ordonez de Pablos
Department of Business Administration, The University of Oviedo, Oviedo, Spain

Paraskevi Papadopoulou
Department of Natural Sciences, Deree-The American College of Greece, Athens, Greece

Sofia Konstantinopoulou
Pulmonary Medicine, Division of Pediatrics, Sheikh Khalifa Medical City, PureHealth, Abu Dhabi, United Arab Emirates; Adjunct Assistant Professor of Pediatrics, Khalifa University, Abu Dhabi, United Arab Emirates

Sarah Abdulrahman Alajlan
Clinical Pharmacy Department, Almaarefa University, Riyadh, Saudi Arabia

Series Editors

Miltiadis Lytras
Patricia Ordonez de Pablos

ELSEVIER

ACADEMIC PRESS
An imprint of Elsevier

Academic Press is an imprint of Elsevier
125 London Wall, London EC2Y 5AS, United Kingdom
50 Hampshire Street, 5th Floor, Cambridge, MA 02139, United States

ISBN: 978-0-443-40572-3

For Information on all Academic Press publications
visit our website at https://www.elsevier.com/books-and-journals

Publisher: Megan Ball
Acquisitions Editor: Linda Buschman
Editorial Project Manager: Soumya Yadav
Production Project Manager: Aishwarya R.
Cover Designer: Arumugam Kothandan

Printed in England by CPI Group (UK) Ltd
Croydon CR0 4YY
United Kingdom

Typeset by MPS Limited, Chennai, India

Contents

List of contributors

Sarah Abdulrahman Alajlan Clinical Pharmacy Department, AlMaarefa University, Riyadh, Saudi Arabia

Huda Aldhanhani Pediatric Infectious Diseases Consultant, Sheikh Khalifa Medical City, SEHA, PureHealth, Abu Dhabi, United Arab Emirates

Luluh Aldhubayi College of Computer and Information Sciences, King Saud University, Riyadh, Saudi Arabia; AI Center of Advanced Studies (Thakaa), King Saud University, Riyadh, Saudi Arabia

Hani Alhashmi Senior Medical Director, Pfizer Saudi Arabia, Riyadh, Saudi Arabia; Medical Affairs, Pfizer Biopharmaceuticals, Riyadh, Saudi Arabia

Mohammed Alhefzi College of Medicine, Alfaisal University, Riyadh, Saudi Arabia; Saudi Association for Health Informatics (SAHI), Riyadh, Saudi Arabia

Lamyaa Munahi AlQahtani Faculty of Pharmaceutical Sciences graduate, Monash University, Melbourne, VIC, Australia

Babar Bashir Chaudhri Department of Cardiac and Thoracic Surgery, King's College Hospital London, Dubai, United Arab Emirates

Patricia Ordonez de Pablos Department of Business Administration, The University of Oviedo, Oviedo, Spain

Islam Elsaeed Hassan Elkholy Learning & Development, International Coaching Federation, Riyadh, Riyadh, Saudi Arabia

Sofia Konstantinopoulou Pulmonary Medicine, Division of Pediatrics, Sheikh Khalifa Medical City, PureHealth, Abu Dhabi, United Arab Emirates; Adjunct Assistant Professor of Pediatrics, Khalifa University, Abu Dhabi, United Arab Emirates

Chaido-Charalampia Lytra Medical School, University of Patras, Patras, Greece

Miltiadis Lytras Computer Science Department, College of Engineering, Effat University, Jeddah, Saudi Arabia

Paraskevi Papadopoulou Department of Natural Sciences, Deree-The American College of Greece, Athens, Greece

Kantiana Patra Statistics and Insurance Science at the University of Piraeus, Piraeus, Greece; The American College of Greece, Athens, Greece

Abdullah Saeed Ministry of Health, Abha, Asir, Saudi Arabia

Constantine A. Stratakis Research Institute, HCA Hospital for Endocrine Surgery, Tampa, FL, United States; ASTREA Health, Athens, Greece; Medical Genetics, H. Dunant Hospital, Athens, Greece; IMBB, FORTH, Human Genetics and Precision Medicine, Heraklion, Greece; Pediatrics, University of Athens Medical School, Athens, Greece

Khizra Sultana King Saud Bin Abdulaziz University for Health Sciences (KSAU-HS), Riyadh, Saudi Arabia; Ministry of National Guard Health Affairs, Riyadh, Saudi Arabia; King Abdullah International Medical Research Center (KAIMRC), Clinical Trial Management, Riyadh, Saudi Arabia

Preface

The pharmaceutical sector is undergoing a structural transformation in which advances in artificial intelligence (AI), data science, automation, digital health, and computational biology are progressively integrated with established scientific, clinical, regulatory, and organizational processes. This transformation is not adequately understood as the adoption of a new generation of technical tools. It is better interpreted as a reconfiguration of how pharmaceutical knowledge is produced, validated, governed, translated into therapeutic interventions, and sustained across the full lifecycle of medicines and health technologies. The significance of AI therefore extends beyond improvements in prediction, classification, or operational efficiency; it concerns the evolving architecture of evidence, decision-making, accountability, and value creation across pharmaceutical and healthcare systems.

The contributions assembled in this volume examine this transition from complementary scientific and sectoral perspectives. They address the changing foundations of pharmaceutical research and development, the emergence of AI-enabled analytics, new models of drug discovery and clinical research, the implications of digital technologies for manufacturing and supply networks, and the growing importance of data-intensive approaches in diagnostics, medical devices, precision medicine, pharmacovigilance, and patient engagement. The volume also considers domains that are sometimes treated separately from the core discussion of AI, including generic medicines and biosimilars, over-the-counter products, access to healthcare, workforce development, and global health. Bringing these domains into a common analytical frame is important because technological transformation in pharma does not occur uniformly. Different sectors operate under distinct scientific uncertainties, regulatory requirements, economic constraints, infrastructures, and patterns of professional responsibility. The consequences of AI adoption must therefore be evaluated in relation to the institutional context in which particular systems are designed and used.

A central theme of this book is the transformation of evidence generation. Pharmaceutical science has historically depended on carefully structured experimental and clinical evidence, supported by rigorous procedures for validation, reproducibility, quality assurance, and regulatory review. AI introduces new possibilities for integrating heterogeneous data, identifying patterns at scales that exceed conventional analytical methods, supporting trial design and patient stratification, generating or synthesizing evidence, and linking clinical research more closely with real-world data. At the same time, these capabilities introduce methodological questions that cannot be resolved by computational performance alone. Data provenance, representativeness, model validity, interpretability, reproducibility, and the stability of results across populations and settings remain fundamental scientific concerns. The appropriate role of AI is therefore not to displace the epistemic standards of pharmaceutical research, but to extend analytical capacity while preserving the principles through which reliable evidence is distinguished from technically plausible output.

The same principle applies to decision-making across the pharmaceutical value chain. As algorithms contribute to target identification, molecule design, clinical development, manufacturing, regulatory intelligence, safety surveillance, and personalized treatment, the boundary between computational recommendation and accountable professional judgment becomes increasingly significant. This raises questions concerning responsibility, escalation, auditability, and human oversight. In highly regulated environments, a technically accurate model may still be unsuitable if its operation cannot be adequately explained, monitored, validated, or situated within a clear framework of decision rights. The future of AI-enabled pharma consequently depends as much on governance capability as on computational capability. Responsible adoption requires institutions to align technical innovation with quality systems, regulatory expectations, ethical obligations, organizational maturity, and the protection of patient interests.

The volume accordingly gives sustained attention to governance, ethics, trust, and equity. AI systems may reproduce or amplify biases embedded in training data; large-scale data integration can create new challenges for privacy and consent; advanced technologies may widen inequalities between well-resourced and resource-constrained health systems; and automation may alter professional roles in ways that require substantial investment in education and reskilling. These are not secondary considerations to be addressed after innovation has occurred. They are constitutive dimensions of technological design and implementation. Transparency, fairness, data stewardship, cybersecurity, accountability, and meaningful human oversight must be treated as part of the scientific and organizational architecture of AI-enabled pharma. Trust among patients, clinicians, researchers, regulators, and society cannot be assumed as a consequence of technical sophistication; it must be established through demonstrable reliability, explainability, institutional responsibility, and ethical consistency.

Another recurring concern is the relationship between technological capability and organizational transformation. Pharmaceutical organizations may possess advanced analytics or AI tools without achieving corresponding improvements in research productivity, clinical outcomes, regulatory performance, or patient value. Sustainable transformation requires more than isolated pilots. It depends on interoperable data environments, coherent operating models, appropriate governance structures, leadership capable of evaluating technological uncertainty, and a workforce that can collaborate across disciplinary boundaries. Scientists, clinicians, pharmacists, engineers, data specialists, regulatory professionals, and managers increasingly work within shared decision environments in which domain expertise and computational expertise are interdependent. The development of AI literacy and continuous professional learning is therefore a strategic requirement, not merely a training activity.

The long-term perspective adopted throughout the volume is intentionally cautious about technological determinism. The direction of pharmaceutical innovation will not be determined by the availability of more powerful algorithms alone. It will be shaped by choices about evidence standards, institutional design, investment priorities, regulation, access, professional responsibility, and the distribution of benefits and risks. Emerging capabilities in generative AI, digital twins, synthetic biology, advanced automation, connected health technologies, and other computational approaches may substantially alter the organization of pharmaceutical research and care, but their contribution will depend on the extent to which they are integrated into scientifically defensible and socially legitimate systems. Future scenarios for the sector should therefore be understood as contingent pathways rather than inevitable outcomes.

The broader purpose of this volume is to support a more integrated understanding of this transition. The chapters collectively position AI within the scientific, organizational, regulatory, and societal systems that give pharmaceutical innovation its meaning and legitimacy. They also emphasize that progress should be assessed not by the quantity of technology deployed, but by the quality of the evidence produced, the soundness of the decisions supported, the safety and equity of the outcomes achieved, and the capacity of institutions to remain accountable as technologies evolve.

We offer this volume in the belief that the most consequential question for the future of pharma is not how rapidly AI can be adopted, but how wisely it can be integrated into the practices through which medicines are discovered, evaluated, produced, governed, and delivered to society. If this book contributes to more rigorous inquiry, more responsible innovation, and more thoughtful collaboration across the scientific and professional communities shaping that future, it will have fulfilled its purpose.

Miltiadis Lytras, Ahmed M. Shaman, Patricia Ordonez de Pablos, Paraskevi Papadopoulou, Sofia Konstantinopoulou, and Sarah Abdulrahman Alajlan

CHAPTER 1

Introduction: navigating the complex landscape of pharma in times of artificial intelligence

Miltiadis Lytras[1] and Patricia Ordonez de Pablos[2]

[1]Computer Science Department, College of Engineering, Effat University, Jeddah, Saudi Arabia,
[2]Department of Business Administration, The University of Oviedo, Oviedo, Spain

1.1 Key challenges in the pharma industry

1.1.1 The complex environment of modern pharma

The pharmaceutical industry has historically played a critical role in global public health. However, it now operates within an increasingly complex environment shaped by numerous economic, scientific, technological, and regulatory pressures. The global pharmaceutical market was valued at approximately USD 1.48 trillion in 2022 and is projected to exceed USD 2 trillion by 2030. This growth is fueled by rising healthcare demands, an aging population, increased prevalence of chronic diseases, and technological innovation. Yet, behind this growth lies an ecosystem marked by significant operational, ethical, and strategic challenges (Blanco-García, 2020; Coucke, 2021; García-García & Rius-Tarruella, 2025; Hong et al., 2024; Marasigan et al., 2020; Rocha et al., 2020; Seewald et al., 2020).

Pharmaceutical firms face growing difficulties in sustaining innovation while managing escalating research and development (R&D) costs. Estimates suggest it costs between USD 1.5 to 2.8 billion to bring a new drug to market, with timelines extending beyond 10 years. The probability of success remains low, with only 10%–15% of compounds entering clinical trials receiving regulatory approval. Additionally, companies must navigate extensive regulatory frameworks and increasing scrutiny around drug pricing, access, transparency, and supply chain resilience.

Table 1.1 outlines the **five most critical challenges** currently facing the pharmaceutical industry.

These challenges are not isolated; rather, they are interconnected and cumulative. For example, supply chain instability directly impacts both R&D continuity and drug

The Future of Pharma Across All Sectors in the Artificial Intelligence Era. DOI: https://doi.org/10.1016/B978-0-443-40572-3.00011-3

Table 1.1 Major challenges in the pharmaceutical industry.

Challenge area	Description
High R&D costs	Long, expensive drug development cycles with high risk of failure.
Regulatory complexity	Diverse and evolving global regulations requiring full compliance.
Supply chain disruptions	Vulnerabilities exposed by global crises (e.g., COVID-19) and geopolitical risks.
Pricing and affordability	Increasing scrutiny over high prices and the need for equitable access.
Personalization and AI gaps	Rising demand for personalized medicine amid slow AI integration in legacy systems.

affordability, while regulatory delays increase costs and reduce access. AI presents a pathway to address many of these issues, but integration remains inconsistent across organizations.

1.1.2 Market trends and disruptive forces

Several disruptive trends are shaping the future of pharma, with AI, big data, precision medicine, and real-world evidence (RWE) analytics at the forefront. Emerging technologies are enabling pharma companies to make smarter, faster, and more informed decisions—but only if they adapt quickly enough. Traditional siloed processes and rigid hierarchies within firms pose internal barriers to agile innovation.

Regulatory expectations are also evolving. Agencies such as the U.S. Food and Drug Administration (FDA) and European Medicines Agency are increasingly encouraging digital transformation, transparency in clinical trial data, and the adoption of RWE in decision-making. Additionally, global shifts toward value-based care, patient-centered models, and sustainability require pharma to reconsider their entire operational and strategic approach (Abdallah & Nizamuddin, 2023; Charitou et al., 2024; Gavriilidis et al., 2021; Heinrich et al., 2024; Hock et al., 2021; Ladner et al., 2025; Pörtner et al., 2025; Sim et al., 2022; Sowndharya et al., 2025; Stagi et al., 2021; Taifa & Nzowa, 2025; Wang et al., 2024).

Table 1.2 highlights **transformational forces** that intersect with the industry's challenges and are paving the way for a new AI-driven landscape.

These trends reflect a move from traditional "product-centered" pharma toward a "patient-centric, data-driven" paradigm. This shift requires not just technology, but cultural and structural transformation within companies. The challenges and transformative forces discussed above underscore a critical reality: the pharmaceutical sector must evolve rapidly to survive and thrive in the AI era. This evolution requires a deep understanding of the **pharmaceutical value chain**—from R&D and manufacturing to distribution and post-marketing surveillance. In the next section, we explore this value chain in detail and examine how AI can optimize each stage of the pharma lifecycle.

Table 1.2 Transformational trends in pharma.

Trend	Impact on industry
Digital therapeutics & mobile apps	Shifting drug development and patient engagement toward digital and hybrid models.
Artificial intelligence (AI)	Enabling automation, predictive modeling, and smart R&D prioritization.
Real-world evidence	Expanding data sources beyond clinical trials to include observational and registry data.
Personalized medicine	Driving demand for AI-driven diagnostics and targeted therapies.
Regulatory science and AI oversight	Increasing focus on ethical, explainable AI for health applications.

This chapter contributes an integrated framework linking AI use cases to adoption maturity, governance requirements, and cross-sector ecosystem strategy in pharma.

1.2 The pharma value chain—processes, roles, and responsibilities

Understanding the pharmaceutical value chain is essential for grasping how the industry operates and identifying opportunities for AI-driven transformation. From early-stage discovery to patient delivery, the value chain encompasses a range of complex, interdependent functions. Each stage demands strategic coordination, regulatory compliance, and scientific excellence (Gavriilidis et al., 2021; Hey et al., 2024; Seewald et al., 2020; Stagi et al., 2024; Wang et al., 2024; Wölfle et al., 2025; Xu et al., 2022; Yoshiura et al., 2025).

1.2.1 Key processes in the pharma value chain

The pharma value chain (see Table 1.3) comprises a series of stages that collectively ensure the development, manufacturing, distribution, and monitoring of medications. These stages include:

1. **Drug discovery and preclinical research**: Identification of potential drug candidates through high-throughput screening, target validation, and early safety assessments in vitro and in vivo. AI is already playing a pivotal role here by enabling computational chemistry and predictive toxicology.
2. **Clinical trials (Phases I–III)**: Assessment of safety, efficacy, dosing, and side effects in human populations. This phase is resource-intensive and highly regulated. AI and digital tools are now streamlining recruitment, monitoring, and data analysis.
3. **Regulatory submission and approval**: Submission of detailed data to health authorities such as the FDA, EMA, or SFDA (Saudi Food and Drug Authority). This process requires strict adherence to compliance protocols.

Table 1.3 Overview of the pharmaceutical value chain and AI opportunities.

Stage	Core function	AI/tech opportunities
Discovery and preclinical	Molecule identification and early research	Target prediction, virtual screening, toxicity forecasting
Clinical Trials	Testing drug candidates on humans	Patient recruitment, trial monitoring, predictive analytics
Regulatory affairs	Drug approval and compliance	Automated submissions, compliance monitoring, document analytics
Manufacturing	Drug production and quality assurance	Predictive maintenance, digital twins, process optimization
Distribution and logistics	Supply chain coordination and delivery	Inventory forecasting, smart logistics, cold chain monitoring
Marketing and sales	Stakeholder engagement and market education	Sentiment analysis, HCP profiling, chatbots
Post-market surveillance	Long-term monitoring and feedback	Real-world data analysis, adverse event detection

4. **Manufacturing and quality control**: Large-scale production of drugs under Good Manufacturing Practice (GMP). AI can support predictive maintenance, automation, and batch monitoring.
5. **Distribution and supply chain management**: Ensuring timely delivery of medications through global networks. Supply chains must be resilient, secure, and transparent.
6. **Marketing, sales, and medical affairs**: Includes product launch, education of healthcare professionals, and pharmacovigilance (drug safety monitoring). Natural language processing (NLP) and CRM tools are being used here.
7. **Post-market surveillance (Phase IV)**: Long-term safety and efficacy monitoring, including RWE and feedback integration.

Each node of this value chain offers specific entry points for digital transformation. AI can help reduce development costs, optimize timelines, and improve patient outcomes—provided that the right data infrastructure and governance systems are in place.

1.2.2 Critical roles and stakeholders across the value chain

Multiple actors contribute to the functioning of the pharmaceutical industry. These include:

- **Research scientists and R&D specialists**: Drive discovery and innovation.
- **Clinical research associates**: Monitor and coordinate trials on the ground.
- **Regulatory affairs specialists**: Ensure compliance with national and international standards.
- **Manufacturing technicians and engineers**: Maintain production quality and scalability.

- **Pharmacovigilance experts**: Monitor post-market safety and adverse reactions.
- **Medical science liaisons**: Serve as key communicators between pharma and medical communities.
- **Data scientists and AI engineers**: Enable the transformation of traditional pipelines into intelligent systems.

In AI-powered environments, these roles are evolving. Data fluency, ethical AI knowledge, and digital tool proficiency are becoming mandatory competencies for pharma professionals. While the pharmaceutical value chain is deeply complex, it is also full of opportunity. As AI technologies evolve, they are reshaping each segment—from discovery to delivery. The next section explores the **AI ecosystem in pharma**, identifying the core technologies, subindustries, and players that are redefining the sector.

1.3 The AI ecosystem of pharma—subindustries, technologies, and players

The integration of artificial intelligence (AI) into the pharmaceutical industry is not simply an incremental improvement—it represents a structural transformation of how the sector operates. From molecular synthesis to patient engagement, AI is enabling precision, personalization, and speed across all functions. In this section, we examine the ecosystem of AI in pharma by focusing on key subindustries, core AI technologies, and influential players shaping the future of healthcare innovation.

1.3.1 AI evolution in pharma: from tool to strategic enabler

In the early 2000s, AI's role in pharma was limited to data mining and rudimentary predictive analytics. However, recent advances in computational power, algorithmic efficiency, and access to massive healthcare datasets have positioned AI as a strategic enabler. Pharma companies are no longer exploring AI as a pilot—they are embedding it into core operations.

Key developments include:

- **Deep learning**: Used in image recognition, compound screening, and protein folding.
- **NLP**: Facilitates the analysis of clinical documents, medical records, and regulatory submissions.
- **Reinforcement learning**: Applied in drug optimization and adaptive clinical trials.
- **Generative AI and foundation models**: Accelerate synthetic molecule generation and hypothesis testing.

AI is no longer an isolated IT solution. It is embedded in the strategic operating model of leading pharma enterprises, requiring alignment between data science, domain expertise, and regulatory understanding.

Table 1.4 AI-driven transformation in Pharma subindustries.

Subindustry	AI-driven transformation
Drug discovery	Predictive compound screening, in silico trials, AI-generated molecules
Clinical development	Automated monitoring, adaptive trial design, ePROs
Medical imaging and diagnostics	AI-assisted diagnosis, anomaly detection in scans
Manufacturing and supply chain	Digital twins, production optimization, real-time monitoring
Pharmacovigilance	Signal detection, adverse event monitoring
Sales and commercial operations	Predictive sales targeting, AI-powered CRM, chatbots
Regulatory and compliance	Automated documentation review, compliance risk prediction

Table 1.5 Core AI technologies and their strategic applications in pharma.

Technology	Application area	Example use case
Machine learning	Drug discovery, trial analytics	Predictive toxicology, trial dropout prediction
Natural language processing	Medical affairs, compliance	Literature mining, regulatory document analysis
Computer vision	Diagnostics, manufacturing	AI interpretation of pathology scans
Generative AI	Research and development	Novel molecule design, scenario simulations
Digital twins	Manufacturing, patient modeling	Production simulation, digital patient avatars
Federated learning	Multicenter trials, real-world data	Privacy-preserving analysis of decentralized datasets

1.3.2 Subindustries benefiting from AI in pharma

AI's impact transcends traditional silos in pharma (see Table 1.4). Several subindustries and functional areas are experiencing rapid transformation:

Each subindustry has distinct AI use cases, but all benefit from shared infrastructure: robust datasets, scalable cloud computing, and regulatory-grade audit trails.

1.3.3 Prominent AI technologies shaping pharma

Several core technologies (see Table 1.5) form the backbone of AI transformation in pharma:

- **Machine learning**—Enables data-driven decision-making, pattern recognition, and process automation.
- **Computer vision**—Assists in pathology, radiology, and visual inspection of compounds.
- **Natural language generation**—Automatically generates trial summaries and regulatory documents.

- **Digital twins**—Simulated models of manufacturing systems, patient profiles, or supply chains.
- **Federated learning**–Facilitates secure and decentralized data modeling across institutions, preserving privacy.

The convergence of these technologies allows pharma to innovate at unprecedented speed and scale—provided that integration is guided by ethical, secure, and evidence-based practices.

1.3.4 Key industry players and startups driving the ecosystem

Several organizations are leading the AI transformation in pharma. These include both large multinational corporations and specialized startups:

- **Large pharma innovators**:
- **Pfizer**: Deploys AI in drug repurposing and digital trials.
- **Novartis**: Partnered with Microsoft for AI-driven innovation platforms.
- **AstraZeneca**: Leverages AI in target identification and patient stratification.
- **Tech Giants**:
- **IBM Watson Health**: Formerly a pioneer in oncology AI (divested in 2022).
- **Google DeepMind**: Revolutionized protein folding with AlphaFold.
- **Amazon Web Services (AWS)**: Provides cloud-based AI infrastructure for pharma.
- **AI-Focused Startups**:
- **Insilico Medicine**: AI-powered drug discovery and biomarker identification.
- **BenevolentAI**: Knowledge graphs and predictive analytics in early-stage R&D.
- **Owkin**: Federated learning in clinical research, particularly in oncology.

Strategic insight: Collaboration between pharma, AI startups, and cloud tech providers is crucial. No single actor can address all challenges alone.

The AI ecosystem in pharma is expanding across multiple dimensions—technological, organizational, and operational. However, its greatest promise lies in transforming how research and development are executed. The next section explores **AI's role in core pharmaceutical R&D areas**, highlighting real-world use cases and future opportunities.

1.4 State of the art: artificial intelligence in the pharmaceutical industry

The scientific literature on AI in the pharmaceutical industry has expanded rapidly over the past decade, reflecting both the growing maturity of AI technologies and the increasing strategic urgency facing pharma organizations. Contemporary research converges on a shared conclusion: AI is no longer an experimental or peripheral technology in pharma, but a foundational enabler of digital transformation across discovery, development, regulation, commercialization, and patient engagement.

1.4.1 AI as a transformational force across the pharma lifecycle

A dominant stream of research emphasizes AI's end-to-end impact across the pharmaceutical value chain. Reviews and empirical studies consistently demonstrate that machine learning, deep learning, and data-driven modeling significantly accelerate drug discovery by enabling rapid screening of large compound libraries, predicting drug–target interactions, and optimizing lead compound selection (Kolluri et al., 2022; Selvaraj et al., 2022; Tiwari et al., 2023). These advances address one of pharma's most persistent challenges: high R&D costs combined with low clinical success rates.

Beyond discovery, AI-driven analytics increasingly shape clinical development. Studies highlight AI's role in patient stratification, adaptive trial design, synthetic control arms, and real-time monitoring, enabling more efficient and ethical trials (Kaitin, 2019; Malheiro et al., 2025; Sankar & Alam, 2024). Collectively, this body of work signals a shift from static, protocol-driven trials toward data-adaptive clinical experimentation.

1.4.2 From digital tools to strategic digital transformation

More recent scholarship moves beyond technical use cases to frame AI as a **strategic driver of pharmaceutical digital transformation**. Harrer et al. (2024) and Miozza (2025) argue that AI adoption is inseparable from cloud computing, big data, and organizational readiness, positioning AI as a catalyst for new operating models, digital health offerings, and ecosystem-based innovation. This perspective reframes AI not as an isolated capability, but as a core element of pharma's strategic architecture.

The literature also highlights AI's growing role in downstream activities such as pharmaceutical marketing, sales, and patient engagement. AI-enabled commercial analytics, behavioral modeling, and personalization strategies are transforming how pharma organizations interact with healthcare professionals and patients, improving engagement while raising new governance challenges (Khanna et al., 2020; Sabapathy, 2025).

1.4.3 Data foundations and the centrality of FAIR principles

A critical enabling theme across the state of the art is data quality and governance. Research strongly emphasizes that AI performance in pharma is constrained less by algorithmic sophistication than by data fragmentation, poor interoperability, and limited reuse of research outputs. The implementation of FAIR (findable, accessible, interoperable, reusable) data principles is repeatedly identified as a prerequisite for scalable AI adoption (Wise et al., 2019). FAIR-aligned data infrastructures enable AI systems to learn across studies, organizations, and RWE sources, accelerating innovation while supporting reproducibility and regulatory confidence.

1.4.4 Ethical, legal, and regulatory dimensions

A substantial and growing body of literature focuses on the ethical, legal, and regulatory implications of AI in pharma. Multiple studies underline that trust, transparency, and accountability are decisive factors for successful AI deployment (Abramova et al., 2025). Key concerns include algorithmic bias, data privacy, explainability, and compliance with regulations such as GDPR and emerging AI governance frameworks.

Explainable AI (XAI) emerges as a particularly critical theme in regulated environments. Research shows that interpretability is not merely a technical preference but a regulatory necessity, especially for GxP validation, regulatory submissions, and clinical decision support (Nair, 2025). Without explainability, AI systems risk regulatory rejection and organizational mistrust.

Legal scholarship further highlights unresolved challenges around intellectual property rights, liability, and ownership of AI-generated inventions. The convergence of software, medical devices, and pharmaceuticals—accelerated by AI—demands new regulatory and IP frameworks capable of addressing hybrid innovations (Lal et al., 2024; Opderbeck, 2019).

1.4.5 Toward patient-centric and personalized pharma

Finally, the state of the art reflects a decisive shift toward patient-centric and personalized medicine. AI-enabled pharmacogenomics, digital biomarkers, and real-world data analytics support tailored therapies, improved adherence, and outcome-driven care models (Dovzhuk et al., 2025; Serrano et al., 2024). This transition aligns pharmaceutical innovation more closely with societal expectations for equity, transparency, and value-based healthcare.

1.4.6 Synthesis and research gap

Taken together, the literature establishes AI as a transformative force reshaping pharma's scientific, operational, and strategic foundations. However, a critical gap remains: while technical capabilities are advancing rapidly, organizational integration, governance maturity, and ethical alignment often lag behind. The most advanced studies increasingly call for **holistic frameworks** that integrate AI technologies with data governance, regulatory strategy, human capital development, and ecosystem collaboration. Addressing this gap is essential for translating AI potential into sustainable pharmaceutical innovation.

1.5 Core AI-powered R&D domains in pharma

The R&D function lies at the heart of pharmaceutical innovation. In this section, we delve into how AI is revolutionizing each phase of the pharmaceutical R&D pipeline—from drug discovery to clinical validation and beyond (see Table 1.6). AI not only accelerates timelines

Table 1.6 AI-enhanced functions across pharma R&D lifecycle.

R&D stage	AI capability	Impact
Target discovery	ML-driven pattern recognition from omics data	Faster identification of viable targets
Lead compound generation	Generative AI to design novel molecules	Larger candidate pools, optimized pharmacodynamics
Preclinical toxicology	Predictive toxicology modeling	Reduced late-stage attrition and ethical gains
Clinical trials	Adaptive trial design, digital twins	Reduced cost, better patient outcomes
Regulatory affairs	NLP and RPA (robotic process automation) for documents	Faster, more accurate submission and compliance

and reduces costs but also brings new methodologies that shift the very paradigm of research in the life sciences.

1.5.1 Drug discovery and target identification

AI enables rapid hypothesis generation and testing at a scale unimaginable in traditional drug discovery models.

- **Target discovery**: AI models analyze genomic, proteomic, and metabolomic data to suggest viable drug targets. Algorithms can identify biomarkers and pathways with high therapeutic potential.
- **Compound generation**: Deep learning models such as variational autoencoders and generative adversarial networks design novel drug-like molecules with optimized pharmacokinetics and reduced toxicity.
- **High-throughput screening**: AI prioritizes compounds for laboratory screening, dramatically reducing wet-lab experimentation.

Example: DeepMind's AlphaFold has enabled accurate protein structure prediction, streamlining target validation and design.

1.5.2 Preclinical development and safety profiling

AI tools are increasingly integrated into animal testing and in silico modeling.

- **Toxicology prediction**: Machine learning algorithms predict adverse events and organ toxicity based on chemical structure and exposure models.
- **In silico simulations**: Virtual organ models and pharmacokinetic simulations replace some in vivo testing, making preclinical phases faster and more ethical.

AI reduces the need for animal models and ensures better selection of viable compounds.

1.5.3 Clinical trial design and optimization

One of the most transformative areas of AI in pharma R&D lies in clinical trials:

- **Patient stratification**: NLP and ML mine EHRs (electronic health records) to identify trial-eligible patients and predict their response based on genetic and demographic markers.
- **Protocol optimization**: AI evaluates previous trial data to suggest trial endpoints, population size, and site selection, reducing failure rates and improving ROI.
- **Synthetic control arms**: Instead of traditional placebo groups, AI generates matched virtual cohorts using historical data—boosting ethics and efficiency.

1.5.4 Biomarker discovery and companion diagnostics

AI models help uncover molecular and digital biomarkers that indicate disease progression or therapeutic efficacy.

- **Omics data integration**: AI integrates transcriptomics, metabolomics, and epigenetic data to identify actionable biomarkers.
- **RWE**: AI analyzes data from wearable devices and mobile apps to create digital biomarkers used in companion diagnostics.

1.5.5 Regulatory submission and compliance automation

Regulatory processes are increasingly being assisted by AI:

- **Document automation**: NLP-based systems extract and organize regulatory data for submission.
- **Clinical narrative generation**: NLG (Natural Language Generation) automates the drafting of clinical summaries, helping reduce submission timelines.

Pharma R&D is evolving from a sequential, siloed model to a data-integrated, AI-augmented system. Algorithms now inform decisions that were once based solely on human judgment, enhancing reproducibility, minimizing bias, and accelerating development timelines. While AI is transforming R&D processes, it also demands robust ecosystems that support technology deployment, data integrity, and regulatory compliance. In the next section, we will explore the **current AI in the Pharma ecosystem**, examining partnerships, infrastructure, and value chain alignment.

1.6 The current AI in pharma ecosystem: infrastructure, players, and integration models

As AI gains momentum in pharmaceutical innovation, an entire ecosystem has emerged to support its implementation—from technology providers and research organizations to cloud platforms, data

Table 1.7 Snapshot of the current AI in pharma ecosystem.

Ecosystem element	Examples	Function
Infrastructure providers	AWS, Azure, Snowflake	Host data and scale AI workloads
Drug discovery startups	Atomwise, Insilico Medicine, Deep Genomics	Generate leads and predict compound behavior
CROs with AI capabilities	IQVIA, Parexel, Labcorp	Enhance trial operations and analytics
Academic/nonprofit consortia	Open Targets, NIH, MIT J-Clinic	Contribute research tools and public data repositories
AI governance and ethics tools	Monitaur, Fiddler AI, IBM AI Governance Suite	Monitor bias, fairness, and transparency of deployed models

integrators, and regulatory technology vendors. This ecosystem (see Table 1.7) is not a peripheral layer but a foundational enabler of AI transformation across pharma.

1.6.1 Infrastructure foundations for AI in pharma

The AI ecosystem in pharma is built on a sophisticated digital infrastructure that enables real-time data access, model deployment, and secure information sharing. Key components include:

- **Cloud computing platforms**: Scalable, secure, and compliant environments provided by AWS, Azure, and Google Cloud to store and process large clinical and genomic datasets.
- **Data lakes and warehouses**: Systems like Snowflake or Redshift aggregate structured and unstructured data from lab systems, EHRs, and real-world sources.
- **APIs and interoperability layers**: Middleware that ensures seamless integration across systems such as LIMS (Laboratory Information Management Systems), CDMS (Clinical Data Management Systems), and CRM (Customer Relationship Management) platforms.

AI cannot thrive without robust infrastructure—organizations must first modernize their data and cloud environments before deploying AI at scale.

1.6.2 The landscape of AI vendors and key players

The AI in pharma space includes startups, tech giants, academic institutions, and CROs (Contract Research Organizations) playing synergistic roles:

- **AI-native startups**: Companies like BenevolentAI, Atomwise, and Recursion Pharmaceuticals specialize in AI-driven drug discovery and prediction.
- **Big tech collaborations**: Microsoft, IBM Watson Health, and Google DeepMind partner with pharma firms for AI-powered solutions ranging from molecule design to predictive diagnostics.

- **Academic and research alliances**: Universities and nonprofits collaborate through initiatives such as Open Targets and the NIH All of Us Research Program, contributing algorithms and datasets.
- **CROs with AI capabilities**: IQVIA, Parexel, and Labcorp increasingly embed AI into protocol design, patient recruitment, and data monitoring.

Strategic partnerships often combine pharma's regulatory know-how with tech companies' data science and computational horsepower.

1.6.3 Integration Models And Business Alignment

Successful deployment of AI is not purely technical; it involves aligning innovation with business models. Integration strategies include:

- **Embedded AI Platforms**: Pharma companies are integrating AI within existing R&D workflows, such as automated trial monitoring or adverse event detection.
- **Center of Excellence (CoE) Models**: Establishing cross-functional AI teams to manage internal capability development, vendor engagement, and model validation.
- **AI-as-a-Service (AIaaS)**: Subscription-based models offered by providers for use in niche applications like molecule screening or regulatory document processing.

Organizations must develop structured AI governance frameworks to ensure data integrity, explainability, and performance monitoring.

A strong AI ecosystem amplifies the capabilities of pharma companies. By integrating AI through internal development or external partnerships, companies can achieve better decision-making, faster development cycles, and increased market responsiveness. However, this integration also raises new expectations around transparency, reproducibility, and compliance. With a deep understanding of the infrastructure and actors shaping AI in pharma, we now shift focus to the **core areas of AI-powered R&D**, where the true value of the ecosystem is realized. The next section will detail use cases, value creation, and translational research powered by AI.

1.7 AI readiness and adoption maturity in pharma: from pilots to AI-at-scale

The rapid growth of AI use cases across the pharmaceutical value chain has created an important managerial reality: the difference between "AI experimentation" and "AI-driven transformation" is not the sophistication of algorithms, but organizational readiness and adoption maturity. While many companies can deploy machine learning models in discovery or trial analytics, fewer can operationalize AI at scale in ways that are compliant, trusted, and strategically embedded across functions. In regulated environments, "readiness" must be understood as a multidimensional capability that includes data foundations, governance, operating model design, and decision ownership. As a result, pharma organizations increasingly differentiate themselves not by whether they use AI, but by how systematically they mature from isolated initiatives to repeatable, enterprise-grade AI.

1.7.1 AI readiness: data, compliance, and the operating model

AI readiness in pharma begins with data, but it is sustained through compliance and organizational design. Data readiness is not only a question of availability; it is also a question of interoperability, quality, representativeness, and traceability across the full lifecycle. AI models in drug discovery may require large, well-curated omics datasets, while clinical development depends on integrated trial data, EHRs, and RWE. Manufacturing and quality domains add further complexity through sensor streams, batch records, and GxP documentation. Without a harmonized data layer—supported by standard terminologies, metadata management, and robust governance—AI initiatives remain fragile, difficult to validate, and hard to scale.

Compliance readiness is equally critical. In pharma, AI systems must operate within regulated expectations for Good Practices (GxP) and documented change control. This transforms "model deployment" into a disciplined capability: organizations must maintain audit trails, explain the intended use of models, validate performance against risk-relevant thresholds, and monitor model drift over time. In practice, this means the AI life cycle must be treated as part of the quality system rather than as an external technical activity. Organizations that neglect this alignment may achieve short-term proofs of concept, but they struggle to institutionalize AI in high-impact workflows such as clinical trial optimization, pharmacovigilance signal detection, and regulatory submissions.

Finally, organizational readiness requires the right operating model. Many pharma organizations begin with a centralized AI CoE to build critical skills and reusable components. However, as maturity grows, a hybrid model often becomes more effective: a central team maintains shared platforms, governance, and model standards, while embedded analytics teams within R&D, clinical operations, manufacturing, and commercial functions ensure business alignment and rapid adoption. Crucially, readiness also depends on decision ownership. AI insights do not create value unless decision rights are explicit—who acts on model outputs, how exceptions are escalated, and how accountability is maintained when human judgment and algorithmic recommendations diverge.

1.7.2 Adoption maturity model: from experimentation to AI-native pharma

Pharma's AI adoption can be conceptualized as a maturity progression, where each stage brings increased value but also increased requirements for governance, integration, and trust. At early stages, organizations typically run pilots in isolated domains—such as predictive toxicology or recruitment optimization—often supported by external vendors. These pilots create initial enthusiasm but may remain disconnected from enterprise systems.

As maturity progresses, organizations begin functional adoption, where AI is deployed repeatedly within one or two value chain areas (e.g., clinical operations and pharmacovigilance). At this stage, repeatability improves and teams develop domain-specific patterns. However, data silos and inconsistent governance can still limit scalability.

Enterprise integration represents a decisive step change. Here, AI is anchored in shared platforms, common data products, consistent validation practices, and cross-functional governance. Models are monitored systematically, integrated into workflows, and linked to measurable operational and strategic outcomes. Adoption also spreads beyond R&D into manufacturing, quality, supply chain, and commercial operations, enabling a more holistic transformation of the organization.

The highest maturity is reached when organizations evolve toward an AI-native pharma model. In this stage, the enterprise becomes capable of continuous learning loops: RWE informs R&D priorities, manufacturing and supply chain analytics feed into risk sensing, and performance monitoring becomes real-time and predictive. Importantly, AI-native does not mean "fully automated." It means the organization is designed to collaborate with AI systems: workflows, roles, and governance are intentionally structured for human–AI complementarity, ensuring accountability, ethical decision-making, and strategic coherence.

1.7.3 Value realization and KPI logic for AI programs

A common limitation in AI adoption is the inability to define and measure value beyond narrow technical metrics. In pharma, value realization must be linked to measurable outcomes that matter across scientific, operational, regulatory, and societal dimensions. This requires a KPI logic that spans three layers.

First, organizations must track **business and mission outcomes**. In R&D, this may include cycle-time reduction in target identification, improved probability-of-success indicators, or decreased late-stage attrition. In clinical development, metrics may include faster recruitment, reduced protocol amendments, improved site performance, and earlier detection of safety signals. In manufacturing and supply chain, outcomes include yield improvement, reduced deviations, higher overall equipment effectiveness, and stronger cold-chain reliability. In commercial and medical affairs, value can include faster insight generation, improved segmentation accuracy, better HCP engagement quality, and more consistent compliance in communications.

Second, organizations must track **adoption and decision impact metrics**. AI programs fail when models exist but are not used. Therefore, adoption metrics—such as active usage of decision support tools, decision-cycle time reduction, percentage of workflows AI-assisted, and rate of human override—provide early signals of whether AI is shaping decisions or merely producing reports.

Third, organizations need **sustainability and risk metrics** that reflect long-term performance and trustworthiness. These include model drift frequency, retraining intervals, bias monitoring signals, explainability coverage for high-risk decisions, and audit-readiness indicators. In regulated contexts, these KPIs represent operational resilience: they ensure AI systems remain stable, valid, and defensible over time.

Together, these metrics establish a pragmatic reality: AI in pharma becomes transformational when it is measured as an organizational capability, not as a collection of models. The maturity of AI is visible not only in predictive accuracy but also in decision quality, operational consistency, governance discipline, and sustained value delivery (Table 1.8).

Having established the readiness requirements and maturity pathways for AI adoption, the chapter now turns to a synthesis of the key takeaways and forward-looking reflections on how pharma organizations can build resilient, responsible, and scalable AI capabilities across the sector.

Executive Warning: Why Most AI-in-Pharma Programs Fail (and How to Prevent It)

AI programs in pharma rarely fail because the models are inaccurate. They fail because the organization is not ready to operationalize AI responsibly, repeatedly, and at scale. In regulated, high-stakes environments, "good pilots" can quickly become expensive dead ends unless executive teams design the conditions for adoption, trust, and governance.

The most common failure modes include:

The pilot trap (innovation without scale): Organizations run many experiments but lack a standardized pathway to production (validation, monitoring, ownership, retraining, and audit evidence). Pilots generate insights, but decision-making remains unchanged.

Data fragmentation and weak foundations: AI is deployed on incomplete, biased, or poorly governed datasets. Interoperability gaps between R&D, clinical operations, manufacturing, and RWE sources prevent models from being reused and trusted across the enterprise.

Compliance misalignment (AI outside the quality system): Models are treated as "IT deliverables," not as regulated assets. This creates weak change control, limited traceability, and insufficient documentation—leading to regulatory friction and stalled deployment.

Low adoption: models that nobody uses: AI outputs are delivered as dashboards or reports rather than embedded into workflows. Decision rights are unclear, incentives are misaligned, and teams default to manual processes when time pressure rises.

Opaque AI and trust erosion: Black-box outputs, limited explainability, and weak accountability mechanisms reduce clinician, regulator, and internal stakeholder trust. This is amplified in high-risk use cases such as trial optimization, safety surveillance, and regulatory documentation.

Over-automation and responsibility gaps: Organizations unintentionally create "automation bias," where AI outputs override human judgment, or they create ambiguity about liability and escalation when AI and expert judgment conflict.

Prevention logic for executives: To avoid these failure modes, pharma leaders should treat AI as a governed enterprise capability: build FAIR-aligned data foundations, embed AI within GxP-ready operating models, define decision ownership, implement monitoring and explainability standards, and measure adoption and decision impact—not only model performance.

Key message: In pharma, AI success is not a technology problem—it is a governance and operating model problem.

Table 1.8 Pharma AI adoption maturity model: capabilities, risks, and indicative KPIs.

Maturity stage	Typical characteristics	Core capabilities	Key risks	Indicative KPIs
Stage 1: Experimentation (pilots)	Isolated pilots in single functions; heavy vendor reliance; limited workflow integration	Basic analytics skills; initial data extraction; sandbox environments	"Pilot trap"; low adoption; unclear ownership; weak validation	# pilots delivered; time-to-prototype; stakeholder satisfaction; limited operational KPI movement
Stage 2: Functional adoption	Repeatable AI use cases within 1–2 domains (e.g., R&D or trials); some process integration	Domain analytics teams; reusable features/models; early governance patterns	Data silos; inconsistent standards; scaling difficulty across functions	% workflows AI-assisted in function; recruitment cycle time; early safety signal detection time; model usage frequency
Stage 3: Enterprise integration	Shared platforms and governance; integration into core systems; cross-functional value focus	Data products; standardized validation; monitoring/drift controls; clear decision rights	Governance overload; change resistance; talent bottlenecks; integration complexity	decision-cycle time reduction; reduction in deviations; improvement in trial execution KPIs; audit readiness indicators
Stage 4: AI-native pharma	Continuous learning loops across value chain; predictive monitoring embedded enterprise-wide; mature human–AI collaboration	end-to-end data architecture; responsible AI controls; operating model optimized for AI; strategic alignment across domains	Over-automation bias; trust erosion if governance fails; ethical and reputational risks	cycle-time reductions across pipeline; late-stage attrition reduction; drift/bias monitoring stability; adoption + decision impact measures sustained

1.8 Cross-sector convergence: how AI is blurring the boundaries between pharma, healthcare, and technology

AI is accelerating a fundamental convergence between the pharmaceutical industry, healthcare delivery systems, and the global technology sector. Traditionally, these domains operated with clearly defined boundaries: pharma focused on drug development and commercialization, healthcare providers delivered care, and technology companies supplied tools and infrastructure. In the AI era, these distinctions are increasingly blurred. Data, algorithms, and digital platforms now connect research, clinical practice, manufacturing, and patient engagement into a single, interdependent ecosystem.

This convergence is not merely technological—it is strategic. AI-driven insights generated in one domain (e.g., real-world patient data from healthcare systems) increasingly shape decisions in another (e.g., R&D prioritization in pharma). As a result, competitive advantage is shifting from isolated capabilities toward ecosystem orchestration and cross-sector collaboration.

1.8.1 Pharma–healthcare integration through data and AI

AI enables pharma companies to move closer to healthcare delivery by leveraging RWE, EHRs, and digital biomarkers. These data sources allow continuous learning beyond controlled clinical trials, enabling pharma organizations to:

- Refine indications and patient stratification
- Monitor long-term safety and effectiveness
- Support value-based care and outcomes-driven reimbursement models

Healthcare providers, in turn, benefit from AI-enabled decision support tools co-developed with pharma, particularly in oncology, rare diseases, and chronic care management. This bidirectional data flow transforms pharma from a product-centric actor into a long-term partner in patient outcomes.

Strategic implication: Pharma organizations must develop capabilities in healthcare data governance, interoperability, and clinical AI collaboration—areas traditionally outside their core competencies.

1.8.2 The expanding role of technology firms and platforms

Technology companies now play a decisive role in shaping AI adoption in pharma. Cloud hyperscalers, AI platform providers, and data infrastructure firms supply the computational backbone required for large-scale modeling, federated learning, and regulatory-grade analytics. At the same time, AI-native startups introduce specialized capabilities—such as generative chemistry, digital twins, and synthetic control arms—that challenge traditional outsourcing models.

This shift creates a new competitive dynamic:

- Pharma companies compete on scientific and regulatory expertise
- Technology firms compete on scalability, speed, and algorithmic innovation
- Value is created through partnerships rather than vertical integration

Strategic implication: Pharma leaders must develop **partner orchestration capabilities**, including vendor governance, IP management, and joint innovation frameworks, rather than attempting to internalize all AI capabilities.

1.8.3 Toward an AI-enabled health innovation ecosystem

The convergence of pharma, healthcare, and technology is giving rise to AI-enabled health innovation ecosystems. These ecosystems are characterized by:

Shared data assets and interoperable platforms
Cocreation between pharma, providers, regulators, and tech firms
Continuous feedback loops between discovery, care delivery, and outcomes

In such ecosystems, success depends less on ownership and more on trust, governance, and alignment of incentives. Regulatory bodies increasingly act as ecosystem participants rather than external gatekeepers, shaping standards for AI validation, transparency, and post-market monitoring.

Strategic implication: Future-leading pharma organizations will be those that can operate effectively within ecosystems—balancing collaboration with control, innovation with compliance, and speed with responsibility.

Executive Insight: From Pharma Company to Ecosystem Orchestrator

Key message: In the AI era, pharmaceutical companies are no longer standalone innovators. They are becoming ecosystem orchestrators—coordinating data, technology, partners, and regulatory expectations across sectors.

Implications for leaders:

- Strategy must extend beyond the firm's boundary
- AI governance must span partners and platforms
- Competitive advantage lies in integration, not isolation (Table 1.9)

Failure Modes and Strategic Risks of AI Adoption Across the Pharma Ecosystem

While AI offers transformative potential across pharma, healthcare, and technology ecosystems, real-world deployments reveal recurring failure modes that undermine value creation. Understanding these risks is essential for executives seeking sustainable and responsible AI adoption.

Key failure modes include:

Technology-first adoption without strategic fit: Organizations deploy AI tools without clearly defined strategic questions, resulting in fragmented pilots that fail to influence core decisions.

Data fragmentation and interoperability gaps: Siloed datasets across pharma, healthcare providers, and partners limit model accuracy and reduce trust in AI outputs.

Over-automation and erosion of human judgment: Excessive reliance on algorithmic recommendations can lead to automation bias, particularly in high-stakes areas such as clinical trial design and regulatory decision-making.

Opaque models and regulatory friction: Black-box AI systems struggle to meet regulatory expectations for explainability, auditability, and accountability.

Ethical and trust deficits: Bias in training data, weak governance, and unclear accountability can erode trust among regulators, clinicians, patients, and partners.

Executive takeaway: AI failure in pharma is rarely a technical issue alone. It is most often a **strategic, organizational, or governance failure**. Successful organizations proactively design controls, escalation mechanisms, and human–AI collaboration models to mitigate these risks.

Table 1.9 Cross-sector AI convergence in pharma.

Converging sector	Role in AI-driven pharma	Strategic impact
Healthcare providers	Source of real-world data and clinical insight	Enables outcome-based innovation and adaptive therapies
Technology platforms	Cloud, AI tooling, and scalable infrastructure	Accelerates experimentation and enterprise deployment
AI startups	Specialized algorithms and niche innovation	Increases speed and diversity of solutions
Regulators	Standards, validation frameworks, oversight	Shapes trust, safety, and adoption at scale
Patients and digital health	Continuous data generation and engagement	Drives personalization and patient-centric models

1.9 The pharma organization of 2035: a vision for AI-native, responsible, and adaptive enterprises

Looking ahead, the full impact of AI on pharma will not be defined by isolated use cases, but by the emergence of **AI-native organizations**—enterprises designed from the ground up to sense, decide, and adapt through intelligent systems. By 2035, leading pharmaceutical organizations will operate fundamentally differently from today's firms.

1.9.1 From pipeline management to continuous intelligence

Future pharma organizations will replace linear R&D pipelines with **continuous intelligence loops**. AI systems will integrate discovery data, RWE, clinical outcomes, and market signals in near real time. Strategy, R&D prioritization, and portfolio management will become adaptive processes rather than fixed plans.

AI will not eliminate uncertainty—but it will make uncertainty **explicit, measurable, and actionable**.

1.9.2 Human-centered AI as the operating norm

Contrary to fears of automation dominance, the pharma organization of 2035 will be deeply human-centered. AI will handle scale, speed, and complexity, while humans retain authority over:
Ethical judgment
Clinical responsibility
Strategic trade-offs
Societal impact

Roles across R&D, regulatory affairs, and commercial functions will evolve toward **AI-augmented decision-making**, requiring strong analytical literacy and governance awareness.

1.9.3 Responsible AI as a source of competitive advantage

By 2035, responsible AI will no longer be a compliance requirement—it will be a **strategic differentiator**. Organizations that embed transparency, fairness, explainability, and accountability into AI systems from the outset will:
Achieve faster regulatory approvals
Build stronger trust with healthcare systems and patients
Enable scalable ecosystem partnerships

AI governance will be embedded into enterprise risk management, quality systems, and board-level oversight (Table 1.10).

Table 1.10 Characteristics of the pharma organization: today versus 2035.

Dimension	Today	Pharma organization of 2035
Strategy	Periodic, document-based	Continuous, AI-informed
R&D model	Sequential pipeline	Adaptive intelligence loops
Decision-making	Experience-driven	Human–AI collaborative
Data use	Fragmented	Integrated and interoperable
AI governance	Emerging	Embedded and strategic
Competitive advantage	Scale and IP	Ecosystem orchestration

Strategic reflection: The future of pharma will belong not to the most automated organizations, but to those that combine **intelligence, responsibility, and adaptability** at scale.

1.10 Discussion and key takeaways: the evolution of AI in pharma

The integration of AI into the pharmaceutical sector marks a transformative era—one where traditional models of drug development, clinical trials, and commercial strategies are being redefined by data-driven insights, automation, and computational power. This chapter has outlined a journey across the multifaceted landscape of pharma, detailing its challenges, value chains, innovation networks, and AI-driven reinvention.

1.10.1 Lessons from industry evolution

The pharmaceutical industry, once considered conservative in its adoption of digital technologies, is now undergoing a radical shift. AI's impact extends across:

- **R&D**: Accelerated identification of drug targets, virtual screening of compounds, and predictive modeling for toxicity and efficacy.
- **Clinical trials**: Streamlined patient recruitment, adaptive trial designs, and real-time monitoring enabled by AI and wearable tech.
- **Manufacturing and supply chain**: Predictive maintenance, demand forecasting, and AI-driven quality assurance improve agility and cost-efficiency.
- **Commercial operations**: Personalized marketing, sales forecasting, and automated regulatory submissions enhance compliance and responsiveness.

AI allows pharma firms to move from reactive models to **proactive**, **predictive**, and **personalized** healthcare solutions.

1.10.2 Ethical, regulatory, and human capital considerations

With these advances come profound ethical and regulatory concerns:

- **Bias and fairness**: AI models trained on unrepresentative datasets may exacerbate inequalities in healthcare delivery.
- **Transparency and explainability**: The "black-box" nature of some algorithms can challenge regulatory approval and clinician trust.
- **Regulatory compliance**: Agencies such as the FDA, EMA, and SFDA are evolving frameworks to address AI integration in clinical and commercial domains.
- **Human capital and talent**: Cross-disciplinary education is vital. Pharma professionals must now possess competencies in data science, regulatory strategy, AI ethics, and clinical knowledge.

Ensuring AI adoption in pharma remains **human-centered**, **responsible**, and **inclusive** is essential for long-term sustainability. In Table 1.11, we provide an overview of significant strategic takeaways and future-ready priorities.

The pharmaceutical sector is not merely adapting to AI—it is evolving with it. The "future of pharma" lies in intelligent, adaptive ecosystems where AI not only supports but drives scientific and strategic decision-making. Organizations that proactively embrace AI, while upholding ethics and human values, will be best positioned to lead in the decades ahead.

1.10.3 Executive synthesis: strategic principles for AI-driven pharma transformation

The analysis presented in this chapter demonstrates that AI is no longer an auxiliary technology within the pharmaceutical industry but a foundational capability reshaping how value is created, governed, and sustained. The transition toward AI-enabled pharma is not defined by algorithmic sophistication alone; it is defined by the strategic, organizational, and

Table 1.11 Strategic takeaways and future-ready priorities.

Strategic area	Priority actions	Long-term impact
R&D acceleration	Invest in AI platforms for virtual screening and target identification	Faster, cost-effective drug discovery
Regulatory preparedness	Develop internal AI governance aligned with global standards	Easier approvals, trust with stakeholders
AI talent development	Cross-train teams in pharma, data science, and ethics	Build internal capability for scalable innovation
Ecosystem collaboration	Forge alliances with tech firms, CROs, and academia	Access to cutting-edge tools and insights
Ethical AI deployment	Integrate fairness, accountability, and transparency into algorithms	Reduced risk, increased societal trust

ethical choices that determine whether AI becomes a source of durable advantage or operational fragility.

First, AI must be understood as an organizational capability rather than a technical asset. Successful pharmaceutical organizations do not treat AI as a collection of isolated tools embedded in R&D or analytics teams. Instead, they institutionalize AI across decision-making structures, operating models, and performance management systems. This shift reframes AI from "innovation support" to "strategic infrastructure," enabling continuous learning across discovery, clinical development, manufacturing, and post-market surveillance.

Second, readiness matters more than speed. While competitive pressure encourages rapid experimentation, premature scaling without data integrity, governance discipline, and regulatory alignment increases risk. Pharma organizations that invest early in data interoperability, FAIR-aligned architectures, validation frameworks, and explainability mechanisms are better positioned to scale AI responsibly. In regulated environments, the ability to explain, audit, and govern AI systems is not a constraint—it is a prerequisite for sustainable adoption.

Third, value realization requires a decision-centric KPI logic. Measuring AI success solely through technical metrics or isolated productivity gains obscures its true impact. Transformational value emerges when AI improves decision quality, reduces uncertainty, shortens learning cycles, and enhances organizational resilience. Leading firms link AI programs directly to strategic outcomes—such as probability-of-success in R&D, clinical trial execution efficiency, regulatory readiness, and patient outcome optimization—while monitoring adoption, trust, and governance performance.

Fourth, ecosystem orchestration is becoming a core leadership competency. AI is accelerating convergence between pharma, healthcare providers, technology platforms, regulators, and patients. Competitive advantage increasingly depends on the ability to coordinate data flows, align incentives, manage partnerships, and govern shared AI systems across organizational boundaries. Pharma companies that operate effectively within ecosystems—rather than attempting full vertical control—are better equipped to innovate at scale while maintaining compliance and trust.

Finally, responsible and human-centered AI is emerging as a strategic differentiator. Ethical design, fairness, transparency, and accountability are not peripheral concerns; they directly influence regulatory acceptance, stakeholder confidence, and long-term scalability. The most future-ready pharmaceutical organizations intentionally design human–AI collaboration models that preserve clinical judgment, ethical responsibility, and societal legitimacy while leveraging AI's capacity for speed and complexity.

Executive reflection: The future of pharma will not be shaped by those who deploy the most AI, but by those who govern it best. Organizations that align AI strategy with data maturity, regulatory discipline, human capital development, and ecosystem collaboration will be positioned to lead in an era where intelligence, responsibility, and adaptability define competitive success.

AI advantage in pharma will be won by organizations that can scale trust as fast as they scale models.

Abbreviations and Acronyms

AI	Artificial intelligence
API	Application Programming Interface
CDSS	Clinical Decision Support Systems
CRM	Customer Relationship Management
CRO	Contract Research Organization
EHR	Electronic Health Records
EMA	European Medicines Agency
FDA	Food and Drug Administration (USA)
GxP	Good Practice (e.g., GMP - Good Manufacturing Practice, GCP - Good Clinical Practice)
IoT	Internet of Things
KPI	Key Performance Indicator
ML	Machine Learning
NLP	Natural Language Processing
R&D	Research and Development
SaaS	Software as a Service
SFDA	Saudi Food and Drug Authority

Learning Activities: Strategic Application of AI Across the Pharma Ecosystem

These learning activities are designed to help students and practitioners translate AI concepts into strategic, ethical, and operational insight, aligned with the chapter's ecosystem perspective.

1. Executive Essay Questions

- Choose one:
  - How does AI transform the pharmaceutical industry from a product-centric model to an ecosystem-oriented innovation system?
  - Discuss the risks of over-automation in AI-driven pharma decision-making and propose governance mechanisms to mitigate them.
  - Why is responsible AI becoming a source of competitive advantage rather than a regulatory constraint in pharma?

2. Ecosystem Strategy Use Case

- **Scenario:** A global pharmaceutical company plans to launch an AI-enabled platform integrating clinical trial data, RWE, and digital biomarkers in collaboration with hospitals and cloud providers.

- **Tasks:**
  - Identify key ecosystem partners and their roles
  - Assess data governance and ethical risks
  - Propose KPIs to monitor value creation and trust

3. **Internet Navigation and Critical Review**
   - Explore two of the following:
     - Insilico Medicine
     - BenevolentAI
     - Owkin
     - Recursion Pharmaceuticals
     - Prepare a short report addressing:
     - Core AI technologies used
     - Position in the pharma ecosystem
     - Regulatory and ethical challenges
4. **Bloom's Taxonomy Learning Tasks** (Table 1.12)
5. **Group presentation**
   - **Topic:** Designing the AI-Native Pharma Organization of 2035
   - Teams develop a 10-slide presentation covering:
     - AI use across the value chain
     - Governance and ethics
     - Human–AI collaboration
     - Ecosystem partnerships

Table 1.12 Learning activities and cognitive skill development based on Bloom's Taxonomy.

Cognitive level	Activity
Remember	Define federated learning, digital twins, and real-world evidence
Understand	Explain how AI reshapes pharma R&D workflows
Apply	Design a high-level AI roadmap for a mid-sized pharma firm
Analyze	Compare two AI adoption models across sectors
Evaluate	Assess ethical risks in AI-enabled clinical trials
Create	Propose a future-ready pharma operating model

AI disclosure

During the preparation of this work the author(s) used Various AI tools in order to Polishing final content. After using this tool/service, the author(s) reviewed and edited the content as needed and take(s) full responsibility for the content of the publication.

References

Abdallah, S., & Nizamuddin, N. (2023). Blockchain-based solution for pharma supply chain industry. *Computers & Industrial Engineering, 177*, 108997. https://doi.org/10.1016/j.cie.2023.108997.

Abramova, R., Filatova, M., & Sazonava, M. (2025). Ethical and practical aspects of AI implementation in the pharmaceutical industry. *International Journal of Pharmaceutical and Healthcare Marketing*.

Blanco-García, E. (2020). Role of business models in funding the biotech industry: Global trends and challenges for cuban biotechnology. *MEDICC Review, 22*(1), 11–16. https://doi.org/10.37757/MR2020.V22.N1.4, https://mediccreview.org/role-of-business-models-in-funding-the-biotech-industry-global-trends-and-challenges-for-cuban-biotechnology/.

Charitou, T., Lallas, E., Gerogiannis, V. C., & Karageorgos, A. (2024). A network modeling and analysis approach for pharma industry regulatory assessment. *IEEE Access, 12*, 46470–46483. https://doi.org/10.1109/ACCESS.2024.3380317, http://ieeexplore.ieee.org/xpl/RecentIssue.jsp?punumber=6287639.

Coucke, P. A. (2021). Pharma industry reinvents itself in the turmoil. Part 1. Challenges. *Revue Medicale de Liege, 76*(3), 216–220. https://www.rmlg.ulg.ac.be/index.php?page=listeArt?date=2021%20Mar&langue=EN.

Dovzhuk, V., Konovalova, L., & Dovzhuk, N. (2025). Prospects for the use of artificial intelligence in personalized medicine, pharmaceutical design and education. *SSP Modern Pharmacy*.

García-García, S., & Rius-Tarruella, J. (2025). Visionary health architects and leaders: The strategic role of medical advisors in modern pharma. *Pharmaceutical Medicine, 39*(2), 87–95. https://doi.org/10.1007/s40290-025-00557-y.

Gavriilidis, G. I., Dimitriadis, V. K., Jaulent, M. C., & Natsiavas, P. (2021). Identifying actionability as a key factor for the adoption of 'intelligent' systems for drug safety: Lessons learned from a user-centred design approach. *Drug Safety, 44*(11), 1165–1178. https://doi.org/10.1007/s40264-021-01103-w, http://rd.springer.com/journal/40264.

Harrer, S., Menard, J., Rivers, M., & Green, D. V. S. (2024). Artificial intelligence drives the digital transformation of pharma. *Artificial Intelligence in Drug Discovery*.

Heinrich, M., Reiken, B., Roether, B., Müller, A., Rumsch, J., & Symma, N. (2024). Consensus statement on the outcome of the european herbal health products summit – which way forward? *Planta Medica, 90*(14), 1052–1055. https://doi.org/10.1055/a-2419-1602.

Hey, C., Hunter, A., Muller, M., Roux, N. L., Bennett, S., Nowok, K., & Oliveira, L. (2024). A future European scientific dialogue regulatory framework: Connecting the dots. *Clinical Therapeutics, 46*(3), 293–299. https://doi.org/10.1016/j.clinthera.2023.12.006, https://www.sciencedirect.com/science/journal/01492918.

Hock, S. C., Siang, T. K., & Wah, C. L. (2021). Continuous manufacturing versus batch manufacturing: Benefits, opportunities and challenges for manufacturers and regulators. *GaBI Journal, 10*(1), 44–56. https://doi.org/10.5639/gabij.2021.1001.004, http://gabi-journal.net/.

Hong, J., Bae, E. Y., Lee, H. J., Lee, T. J., & Clarke, P. (2024). Values, challenges, and responses associated with high-priced potential cures: Perspectives of diverse stakeholders in South Korea. *Cost Effectiveness and Resource Allocation, 22*(1). https://doi.org/10.1186/s12962-024-00527-2, https://resource-allocation.biomedcentral.com.

Kaitin, K. I. (2019). Artificial intelligence and patient-centric approaches to advance pharmaceutical innovation. *Clinical Therapeutics, 41*(9), 1658–1662.

Khanna, V., Ahuja, R., & Popli, H. (2020). Role of artificial intelligence in pharmaceutical marketing: A comprehensive review. *Journal of Advanced Scientific Research, 11*(3), 1–8.

Kolluri, S., Lin, J., Liu, R., Zhang, Y., & Zhang, W. (2022). Machine learning and artificial intelligence in pharmaceutical research and development: A review. *The AAPS Journal, 24*(4), 1–18.

Ladner, T., Weh, C., Dhillon, A., Giffard, M., & Iacovelli, D. (2025). Data computation platform (DCP): Empowering pharma 4.0 innovation through GxP-compliant and scalable software platform enabling advanced data analytics and real-time process monitoring in regulated environments. *Journal of Intelligent Manufacturing*. https://doi.org/10.1007/s10845-025-02574-9.

Lal, S., Singh, B., & Kaunert, C. (2024). Role of artificial intelligence (AI) and intellectual property rights (IPR) in transforming drug discovery and development in the life sciences. *Library of Progress*.

Malheiro, V., Santos, B., & Figueiras, A. (2025). The potential of artificial intelligence in pharmaceutical innovation: From drug discovery to clinical trials. *Pharmaceuticals, 18*(2), 1–22.

Marasigan, K., Doshi, S., & Fung, S. (2020). Pharma collaboration for transparent medical information (phactMI™) benchmark study: Results of organizational structure and resourcing of medical information services in support of building departmental strategies. *Therapeutic Innovation & Regulatory Science, 54*(6), 1269–1274. https://doi.org/10.1007/s43441-020-00143-1.

Miozza, M. (2025). Digital transformation of the pharmaceutical industry. LUISS University Working Paper.

Nair, S. (2025). Explainable AI in GxP validation: Balancing automation, traceability, and regulatory trust in the pharmaceutical industry. *Clinical Medicine and Health Research Journal, 5*(1), 12–25.

Opderbeck, D. W. (2019). Artificial intelligence in pharmaceuticals, biologics, and medical devices: Present and future regulatory models. *Fordham Law Review, 87*(4), 1749–1786.

Pörtner, L., Riel, A., Schmidt, B., Leclaire, M., & Möske, R. (2025). Data management maturity model—process dimensions and capabilities to leverage data-driven organizations towards industry 5.0. *Applied System Innovation, 8*(2), 41. https://doi.org/10.3390/asi8020041.

Rocha, Md. M., de Andrade, E. P., Alves, E. R., Cândido, J. C., & Borio, Md. M. (2020). Access to innovative medicines by pharma companies: Sustainable initiatives for global health or useful advertisement? *Global Public Health. 15*(6), 777–789. https://doi.org/10.1080/17441692.2020.1729391, http://www.tandf.co.uk/journals/titles/17441692.asp.

Sabapathy, G. (2025). Artificial intelligence in pharmaceutical commercial operations: Transforming sales performance and patient engagement in the digital era. *Journal of Computer Science and Technology Studies, 7*(1), 45–60.

Sankar, R., & Alam, M. N. (2024). Artificial intelligence in drug development and delivery: Opportunities, challenges, and future directions. *Journal of Angiotherapy, 8*(2), 1–14.

Seewald, M. J., Plumb, J. M., Gutierrez, B., Liwing, J., Tepie, M. F., Hammer, M., LoCasale, R., Khosla, S., Yin, D., Pashos, C. L., & Nagy, M. (2020). Strengthening pharma's contract with society: The value of trusted partnerships between pharma and healthcare facilitated by real-world data. *Journal of Comparative Effectiveness Research, 9*(3), 155–159. https://doi.org/10.2217/cer-2019-0183, https://becarispublishing.com/loi/cer.

Selvaraj, C., Chandra, I., & Singh, S. K. (2022). Artificial intelligence and machine learning approaches for drug design: Challenges and opportunities for the pharmaceutical industries. *Molecular Diversity, 26*(5), 1897–1915.

Serrano, D. R., Luciano, F. C., Anaya, B. J., Ongoren, B., & Kara, A. (2024). Artificial intelligence applications in drug discovery and drug delivery: Revolutionizing personalized medicine. *Pharmaceutics, 16*(3), 1–28.

Sim, C., Zhang, H., & Chang, M. L. (2022). Improving end-to-end traceability and pharma supply chain resilience using blockchain. *Blockchain in Healthcare Today, 5*. https://doi.org/10.30953/bhty.v5.231, https://blockchainhealthcaretoday.com/index.php/journal/article/view/231.

Sowndharya, M., Joga, R., Gandhi, K., Vijay, G. K., Waikar, S., Yerram, S., Raghuvanshi, R. S., & Srivastava, S. (2025). Navigating the trends in USFDA authorized generic approvals (2019–2024): Enhancing healthcare accessibility and affordability. *Therapeutic Innovation and Regulatory Science*. https://doi.org/10.1007/s43441-025-00806-x, https://www.springer.com/journal/43441.

Stagi, L., Bocchi, I., Bernardini, D., Ciappa, M., Dellon, S., Castiglione, G. N., Romano, S., Fabrizi, E., Mattavelli, A., Grisoni, I., Finizia, G., & Bonato, S. (2024). The evolution of the pharmacovigilance department in the pharmaceutical industry: Results of an Italian national survey. *Therapeutic Advances in Drug Safety, 15*. https://doi.org/10.1177/20420986241293296, https://journals.sagepub.com/home/TAW.

Stagi, L., Bocchi, I., Bianco, S., Sirizzotti, G., Bernardini, D., Calderazzo, V., Pirisino, G., Grisoni, I., & Romano, S. (2021). Pharmacovigilance and the digital world in Italy: Presentation of the results of a national survey. *Therapeutic Advances in Drug Safety, 12*. https://doi.org/10.1177/2042098620985991.

Taifa, I. W. R., & Nzowa, J. S. (2025). Implementing supply chain management 4.0: Potential driving forces and strategies from an empirical study of pharmaceutical industries. *Engineering Reports, 7*(6). https://doi.org/10.1002/eng2.70190, https://onlinelibrary.wiley.com/journal/25778196.

Tiwari, P. C., Pal, R., & Chaudhary, M. J. (2023). Artificial intelligence revolutionizing drug development: Exploring opportunities and challenges. *Drug Development Research, 84*(6), 765–780.

Wang, Z., Tang, S., Guo, G., Yang, Y., He, D., Yang, L., Han, M., & Hou, Y. (2024). Adaptive quality control with uncertainty for a pharmaceutical cyber-physical system based on data and knowledge integration. *IEEE Transactions on Industrial Informatics, 20*(3), 3339–3350. https://doi.org/10.1109/tii.2023.3306355.

Wise, J., de Barron, A. G., Splendiani, A., & Balali-Mood, B. (2019). Implementation and relevance of FAIR data principles in biopharmaceutical R&D. *Drug Discovery Today, 24*(4), 933–938.

Wölfle, R., Saur-Amaral, I., & Teixeira, L. (2025). Information model for pharmaceutical smart factory equipment design. *Information (Switzerland), 16*(5). https://doi.org/10.3390/info16050412, http://www.mdpi.com/journal/information/.

Xu, Q., Ahmadi, E., Amini, A., Rus, D., & Lo, A. W. (2022). Identifying and mitigating potential biases in predicting drug approvals. *Drug Safety, 45*(5), 521–533. https://doi.org/10.1007/s40264-022-01160-9, https://www.springer.com/journal/40264.

Yoshiura, H., Kawata, Y., & Sengoku, S. (2025). Open innovation and regulatory challenges in new modality development: The pivotal role of contract development and manufacturing organisations in advancing antibody drugs. *Therapeutic Innovation & Regulatory Science, 59*(1), 63–70. https://doi.org/10.1007/s43441-024-00701-x.

CHAPTER 2

Disrupting technologies for future pharma: from analytics to super intelligence

Miltiadis Lytras

Computer Science Department, College of Engineering, Effat University, Jeddah, Saudi Arabia

2.1 Introduction—the current state of technology in the pharma lifecycle

The pharmaceutical industry is experiencing a profound transformation driven by technological innovation across its entire value chain. From early-stage discovery to post-market surveillance, technology has embedded itself as a core enabler of speed, precision, safety, and personalization. Digital disruption has not merely optimized processes—it is redefining what is possible in pharma (Artico et al., 2022; Basu & Heumann, 2024; Faridi & Malik, 2020; Harrer et al., 2023).

Pharma is no longer an isolated sector operating in silos. It has become an interconnected ecosystem, increasingly reliant on digital tools, data analytics, and intelligent automation (Argiyantari et al., 2020; Busquets et al., 2024; Chircu et al., 2017; Gong et al., 2025; Kumar et al., 2020; Malviya et al., 2023; Phiri et al., 2025; Polshettiwar et al., 2024; Ramos et al., 2020; Reed, 2024). Pharmaceutical companies are adopting emerging technologies not only to address inefficiencies and regulatory demands but also to fuel scientific discovery, enhance patient outcomes, and expand access to life-saving therapies. This dynamic environment is further intensified by global challenges such as pandemics, chronic disease burdens, aging populations, and climate-related health threats, all of which call for a faster, smarter, and more responsive pharmaceutical infrastructure (Hull & Coutts, 2021; Hütten, 2021; Johnson & Uwaoma, 2023; Jones et al., 2024; Malviya et al., 2024).

2.1.1 Key stages in the pharma lifecycle empowered by technology

To appreciate the magnitude of disruption and the need for future-proofing, it is crucial to map out how technology supports each major stage of the pharmaceutical lifecycle (Kumar et al., 2020; Malheiro et al., 2023; Stagi et al., 2024; Steinwandter et al., 2019; Williams et al., 2022).

As shown in Table 2.1, technologies such as artificial intelligence (AI), IoT, and blockchain are already embedded into all critical stages of the pharma value chain, laying the groundwork for more disruptive applications in the future.

The Future of Pharma Across All Sectors in the Artificial Intelligence Era. DOI: https://doi.org/10.1016/B978-0-443-40572-3.00008-3

Table 2.1 Technology applications across the key stages of the pharmaceutical lifecycle.

Stage	Technology applications
Drug discovery and preclinical	AI-driven target identification, high-throughput screening, molecular simulation, omics data integration
Clinical trials	Remote monitoring, eConsent, virtual trials, wearable health devices, real-world data integration
Manufacturing	IoT-enabled smart factories, predictive maintenance, digital twins, automated quality control
Supply chain and distribution	Blockchain for traceability, AI for demand forecasting, robotics in logistics, cold chain optimization
Pharmacovigilance and post-market surveillance	NLP for adverse event detection, social media mining, machine learning in signal detection
Commercialization and access	CRM automation, predictive marketing, dynamic pricing models, AI-based health economics analysis

2.1.2 The rise of integrated tech-pharma platforms

One notable shift is the convergence of multiple technologies into holistic platforms. For instance, companies like Pfizer and Roche are investing in integrated AI-cloud infrastructures that combine genomic insights, real-world evidence (RWE), and predictive analytics to accelerate precision medicine. Meanwhile, Microsoft's Project Hanover demonstrates how cognitive computing platforms are directly contributing to clinical oncology decision support. This integration eliminates barriers between departments (e.g., R&D, regulatory affairs, marketing) and promotes seamless data flows.

Cloud platforms now serve as the backbone for managing pharmaceutical pipelines, enabling:

- Federated data sharing for global collaboration
- Real-time dashboards for trial monitoring
- AI augmentation for risk-benefit analysis in regulatory submissions
- ML-powered diagnostics for companion drug development

This shift marks the evolution from tool-based digital transformation to orchestrated digital ecosystems, where intelligent systems learn, adapt, and improve continuously across the pharma lifecycle.

2.1.3 Current pain points despite digital maturity

Despite impressive adoption, several structural and systemic challenges remain:

- Data silos between clinical, regulatory, and commercial units
- Compliance complexity due to fragmented global regulatory landscapes
- Interoperability gaps across platforms and devices

- Ethical AI concerns, particularly around data privacy and algorithmic bias
- High cost of entry for mid-sized pharmaceutical firms

These hurdles underscore the importance of moving beyond digital adoption and toward future-proof design thinking. That means designing technologies and platforms not only for current operational optimization but also for scalability, adaptability, and long-term resilience.

2.1.4 Strategic objectives of tech integration in pharma

Organizations that succeed in digital transformation adopt a long-view approach aligned with five strategic imperatives:

- **Acceleration of drug development:** Shortening the time from molecule to market
- **Enhancement of patient outcomes:** Enabling individualized therapies through AI
- **Operational resilience:** Automating mission-critical functions for continuity and efficiency
- **Regulatory intelligence:** Proactive adaptation to compliance and safety protocols
- **Scalable innovation:** Creating a foundation for integrating future technologies (quantum, AGI, etc.)

Table 2.2 identifies the alignment between strategic objectives and the digital technologies that support them. These pillars will guide future investments in disruptive pharma technologies.

The technologies supporting today's pharma lifecycle have delivered measurable results—but what lies ahead is even more transformative. In the next section, we provide a systematic review of the ten most disruptive and promising technologies that will shape the future of pharma over the next decade.

2.2 Disruptive technologies of the next pharma evolution

The future of pharma is being built at the intersection of data, intelligence, and automation. As we stand on the threshold of an AI-powered scientific renaissance, a new cohort of

Table 2.2 Strategic objectives of technology integration and their supporting digital enablers in pharma.

Strategic objective	Digital enablers
Accelerated development	AI simulations, digital twins, federated learning
Patient-centric personalization	Genomics, AI-powered diagnostics, digital biomarkers
Resilience and risk mitigation	Predictive maintenance, edge computing, cybersecurity
Regulatory intelligence	NLP for regulatory text, AI audit trails, automatic compliance updates
Scalability and future integration	Modular architectures, cloud-native solutions, AI lifecycle management systems

technologies is set to redefine every aspect of the pharmaceutical value chain. This section systematically introduces ten of the most disruptive technologies, each playing a foundational role in shaping the pharma industry of tomorrow (Gong et al., 2025; Kumar et al., 2020; Malheiro et al., 2023).

2.2.1 Artificial intelligence and machine learning

AI and ML are central to the future of pharma, enabling predictive analytics, intelligent automation, and adaptive learning systems. In drug discovery, AI algorithms are already identifying promising molecular structures in silico, reducing R&D timelines significantly. In clinical trials, AI enhances protocol design, patient recruitment, and real-time monitoring, driving both speed and precision.

Key impact: AI will power autonomous decision-making in drug design, risk prediction, and personalized treatment pathways.

2.2.2 Quantum computing

Quantum computing introduces new paradigms in molecular modeling, enabling the simulation of complex biochemical interactions at unprecedented speed. It has the potential to crack protein folding mysteries, accelerate compound screening, and unlock new drug targets.

Key impact: Quantum-enabled discovery will drastically shorten drug development cycles and unlock drugs once deemed too complex.

2.2.3 Synthetic biology

By engineering cells and genetic materials, synthetic biology allows pharma companies to design novel biologics, vaccines, and gene therapies. With platforms like CRISPR-Cas and mRNA becoming mainstream, synthetic biology is rewriting the rules of what medicine can be.

Key impact: Tailored biologics and gene-based treatments will emerge as front-runners in disease prevention and management.

2.2.4 Digital twins

Digital twins—virtual representations of biological systems—offer powerful modeling and simulation tools for understanding drug-body interactions. In pharma, they support personalized therapy optimization, trial simulation, and adverse event forecasting.

Key impact: Digital twins will facilitate hyper-personalized treatment design and real-time clinical decision support.

2.2.5 Blockchain technology

Blockchain offers immutable, transparent, and decentralized data systems, ensuring traceability across the drug lifecycle. It addresses issues of counterfeiting, supply chain fraud, and regulatory compliance.

Key impact: Secure, verifiable transactions and product traceability will enhance trust and safety in the pharma ecosystem.

2.2.6 Internet of Medical Things (IoMT)

IoMT encompasses wearable devices, smart diagnostics, and connected sensors that monitor patient health in real time. These devices generate continuous health data critical for R&D, clinical trials, and remote patient care.

Key impact: Continuous patient feedback loops will transform RWE and adherence monitoring.

2.2.7 Extended reality (XR: AR/VR/MR)

XR technologies support immersive training, virtual lab simulations, and enhanced surgical planning. In pharma, VR is being tested for simulating molecule behavior, educating patients, and accelerating regulatory walkthroughs.

Key impact: XR will enhance pharma education, design prototyping, and immersive regulatory compliance.

2.2.8 Autonomous robotics

Autonomous robots support precision manufacturing, high-throughput screening, and smart warehousing. They are essential in cleanroom operations, 24/7 production lines, and real-time inventory management.

Key impact: Hyper-efficient, zero-error production processes will be achieved through robotic integration.

2.2.9 5G and edge computing

5 G offers ultra-low latency communication necessary for real-time remote diagnostics, AR surgeries, and decentralized trials. When paired with edge computing, it enables data processing at the source—enhancing privacy and responsiveness.

Key impact: Fast, local data analytics will unlock real-time intervention and decentralized pharma operations.

2.2.10 Generative artificial intelligence and superintelligence

Generative AI models, such as those used in protein structure prediction or scientific literature synthesis, create novel knowledge and compounds. When augmented toward artificial superintelligence, these systems may independently design new drug categories.

Key impact: Self-improving AI systems will reshape R&D pipelines, knowledge discovery, and regulatory submissions (Table 2.3).

2.2.11 Strategic taxonomy of disruptive technologies in pharma: from foundational infrastructure to frontier intelligence

While the ten disruptive technologies presented in Sections 2.1–2.10 are all relevant to the future of the pharmaceutical ecosystem, they do not mature at the same pace, they do not carry the same strategic weight, and they do not demand the same governance intensity. A key risk in technology-driven transformation is treating all innovations as equal and pursuing "parallel adoption" without prioritization. In reality, pharma leaders must differentiate between technologies that enable enterprise readiness, those that accelerate performance and integration, and those that trigger paradigm shifts—often accompanied by higher uncertainty and risk.

Table 2.3 The ten most disruptive technologies shaping the future of pharma: current contributions and future potential.

Technology	Core contribution to pharma	Future potential
AI/ML	Predictive models, automation, diagnostics	Self-learning drug design and adaptive trials
Quantum computing	Molecular simulations, optimization problems	Real-time biochemical interaction modeling
Synthetic biology	Novel therapies, vaccine design	Personalized and programmable biologics
Digital twins	Virtual simulations, treatment prediction	Real-time patient-model integration
Blockchain	Supply chain integrity, compliance	Smart regulatory contracts and data-sharing networks
IoMT	Continuous patient monitoring, data collection	Real-world evidence and real-time drug efficacy tracking
XR (AR/VR/MR)	Training, molecule visualization, regulatory reviews	Full immersive simulations for drug development and patient care
Autonomous robotics	Precision manufacturing, logistics	Fully automated pharma production pipelines
5 G + edge computing	Decentralized data processing	Instant feedback in clinical and real-world settings
Generative AI/ superintelligence	Knowledge generation, design of new molecules	Autonomous pharma intelligence and innovation agents

To support strategic decision-making, this chapter proposes a taxonomy that clusters disruptive technologies into three categories based on their role in transformation, required organizational capabilities, and typical time-to-value. This taxonomy helps executives, regulators, and innovation leaders to (a) sequence investments, (b) align adoption with digital maturity, and (c) anticipate governance and capability requirements.

2.2.11.1 Category A: foundational technologies (enterprise readiness and "AI-Ready Pharma")

Foundational technologies create the minimum viable architecture for digital and AI-enabled pharma. They establish connectivity, data capture, data movement, and compute capacity—without which higher-order capabilities remain fragmented or nonscalable. In practice, these technologies determine whether an organization can move from isolated pilots to repeatable deployment.

Key characteristics:

Build interoperable data flows across the lifecycle (R&D → trials → manufacturing → supply chain → post-market)

Enable real-time monitoring and analytics at scale

Form the base layer for AI validation, auditability, and continuous improvement

Typical examples in this chapter:

AI/ML (as operational intelligence and analytics capability)

IoMT (as a real-world data capture and patient monitoring infrastructure)

5 G and edge computing (as low-latency connectivity and distributed processing for decentralized trials and monitoring)

2.2.11.2 Category B: acceleration technologies (scale, trust, automation, and integration)

Acceleration technologies build on the foundational layer and drive measurable value through optimization, operational automation, transparency, and cross-functional integration. These technologies enable "AI-at-scale" by improving reliability, repeatability, and trust across enterprise workflows.

Key characteristics:

Increase speed and quality of execution (e.g., manufacturing, trials, logistics)

Enable simulation and decision support in complex systems

Strengthen trust, traceability, and organizational adoption

Typical examples in this chapter:

Digital twins (simulation and predictive decision support)

Blockchain (traceability, consent, and compliance transparency)

Autonomous robotics (automation and precision at scale)

XR (AR/VR/MR) (training, prototyping, and immersive compliance/education pathways)

2.2.11.3 Category C: frontier technologies (paradigm shift and discontinuous innovation)

Frontier technologies are those with the potential to redefine the structure of pharmaceutical innovation itself—compressing discovery timelines, changing how evidence is generated, and enabling new therapeutic modalities. They are high-upside, but typically require stronger governance, new regulatory thinking, and significant organizational readiness to avoid high-cost experimentation without scalable outcomes.

Key characteristics:

Introduce discontinuous innovation (new discovery paradigms; new evidence models)

Require new operating models and oversight frameworks

Carry higher uncertainty, higher strategic impact, and higher governance requirements

Typical examples in this chapter:

Quantum computing (new paradigms in molecular simulation and optimization)

Synthetic biology (programmable biologics and next-generation modality design)

Generative AI and superintelligence (autonomous scientific reasoning and knowledge generation) (Table 2.4).

2.2.11.4 Strategic takeaway

This taxonomy highlights a practical principle for future-proofing pharma: disruption must be sequenced. Foundational technologies establish the conditions for trust and scale; acceleration technologies translate readiness into operational value; and frontier technologies unlock discontinuous innovation—but only when the organization is mature enough to adopt them responsibly.

This structured view also strengthens the chapter's central argument: the future of pharma depends not on adopting the most technologies, but on building the right architecture, governance, and human capabilities to turn technology into sustainable value.

Table 2.4 Strategic taxonomy of disruptive technologies in pharma: role, horizon, and adoption logic.

Category	Technologies (from this chapter)	Primary strategic role	Typical time-to-value	Adoption logic / executive focus
A. Foundational	AI/ML, IoMT, 5 G + Edge Computing	Build enterprise readiness, data capture, connectivity, and analytics backbone	Short-term	Prioritize interoperability, data governance, and scalable platforms; create "AI-ready" workflows
B. Acceleration	Digital Twins, Blockchain, XR, Autonomous Robotics	Scale and integrate operations; enable trust, automation, simulation, and operational performance	Mid-term	Select high-impact use cases; embed into workflows; define KPIs for adoption and decision impact
C. Frontier	Quantum Computing, Synthetic Biology, Generative AI / Superintelligence	Enable paradigm shifts in discovery, modality design, and scientific knowledge generation	Longer-term	Invest selectively; run governed experiments; design oversight, validation, and regulatory engagement early

Source: The authors.

While all ten technologies hold immense promise, not all will mature at the same pace. In the next section, we identify four of these technologies that are expected to lead pharma's immediate future—and propose scenarios for their adoption and impact.

2.2.12 Governing disruption: executive decision logic for sequencing, risk, and value in tech-driven pharma

The rapid expansion of disruptive technologies in pharma introduces a paradox for executive leadership: while innovation velocity is accelerating, the cost of poor sequencing, weak governance, or misaligned adoption is rising just as fast. Many pharma organizations fail not because they invest too little in technology, but because they invest without a coherent decision logic that aligns technological ambition with organizational maturity, regulatory exposure, and strategic intent.

This section introduces an executive governance perspective that reframes disruptive technologies not as isolated innovations, but as managed strategic assets that require explicit prioritization, ownership, and escalation pathways.

2.2.12.1 *From technology adoption to strategic sequencing*

One of the most common pitfalls in tech-enabled pharma transformation is parallel adoption—deploying AI, blockchain, digital twins, robotics, and advanced analytics simultaneously across functions without a unifying roadmap. This often leads to fragmented pilots, duplicated investments, and regulatory friction.

A future-proof approach requires sequenced adoption, where:

Foundational technologies are stabilized before acceleration technologies are scaled

Acceleration technologies demonstrate repeatable value before frontier technologies are operationalized

Each wave is governed by explicit readiness criteria rather than hype or vendor pressure

Sequencing is not about slowing innovation—it is about protecting value creation by ensuring that each technological layer has the data integrity, human capability, and governance maturity it requires.

2.2.12.2 *Decision rights, accountability, and the human-in-the-loop*

As technologies become more autonomous, the question of who decides becomes as important as what is deployed. AI-driven insights, digital twin simulations, and generative models increasingly influence decisions in areas such as trial design, manufacturing optimization, and regulatory documentation.

However, regulated environments demand clear accountability boundaries:

Which decisions can be automated?

Which decisions must remain human-led?

When AI and expert judgment diverge, who escalates—and how?

Leading pharma organizations explicitly define human-in-the-loop and human-on-the-loop models, ensuring that:

AI supports decisions, but does not replace clinical, ethical, or regulatory responsibility

Escalation paths exist for high-risk or ambiguous outputs

Governance bodies understand both the scientific and algorithmic dimensions of decisions

This preserves trust, reduces automation bias, and aligns technology deployment with ethical and regulatory expectations.

2.2.12.3 Executive risk lens: innovation, compliance, and reputation

Disruptive technologies introduce a new risk profile for pharma leaders—one that blends innovation risk with compliance, reputational, and societal risk. Frontier technologies such as generative AI, synthetic biology, and quantum-enabled discovery magnify this exposure because their regulatory interpretation often lags behind technical capability.

Effective governance therefore requires risk-tiered oversight:

Low-risk use cases (e.g., internal analytics, training simulations) can follow lightweight governance

Medium-risk use cases (e.g., trial optimization, supply chain automation) require validation and monitoring

Table 2.5 Executive governance logic for disruptive technologies in pharma.

Governance dimension	Key executive question	Strategic response
Sequencing	Are we adopting technologies in a maturity-aligned order?	Align adoption with foundational → acceleration → frontier roadmap
Decision rights	Who owns decisions influenced by AI and advanced systems?	Define human-in-the-loop escalation and accountability
Risk exposure	What is the regulatory and ethical risk of each use case?	Apply tiered governance based on use-case criticality
Value realization	Are technologies changing decisions or just producing insights?	Track adoption and decision-impact KPIs
Trust and reputation	Can outputs be explained to regulators, clinicians, and patients?	Embed explainability, auditability, and transparency by design

Source: The authors.

High-risk use cases (e.g., patient-facing AI, regulatory submissions, autonomous design systems) demand board-level visibility and continuous oversight

This tiered approach allows innovation to proceed without exposing the organization to uncontrolled regulatory or ethical fallout (Table 2.5).

2.2.12.4 Strategic takeaway

Disruptive technologies do not fail because they are too advanced. They fail because organizations deploy them without decision discipline, sequencing logic, and governance clarity. Future-proof pharma leaders will distinguish themselves not by technological ambition alone, but by their ability to govern innovation responsibly, transparently, and at scale.

Why Tech-First Transformations Fail in Pharma (and What Leaders Must Do Differently)

Despite unprecedented investment in AI, advanced analytics, and automation, many pharmaceutical organizations struggle to convert technological innovation into sustained strategic advantage. Evidence from industry practice suggests that failure is rarely caused by weak algorithms or immature tools. Instead, breakdowns mainly occur at the organizational, governance, and leadership levels.

Common failure patterns:

Innovation without decision impact: Technologies are deployed as dashboards, pilots, or proofs of concept that generate insights but do not materially influence core decisions in R&D, clinical operations, manufacturing, or regulatory strategy.

Parallel adoption without sequencing: Organizations attempt to implement AI, digital twins, blockchain, and advanced automation simultaneously, without stabilizing data foundations or operating models first—resulting in fragmentation and dilution of value.

AI outside the quality and compliance system: Advanced analytics and machine learning models are treated as IT tools rather than regulated assets, leading to weak validation, limited traceability, and regulatory friction.

Unclear accountability and escalation paths: When AI-generated recommendations conflict with expert judgment, responsibility becomes ambiguous—eroding trust and increasing operational risk.

Technology-centered, not human-centered design: Systems are optimized for performance metrics rather than for clinician adoption, regulatory interpretability, or ethical transparency.

What successful leaders do differently

Future-proof pharma organizations reverse these patterns by:

Governing AI and emerging technologies as enterprise capabilities, not experiments

Sequencing adoption based on organizational readiness, not vendor maturity

Embedding AI governance within GxP, risk management, and executive oversight

Defining explicit human–AI decision boundaries

Measuring success through decision quality and adoption, not model accuracy alone

Executive message: In pharma, technology does not transform organizations—governance does. Disruptive technologies succeed only when leaders design the conditions under which innovation can be trusted, scaled, and sustained.

2.2.13 Mini case vignette (anonymized)—from artificial intelligence enthusiasm to enterprise discipline

2.2.13.1 Background

A global, research-intensive pharmaceutical organization (hereafter *PharmaCo*) launched an ambitious digital transformation program aimed at accelerating drug discovery and clinical development through AI and advanced analytics. Over a three-year period, the company invested heavily in AI platforms, external partnerships, and data science talent.

2.2.13.2 Initial outcomes

Within the first 18 months:

Over 40 AI pilots were launched across R&D, clinical trials, manufacturing, and regulatory affairs

Multiple vendors delivered promising predictive models for target identification and trial optimization

Executive leadership reported strong innovation visibility but limited measurable impact on cycle time, cost, or approval outcomes

Despite technical success, adoption stalled. Scientists and clinicians remained hesitant, regulatory teams raised concerns about explainability, and business leaders struggled to prioritize which initiatives should scale.

2.2.13.3 The turning point

A strategic review revealed that the organization lacked:

A unified AI governance model

Clear decision ownership for AI-influenced outcomes

Alignment between AI initiatives and regulated quality systems

In response, *PharmaCo* restructured its approach:

Introduced a tiered AI governance framework aligned with regulatory risk

Consolidated pilots into a sequenced enterprise roadmap

Embedded AI validation and monitoring into existing GxP processes

Defined explicit human-in-the-loop escalation rules for high-impact decisions

2.2.13.4 Results after realignment

Within 24 months of governance redesign:

AI-supported trial design reduced recruitment timelines by double digits

Regulatory confidence improved due to traceable and explainable AI outputs

Decision-cycle times in R&D have been shortened, with higher adoption by domain experts

Executive oversight shifted from "tracking pilots" to "managing AI as a strategic asset"

2.2.13.5 Key lesson

The transformation succeeded not because the technology improved—but because leadership reframed AI from innovation theatre to decision infrastructure.

Strategic insight: Pharma organizations do not become future-proof by deploying more AI. They become future-proof by deciding how AI is allowed to decide.

2.3 Future-proof tech-pharma scenarios: Strategic implementation pathways

To build a future-proof pharmaceutical ecosystem, stakeholders must not only understand emerging technologies but also envision how these tools will be strategically embedded across the pharma value chain. This section focuses on four breakthrough technologies—AI, digital twins, synthetic biology, and blockchain—and provides structured, actionable scenarios for their implementation.

2.3.1 Artificial intelligence: The autonomous pharma intelligence layer

AI is no longer just a tool—it is becoming a strategic intelligence layer embedded across R&D, clinical operations, and market access. Pharma companies of the near future will employ AI not merely to process data, but to generate hypotheses, design experiments, optimize molecules, and personalize therapies.

Scenario: Autonomous Drug Discovery Units (ADDUs)
- AI algorithms autonomously scan molecular libraries, identify viable drug candidates, and simulate their biological behavior
- Collaboration between cloud-based AI labs and pharma R&D units allows instant iteration and redesign of chemical compounds
- Integrated real-world data (EHRs, wearables) trains models to personalize drug interactions for diverse populations

Impact: Shrinking drug discovery from 12 years to 3–4 years, while reducing costs by up to 40%.

2.3.2 Digital twins: Personalized pharma meets systems biology

Digital twins offer a living model of individual physiology and disease progression, enabling simulation-based medicine and ultra-precise treatment design.

Scenario: Digital twin-enabled clinical trials
- Patients participating in trials are paired with their digital twins, simulating drug response before actual administration
- Trial arms are dynamically adapted based on real-time twin feedback, improving safety and minimizing adverse events
- Regulatory agencies begin accepting twin simulations as part of submission packages

Impact: Reduced trial size by 30%, increased inclusion of underrepresented groups, and accelerated regulatory approval timelines.

2.3.3 Synthetic biology: Designing biologics with programmed precision

Synthetic biology will transition from cutting-edge research to a core pharmaceutical platform, supporting everything from mRNA vaccines to cell-based therapies and programmable antibodies.

Scenario: Distributed biomanufacturing networks
- Pharma firms develop modular biomanufacturing pods near healthcare hubs
- Therapies like CAR-T cells and mRNA vaccines are synthesized locally using open-source genetic designs
- Patients can receive personalized treatments within 24 hours of diagnosis

Impact: Democratization of biologics access, faster production cycles, and reduced supply chain vulnerabilities.

2.3.4 Blockchain: reinventing trust and compliance in pharma

In an industry plagued by counterfeiting, data silos, and regulatory complexity, blockchain offers a path to transparent, tamper-proof transactions.

Scenario: Blockchain-based global drug ledger
- Every batch of a pharmaceutical product is tracked on a blockchain from manufacturing to dispensing.
- Clinical trial data, consent forms, and adverse event logs are stored securely and transparently.
- Patients, regulators, and providers access validated data in real time.

Impact: Eliminates fraud, enhances regulatory visibility, and establishes a decentralized audit trail.

Strategic alignment considerations for pharma leaders

For these technologies to scale, pharma leaders must align their vision, investment, and digital capabilities:

- **Innovation mindset**: Future scenarios demand bold leadership and a willingness to reimagine current models
- **Interdisciplinary collaboration**: AI experts, biologists, ethicists, and data architects must codesign the future
- **Digital maturity roadmaps**: Companies should assess readiness across data infrastructure, skills, and culture

Having explored plausible future scenarios for four pivotal technologies, we now move toward constructing a value-based framework to guide pharma's transformation. This framework aligns technology adoption with outcomes, ethics, patient needs, and business sustainability.

2.4 A value-based framework for next-generation tech-enabled pharma

The convergence of emerging technologies with pharmaceutical innovation demands more than isolated use cases—it calls for a comprehensive, value-based framework that prioritizes outcomes, accessibility, sustainability, and patient-centered design. This section introduces a multi-layered framework that aligns technological capability with ethical responsibility, business performance, and public health objectives.

2.4.1 Core dimensions of the framework

To systematize the transformation of pharma, our framework is built on six foundational pillars:

2.4.1.1 Outcome-centric innovation

Definition: Prioritize innovations that directly improve patient outcomes, reduce side effects, and optimize health system efficiency.

- **Examples**: AI-based early diagnostics, real-time disease progression monitoring, pharmacogenomics-informed treatment paths.
- **Rationale**: Technology must serve clear clinical and therapeutic goals—not just novelty.

2.4.1.2 Personalization at scale

Definition: Integrate individualized care models powered by AI, digital biomarkers, and genomics into large-scale pharmaceutical operations.

- **Examples**: Digital twins in precision oncology, tailored dosage algorithms for chronic diseases.
- **Rationale**: Personalization reduces waste, increases efficacy, and enhances trust in pharmaceutical interventions.

2.4.1.3 Transparent and ethical technology governance

Definition: Ensure technologies are used in ways that are transparent, auditable, explainable, and aligned with public trust.

- **Examples**: Blockchain-based data sharing, AI models with explainable outputs, and ethical AI auditing boards.
- **Rationale**: Trust and compliance are essential in healthcare, where the stakes are life and death.

2.4.1.4 Lifecycle integration and automation

Definition: Seamlessly connect R&D, manufacturing, clinical trials, regulatory compliance, and post-market surveillance using intelligent automation.

- **Examples**: Digital R&D platforms, AI-powered regulatory compliance dashboards, smart packaging for adherence tracking.
- **Rationale**: Siloed operations limit innovation; integration multiplies its impact.

2.4.1.5 Sustainability and global equity

Definition: Design technologies that minimize environmental impact and maximize access across income and geography.

- **Examples**: Green chemistry innovations, low-cost mRNA platforms, distributed biomanufacturing.
- **Rationale**: A future-proof pharma industry cannot ignore planetary or social health.

2.4.1.6 Continuous learning and feedback loops

Definition: Build adaptive systems that learn from every treatment, failure, and patient experience to evolve smarter interventions.

- **Examples**: AI-driven post-market surveillance, dynamic treatment protocols updated by global EHR data.
- **Rationale**: Static systems are obsolete in the age of dynamic intelligence (Table 2.6).

Table 2.6 Value-based framework for next-generation technology-enabled pharma.

Pillar	Key objective	Technological enabler	Example use case
Outcome-centric innovation	Improve patient health outcomes	AI, predictive analytics	Early detection of sepsis via wearable sensors
Personalization at scale	Deliver tailored treatments	Digital twins, pharmacogenomics	Adaptive dosing in diabetes management
Ethical technology governance	Ensure transparency and fairness	Blockchain, explainable AI	Auditable AI models in clinical decisions
Lifecycle integration	Remove silos and enhance efficiency	Cloud platforms, intelligent automation	End-to-end automated drug development
Sustainability and equity	Reduce footprint and increase accessibility	Green manufacturing, modular biotech	Mobile vaccine production labs in LMICs
Continuous learning	Evolve systems based on real-world evidence	Machine learning, real-world data platforms	Personalized updates to treatment guidelines

2.4.2 *Strategic application in pharma operations*

This framework enables pharma leaders to map technologies to strategic goals:

- In R&D, outcome-centric innovation means using AI for disease mapping aligned with unmet needs
- In manufacturing, lifecycle integration supports real-time quality control through IoT
- In regulatory affairs, ethical governance ensures traceability and interpretability of AI-generated data
- In patient engagement, personalization and feedback loops enable better adherence and satisfaction

While this framework sets the foundation for transformative, tech-enabled pharma, it is equally important to recognize that no innovation is immune to risk. We now turn to a critical discussion of limitations, ethical concerns, systemic pitfalls, and emerging regulatory challenges—essential for maintaining balance and responsibility in the pursuit of pharmaceutical progress.

2.5 *Limitations, ethical challenges, and governance risks*

As the pharmaceutical sector accelerates into a digitally enhanced future, it's imperative to balance technological ambition with ethical foresight, governance structures, and a robust understanding of limitations. While disruptive technologies hold promise, they also carry risks that, if left unaddressed, can undermine trust, equity, safety, and societal benefit.

2.5.1 Key limitations in current and emerging technologies

Despite their transformative potential, several technologies face inherent limitations in pharmaceutical applications:

- **Data bias and quality gaps:** Algorithms trained on nondiverse or biased datasets can lead to misleading outcomes, especially in genomics or clinical predictions for underrepresented populations.
- **Scalability barriers:** While digital twins or precision medicine platforms work well in pilot programs, replicating them across regions with fragmented infrastructure is a significant challenge.
- **Lack of interoperability:** Disparate platforms used across R&D, manufacturing, and clinical systems often fail to communicate, stalling the end-to-end vision of digital pharma.
- **Resource and cost intensity:** Implementing high-tech solutions like AI drug discovery, autonomous labs, or advanced IoT requires heavy upfront investment—making them inaccessible to many key stakeholders, especially in low- and middle-income countries (LMICs).
- **Human capital shortage:** Many pharmaceutical organizations lack sufficient internal expertise in AI, data science, and digital transformation strategy.

2.5.2 Ethical challenges at the intersection of technology and pharma

AI and automation introduce deep philosophical and operational questions into pharmaceutical decision-making. Key ethical dilemmas include:

2.5.2.1 Algorithmic transparency and accountability

- *Issue*: Many AI models operate as "black boxes" with unclear rationale for decisions (e.g., patient selection criteria, optimal dosage recommendations).
- *Risk*: Lack of explainability erodes trust among clinicians and regulators.

2.5.2.2 Equity and access

- *Issue*: Advanced therapies and diagnostics powered by AI may disproportionately benefit well-funded healthcare systems.
- *Risk*: A new "pharma divide" may emerge, further deepening global health disparities.

2.5.2.3 Data privacy and consent

- *Issue*: Technologies like digital biomarkers and real-time health tracking require constant data collection.
- *Risk*: Without robust consent protocols and data anonymization, patient privacy is at stake.

2.5.2.4 Artificial intelligence ownership and intellectual property

- *Issue*: Who owns an AI-generated drug molecule—the developer, the algorithm provider, or the pharma company?
- *Risk*: Legal ambiguity can slow down innovation or foster monopolies.

2.5.2.5 *Automation and workforce displacement*

- *Issue*: Advanced robotics and AI could phase out traditional roles in labs and logistics.
- *Risk*: Loss of employment opportunities in developing nations, reduced skills diversity in pharma (Table 2.7).

2.5.3 *Governance and regulation: the call for agile oversight*

To future-proof pharma, regulatory innovation must match the pace of technological advancement. Several progressive trends are emerging:

- **Regulatory sandboxes:** Inspired by fintech, these allow pharma companies to test AI solutions under controlled environments with regulatory oversight.
- **International harmonization:** Organizations like the International Council for Harmonisation (ICH) are moving toward global standards for digital health tools.

Algorithm certification systems: Certification Systems: Emerging frameworks suggest that algorithms used in pharma should undergo periodic certification and validation—like medical devices.

- **Ethics-by-design policies:** Embedding ethical considerations at the earliest stages of tech development can help preempt challenges.

2.5.4 *The ethics–innovation paradox*

The central paradox in this discourse is clear: The faster we innovate, the deeper our responsibility becomes. We must accept that technology alone cannot solve every problem. In some cases, over-reliance on automation or blind faith in AI can cause unintended harm.

Thus, the road to future pharma is not just about what we can do, but about what we should do.

Table 2.7 Common risks and mitigation strategies in tech-enabled pharma.

Risk area	Challenge	Mitigation strategy
Data bias	Skewed training datasets	Inclusive data collection; Bias audits
Algorithm opacity	Lack of interpretability	Deploy explainable AI models (XAI)
Access inequality	Uneven tech deployment globally	Global licensing models; public-private partnerships
Consent and privacy	Continuous data harvesting without proper oversight	Blockchain for consent management; data minimization
Talent gaps	Shortage of digital-savvy pharma professionals	Upskilling programs, AI-literacy for nontechnical workers
Regulatory lag	Technologies evolve faster than regulations	Proactive collaboration between tech, pharma, and regulators

Having mapped both the potentials and the pitfalls, it becomes essential to reinforce the core narrative of this book. In the next section, we synthesize how this chapter supports and integrates into the broader goal of redefining pharma across all sectors in the AI era.

2.6 Integrating the chapter into the book's narrative: disruption, alignment, and transformation

This chapter has provided a focused lens on the evolving technological foundations that are rapidly reshaping the pharmaceutical sector. But to truly appreciate the chapter's value, it is essential to frame its insights within the broader narrative of this book: Reimagining the future of pharma across all sectors in the AI era.

2.6.1 Aligning with the book's vision: from silos to ecosystems

The central premise of this book is that pharma can no longer operate in isolated R&D, production, and distribution silos. Instead, tomorrow's pharmaceutical landscape is an interconnected ecosystem—bridging:

- AI and Life Sciences
- Smart Manufacturing and Precision Supply Chains
- Regulatory Science and Real-Time Surveillance
- Healthcare Delivery and Patient-Centric Design

This chapter contributes by offering a technology-centered roadmap that serves as a foundational layer for these transformations.

2.6.2 Framing disruption as an opportunity

Disruption is not an obstacle—it is an accelerator. The ten transformative technologies explored in this chapter are not isolated trends but strategic enablers of:

- Hyper-personalized treatments powered by AI and genomics
- Automated discovery and validation through deep learning and simulation
- Next-generation clinical trials enhanced by synthetic data, RWE, and remote monitoring
- Sustainable production models enabled by green chemistry and smart robotics

This chapter advances the book's broader claim that embracing disruption is the key to long-term pharma sustainability.

2.6.3 From theory to real-world pharma transformation

Throughout this book, case studies and sectoral analyses reveal that technology adoption varies dramatically across geographies, therapeutic areas, and companies. This chapter helps unify these differences by offering:

- A core architecture for identifying where technology fits in the pharmaceutical lifecycle
- A scenario-building approach for future-proofing decision-making
- A value-based model that moves beyond return on investment (ROI) to include ethical, patient-centric, and societal metrics

This systems approach reinforces the book's multidimensional coverage of pharma, touching business strategy, regulatory shifts, medical innovation, and digital policy.

2.6.4 Anchoring the role of the human

While the chapter has focused on disruptive technologies, it firmly supports the book's assertion that humans remain the constant. The workforce of the future must:

- Work alongside intelligent machines, not beneath them
- Continuously upskill in ethical AI, data science, and digital operations
- Design with empathy, ensuring that patient welfare drives innovation

The book argues that without human judgment, empathy, and governance, technology may solve the wrong problems. This chapter's focus on ethical considerations and skill development directly supports this message.

2.6.5 A platform for action, not just insight

In its final purpose, this chapter invites readers—whether they are pharma executives, data scientists, regulators, or students—to take action:

- Build cross-disciplinary partnerships between biotech, AI, and public health
- Design flexible infrastructures to integrate new tools as they emerge
- Educate and reskill the workforce to handle complexity, not just automation
- Advocate for fairness and access in the deployment of new pharmaceutical technologies

These imperatives align with the overarching goal of this volume: To equip the pharmaceutical ecosystem to thrive responsibly and equitably in the AI era.

With a full-circle understanding of technological disruption, innovation scenarios, and systemic risks, we now move to the final section of this chapter. There, we consolidate insights, revisit the strategic opportunities, and emphasize a sustainable, human-driven roadmap for the next evolution in pharma.

2.7 Conclusion: charting a human-centered, technology-enabled future for pharma

The pharmaceutical industry stands at a once-in-a-century inflection point. While previous waves of innovation—from molecular biology to genomics—have incrementally advanced healthcare, the current convergence of AI, big data, robotics, and computational modeling promises to redefine the entire pharma lifecycle. But as this chapter has illustrated, the promise of disruption can only be fulfilled if it is strategic, value-driven, and human-centered.

2.7.1 Summary of key insights

Across the sections of this chapter, we have:

- Mapped the existing technological infrastructure supporting drug discovery, development, and distribution.
- Explored ten powerful disruptive technologies that will shape the next generation of pharma innovation, from synthetic biology to explainable AI.
- Presented real-world, future-proof scenarios demonstrating how AI and related technologies can transform core pharma processes.
- Proposed a value-based, strategic framework that moves beyond efficiency to include ethics, personalization, sustainability, and impact.
- Highlighted risks and ethical concerns, including bias, overdependence on opaque algorithms, and digital inequity.
- Framed the future of pharma not as an arms race of tools, but as a coevolution between smart systems and skilled professionals.

2.7.2 Strategic takeaways for the pharma ecosystem

To translate this vision into reality, stakeholders across the ecosystem—researchers, policymakers, executives, and educators—must consider the following imperatives:

- Embed AI and emerging technologies as long-term capabilities, not temporary fixes.
- Invest in multidisciplinary talent pipelines that blend data science, pharmacology, ethics, and systems thinking.
- Design adaptive infrastructures capable of continuous learning, regulatory alignment, and secure data exchange.
- Reimagine pharma success metrics by embracing patient-centricity, digital access equity, and societal value.

2.7.3 Future outlook: towards Pharma 2040

Looking ahead to 2040, we envision a pharmaceutical sector that is:

- **Deeply personalized**: Treatment pathways tailored to individual patients via digital twins and genomic data.

- **Hyper-efficient**: Drug development cycles cut from years to months through AI-driven simulation and predictive modeling.
- **Globally synchronized**: Real-time data exchange enabling proactive public health responses to emerging diseases.
- **Ethically sound**: Strong governance mechanisms ensuring AI use aligns with medical ethics and public interest.

But this future requires effort such as strategic leadership, ethical foresight, and collaborative innovation.

Disruptive technologies are not the destination—they are the means. The real transformation will come from how the pharmaceutical industry chooses to use them. Will it deepen inequalities or democratize access? Will it isolate experts or foster collective intelligence? The answers will depend on the choices we make today.

This chapter, and indeed this book, is an invitation to rethink pharma as a resilient, intelligent, and inclusive force for global health. The future of pharma is not just about what we invent, but who we become as a result of it.

Learning activities: Strategic mastery of disruptive technologies in future pharma

This enhanced set of learning activities is designed to move learners beyond technology awareness toward strategic judgment, ethical reasoning, and governance capability. The activities reflect the chapter's central message: disruptive technologies only create value in pharma when embedded within coherent operating models, human-centered governance, and ecosystem-aware strategies.

Activity 1: Strategic technology mapping across the pharma lifecycle (executive lens)

Objective: To develop the ability to assess disruptive technologies not as standalone innovations, but as decision-enabling capabilities across the pharma lifecycle.

Task: Select three disruptive technologies discussed in the chapter (e.g., Generative AI, Digital Twins, Synthetic Biology, Blockchain).

For each technology, map its role across at least four lifecycle stages:
Drug discovery and preclinical
Clinical development
Manufacturing and quality
Regulatory affairs or post-market surveillance

Deliverable: A structured table including:
Lifecycle stage

Strategic decision supported
Value created (speed, quality, compliance, personalization, resilience)
Key governance or ethical risks
Required organizational capability (data, talent, operating models)

Learning outcome: Learners demonstrate systems thinking and recognize that technology value emerges through decision impact, not deployment volume.

Activity 2: Mini case analysis—diagnosing failure and redesigning success

Objective: To apply the chapter's insights on why tech-first transformations fail in pharma and how they can be redesigned.

Case material: Use the anonymized mini case vignette presented in this chapter.

Tasks

Identify the three primary failure modes present in the initial transformation phase

Map each failure mode to:
Governance gaps
Operating model weaknesses
Human–AI interaction failures

Propose two concrete corrective actions for each failure mode, aligned with:
Regulatory expectations
Organizational readiness
Ethical AI principles

Deliverable: A 1200–1500-word strategic case memo written as if addressed to the executive committee.

Learning outcome: Learners develop diagnostic and advisory skills required for real-world pharma leadership and consulting roles.

Activity 3: Scenario design—Future Pharma 2040 under technological convergence

Objective: To cultivate foresight and scenario-planning skills under high uncertainty.

Task: In groups, design a Pharma 2040 scenario where at least four disruptive technologies converge (e.g., AI + Digital Twins + IoMT + Quantum Computing).

Each scenario must address:
How decisions are made (human vs AI roles)
How trust is maintained (regulatory, patient, healthcare ecosystem)
How value is measured beyond ROI
How ethical risks are governed

Constraints

One scenario must assume strong regulation
One scenario must assume weak or fragmented regulation

Deliverable: A scenario narrative (1500 words) plus a one-page strategic implications brief.

Learning outcome: Learners understand that future-proofing is about adaptive governance, not predicting technologies.

Activity 4: Role play simulation—the pharma artificial intelligence ethics and governance board

Objective: To experience the ethical and governance tensions of disruptive technologies in pharma.

Roles:

Chief Scientific Officer
Head of Regulatory Affairs
AI Platform Lead
Patient Advocate
Ethics Committee Chair

Scenario: A generative AI system proposes a novel drug candidate and optimized clinical trial design. Early results are promising, but:

Training data transparency is incomplete
Explainability is limited
Long-term safety signals are uncertain

Task: Participants must debate:

Whether to advance, pause, or redesign the program
What safeguards are required
Who retains final decision authority

Deliverable: A joint governance resolution outlining:

Decision rationale
Escalation paths
Accountability allocation

Learning outcome: Learners internalize that ethical leadership is operational, not abstract, in AI-enabled pharma.

Activity 5: Skills inventory and capability roadmap for tech-driven pharma

Objective: To align individual and organizational skill development with future pharma realities.

Task: Identify 10 critical future competencies, spanning:

Technical (e.g., AI-literacy, data governance)
Strategic (e.g., ecosystem orchestration)
Ethical (e.g., responsible AI oversight)
Human (e.g., judgment under uncertainty)
For each skill, specify:
Relevant pharma roles
Enabling technologies
Recommended upskilling pathways

Deliverable: A capability roadmap presented as a table or visual matrix.

Learning outcome: Learners recognize that future pharma success depends on people evolving with technology, not being replaced by it.

Optional capstone assignment (advanced programs)

Title: Designing the Tech-Governed Pharma Organization of the Future

Task: Develop a comprehensive transformation blueprint for a mid-to-large pharmaceutical organization integrating:
At least five disruptive technologies
A clear governance model
Ethical safeguards
Decision-centric KPIs
Evaluation focus
Strategic coherence
Realism under regulation
Human-centered design

Pedagogical note (for editors and instructors):

These learning activities intentionally shift emphasis from what technologies can do to how leaders must decide, govern, and take responsibility in an AI-driven pharmaceutical ecosystem.

References

Argiyantari, B., Simatupang, T. M., & Basri, M. H. (2020). Pharmaceutical supply chain transformation through application of the lean principle: A literature review. *Journal of Industrial Engineering and Management, 13*(3), 475–494.

Artico, F., Edge, A. L., & Langham, K. (2022). The future of artificial intelligence for the biotech big data landscape. *Current Opinion in Biotechnology, 76*.

Basu, S., & Heumann, K. (2024). Data integrity and AI: How pharma can build a data-driven future. *Pharmaceutical Review, 29*(3), 30.

Busquets, J., Ramírez-Peinado, S., Peiró, M., & Camacho, M. (2024). Novartis oncology Spain: Agile innovation and the RWE cell. *Journal of Information Technology Teaching Cases, 14*(2), 247–261.

Chircu, A. M., Sultanow, E., & Sözer, L. D. Gesellschaft fur Informatik (GI) United States. (2017). A reference architecture for digitalization in the pharmaceutical industry. In *Lecture Notes in Informatics (LNI), Proceedings - Series of the Gesellschaft fur Informatik (GI)*2043–2057.

Faridi, M. R., & Malik, A. (2020). Digital transformation in supply chain, challenges and opportunities in SMEs: A case study of Al-Rumman pharma. *Emerging Markets Case Studies, 10*(1), 1–16.

Gong, S. J., Kim, H. R., Park, Y. J., & Kim, J. E. (2025). Recent trends in continuous manufacturing and digitalization in pharmaceutical process development and manufacturing. *Journal of Pharmaceutical Investigation, 55*(3), 397–414.

Harrer, S., Menard, J., Rivers, M., Green, D. V. S., Karpiak, J., Jeliazkov, J. R., Shapovalov, M. V., del Alamo, D., & Sternke, M. C. (2023). Artificial intelligence drives the digital transformation of pharma. In *Artificial Intelligence in Clinical Practice: How AI Technologies Impact Medical Research and Clinics*. Australia: Elsevier, 345–372.

Hull, W., & Coutts, R. (2021). Pci pharma's digital transformation: Reaching new levels of customer experience. *Drug Development and Delivery, 21*(6), 66–69.

Hütten, D. (2021). Digital transformation of the production-based pharmaceutical industry. *Chimica Oggi/ Chemistry Today. 39*(2), 64–65.

Johnson, F. K., & Uwaoma, C. C. (2023). PLS-based evaluation of a digital transformation adoption model for biopharma manufacturing. In *Springer Proceedings in Business and Economics*. Springer Nature United States, 183–192.

Jones, C. H., Madhavan, S., Natarajan, K., Corbo, M., True, J. M., & Dolsten, M. (2024). Rewriting the textbook for pharma: How to adapt and thrive in a digital, personalized and collaborative world. *Drug Discovery Today, 29*(9).

Kumar, S. H., Talasila, D., Gowrav, M. P., & Gangadharappa, H. V. (2020). Adaptations of pharma 4.0 from industry 4.0. *Drug Invention Today, 14*(3), 405–415.

Malheiro, V., Duarte, J., Veiga, F., & Mascarenhas-Melo, F. (2023). Exploiting pharma 4.0 technologies in the non-biological complex drugs manufacturing: Innovations and implications. *Pharmaceutics, 15*(11), 2545.

Malviya, N., Malviya, S., & Saxena, R. (2024). Innovation in pharmaceutical manufacturing: Leveraging human capital to get to industry 5.0 by beyond pharma 4.0. *Pharma Times, 56*(5), 8–20.

Malviya, R., Sundram, S., Fuloria, S., & Meenakshi, D. U. (2023). *Pharmaceutical industry 4.0: Future, Challenges & Application*. River Publishers.

Phiri, V. J., Battas, I., Semmar, A., Medromi, H., & Moutaouakkil, F. (2025). Towards enterprise-wide pharma 4.0 adoption. *Scientific African, 28*.

Polshettiwar, S., Kachhi, M., Dargude, S., Jagdale, S., Bhiote, S., & Polshettiwar, D. (2024). Next frontier in pharma revolution: Synergy of AI, big data, and blockchain technology. *Pharma Times, 56*(9), 21–29.

Ramos, M. V., Beleiro, B. L., Fernandez, M. G., Martinez, M. G., & de Silva Urquijo, J. (2020). Together beyond COVID-19 - A look at the future. *Chimica Oggi/Chemistry Today, 38*(6), 54–57.

Reed, J. (2024). How pharma companies are solving regulatory challenges with AI-based technology. *American Pharmaceutical Review, 27*(2), 56–57.

Stagi, L., Bocchi, I., Bernardini, D., Ciappa, M., Dellon, S., Castiglione, G. N., Romano, S., Fabrizi, E., Mattavelli, A., Grisoni, I., Finizia, G., & Bonato, S. (2024). The evolution of the pharmacovigilance department in the pharmaceutical industry: Results of an Italian national survey. *Therapeutic Advances in Drug Safety, 15*.

Steinwandter, V., Borchert, D., & Herwig, C. (2019). Data science tools and applications on the way to Pharma 4.0. *Drug Discovery Today, 24*(9), 1795–1805.

Williams, C., Kobashi, N., & Weber, N. (2022). *Meeting an Unmet Pharma Need: Pioneering the Way to a Connected Future*. Switzerland: Frederick Furness Publishing, 55–59 ONdrugDelivery.

CHAPTER 3

The role of AI-enabled analytics in healthcare

Kantiana Patra[1,2] and Miltiadis Lytras[3]

[1]Statistics and Insurance Science at the University of Piraeus, Piraeus, Greece, [2]The American College of Greece, Athens, Greece, [3]Computer Science Department, College of Engineering, Effat University, Jeddah, Saudi Arabia

3.1 Introduction

Artificial intelligence (AI) and data analytics have emerged as the most critical driving forces for transforming the healthcare and pharmaceutical industries. AI's capacity to process and interpret vast, complex volumes of data has led to significant advancements, ranging from clinical diagnostics and precision medicine to research and development of new drugs. These technologies are being applied in predictive modeling tools for manufacturing management as well as in rapid diagnostic systems for critical conditions.

Furthermore, artificial intelligence is progressively incorporated into real-time patient monitoring systems via connected devices and advanced biosensors (IoT/IoMT). This digital convergence creates an environment where care and decision-making are increasingly based on automated data analysis.

However, the increasing dependence on these complex AI models introduces significant ethical, legal, and operational challenges. The lack of transparency in models that function as "black boxes" impedes their full implementation, undermining trust and the accountability required in the clinical environment. The issue of regulatory compliance becomes critical, as AI-driven decisions must be fully understandable.

Consequently, explainable artificial intelligence (XAI) is essential. XAI seeks to provide the required transparency and interpretability of algorithmic decisions. The integration of XAI strategies is vital for fostering trust and ensuring ethical compliance in AI systems within the healthcare sector.

The Future of Pharma Across All Sectors in the Artificial Intelligence Era. DOI: https://doi.org/10.1016/B978-0-443-40572-3.00002-2

A/A	References (authors, journal, year)	Article title	Key contribution	Impact on our research model
1.	El-Jlaidi et al., *Lecture Notes in Networks and Systems* (2025)	Artificial intelligence in healthcare: AI-driven diagnostics, tailored medicine, predictive analytics, and robotic surgery	Provides a broad overview of AI's role in key clinical areas and techniques (diagnostics, prediction, personalization).	Provides a strong thematic foundation for defining the state of the art and the comprehensive scope of AI analytics in healthcare.
2.	Somara et al., *Current Stem Cell Reports* (2025)	Artificial intelligence in biotechnology and pharmaceuticals: evolution, applications, and regulatory frontiers	Comprehensive review of AI/ML use in Biotechnology and Pharmaceuticals, emphasizing R&D and necessary regulatory adjustments.	Explores the evolution of AI in pharmaceutical R&D, focusing on innovation and the relevant regulatory landscape.
3.	Maharjan et al., *Int. Journal of Pharmaceutics X* (2025)	Transformative roles of digital twins from drug discovery to continuous manufacturing: pharmaceutical and biopharmaceutical perspectives	Analyzes the advanced concept of digital twins and how this AI technique transforms the pharmaceutical product lifecycle.	Serves as a key example of advanced predictive modeling techniques in pharmaceutical production and manufacturing.
4.	Vitorino et al., *Biochimica Et Biophysica Acta* (2026)	Convergence: multiomics and AI are reshaping the landscape of biomedical research	Explains the use of AI for synthesizing and analyzing complex multiomics data in precision research.	Establishes the necessity of AI analytics for processing complex, high-dimensional datasets in precision diagnostics.
5.	Bhimani et al., *Diagnostic Microbiology* (2026)	Multidrug-resistant pathogens in UTIs: a concise review of epidemiology, diagnostics, and patent landscaping for precision healthcare.	Review on the diagnosis and management of multidrug resistant pathogens, an area where rapid AI diagnostics are critical.	Illustrates a critical clinical application where AI analytics enables rapid and precise diagnostic support.
6.	Chin et al., *Clinica Chimica Acta* (2025)	Advancement of machine learning algorithms in biosensors	Analyzes the evolution of ML algorithms in processing data derived from biosensors.	Explains the technical development of new tools and sensors, which form the basis for continuous patient monitoring and data collection.
7.	Cherradi et al., *Lecture Notes in Networks and Systems* (2025)	Artificial intelligence and connected devices in healthcare: exploring their potential and limitations	Discusses the potential and restrictions of AI when combined with connected devices (IoT, IoMT) in patient care.	Provides necessary context for discussing the opportunities and inherent limitations of connecting AI with real-world IoT devices.
8.	Alshehade et al., *Lecture Notes in Networks and Systems* (2025)	Ethical considerations in the application of artificial intelligence in the pharmaceutical industry	Focuses on the ethical and legal challenges of implementing AI in pharmaceutical R&D (bias, data privacy, transparency).	Offers a crucial perspective on the ethical requirements and challenges of deploying AI systems within the drug industry ecosystem.

9.	Mohammad et al., *Discover Internet of Things* (2025)	Strategies for applying interpretable and explainable AI in real-world IoT applications	Analyzes the necessity of Explainable AI (XAI) strategies in real-world IoT applications.	Supports the proposed framework for building trust and transparency in AI systems through XAI strategies.
10.	Bergen et al., *Nature Communications* (2025)	A large-scale human toxicogenomics resource for drug-induced liver injury prediction	Presents a resource and model for predicting drug toxicity (e.g., liver injury) using genomics and large-scale data analysis.	Presents a specific academic example of predictive analytics used to enhance drug safety and reduce clinical risk during the R&D phase.

3.2 Core applications of artificial intelligence analytics across the value chain

To enable a crucial transition from reactive care to a predictive, proactive prototype, the transformation of healthcare systems depends on AI analytics. AI is essential because its ability to process massive, heterogeneous data enables real-time decision-making, which is critical for modern medicine. Every stage of the value chain is impacted by this change, from early drug research and development (R&D) to clinical operations management.

3.2.1 Artificial intelligence in pharmaceutical R&D and clinical trials

The Pharmaceutical sector encounters a monumental challenge: the expenses and duration involved in order to develop a new drug are prohibitively high. Historically, the process from Phase 1 of clinical trials to final regulatory approval has seen failure rates surpassing 90% (Hay et al., 2014). AI-enabled analytics are vital in addressing this issue and are fundamentally designed to reduce this elevated failure rate (Somara et al., 2025).

AI accomplishes this by shifting the discovery phase from a protracted trial-and-error process to predictive modeling, thus improving the Probability of Success (PoS). Machine learning methods speed up the discovery of promising drug candidates by examining vast biological and chemical datasets and eliminating problematic compounds earlier.

An important application involves utilizing extensive toxicogenomics resources along with AI to predict adverse effects, such as induced liver injury, prior to compounds undergoing human trials (Bergen et al., 2025). This early identification of ineffectiveness ensures that only the safest and most viable molecules proceed to the costly later stages of clinical trials. This selective process substantially increases the overall clinical success rate and simplifies the main obstacles of Industry R2D. Additionally, sophisticated ideas such as Digital Twins allow pharmaceutical firms to create virtual replicas of biological or manufacturing processes, facilitating accurate modeling of continuous production and supply chains (Maharjan et al., 2025).

3.2.2 Precision diagnostics and prognosis

In the clinical setting, AI analytics are revolutionizing precision diagnostics. Machine learning models can analyze diverse data types (e.g., medical imaging, lab results, and electronic health records, EHRs) more effectively than traditional human analysis (El-Jlaidi et al., 2025).

A crucial aspect is the integration of multiomics data. Multiomics refers to the combination of different biological omics data sources and is an analytic approach in which datasets are derived from multiple "omes," such as the genome, proteome, transcriptome, epigenome, metabolome, and microbiome (Choi et al., 2021). AI is the only tool capable of efficiently synthesizing this data to detect subtle biomarkers and molecular patterns that forecast disease trajectory. This is essential for categorizing risk levels. For example, AI assists in the rapid diagnosis of critical conditions, such as detecting multidrug-resistant pathogens in infections, thereby providing immediate support for clinical decision-making (Bhimani et al., 2026). Overall, AI transforms unprocessed clinical information into prognostic insights for individualized therapy.

3.2.3 Optimizing operations and smart hospital management

Beyond clinical and research benefits, AI analytics enhances the operational effectiveness of hospitals (Smart Hospital concept). This involves improving resource distribution (beds, staff), reducing wait times, and managing supply chains. An emerging area where AI provides substantial time savings is clinical documentation. The use of automatic speech recognition (ASR) systems that utilize natural language processing (NLP) techniques enables doctors to verbally record their clinical findings directly, converting speech into organized EHRs. For example, the development of systems like the "Automatic Speech Recognition for Greek Medical Dictation" illustrates the feasibility of this technology even in specialized, complex language contexts, directly aiding doctors in efficiently documenting clinical notes (Georgilas, 2025). The enhanced quality and speed of documentation are fundamental for the functioning of the "Smart Hospital," as they guarantee that data are readily available to support predictive models. Finally, AI is utilized to enhance patient flow, ensuring efficient resource allocation and comprehensive management.

3.2.4 Artificial intelligence in mental and behavioral health

Mental health is a rapidly evolving domain where AI provides options for early detection, risk evaluation, and personalized treatment, particularly in areas with restricted access to specialized practitioners. The worth of AI in this field stems from its ability to analyze complex, nonlinear behavioral data. Key applications include:

- *Voice and text analysis:* Utilizing NLP techniques, AI examines the tone, pitch, and content of speech or written texts. This enables the identification of slight biomarkers associated with conditions like depression, anxiety, or even the early diagnosis of neurodegenerative disorders.

- *Predictive risk modeling:* Machine learning (ML) can analyze a patient's EHRs, combining history, demographics, and social factors, to more accurately forecast the likelihood of suicide or psychotic episodes compared to traditional clinical tools.
- *Personalized therapeutic interventions (chatbots/virtual assistants):* AI-driven chatbots provide cognitive-behavioral therapy and immediate assistance, serving as an initial intervention or a supplement to traditional therapy, thus enhancing patient involvement.

This technological capability improves early intervention and population health management, shifting mental healthcare from the clinical environment into the patient's everyday life.

3.2.5 Data foundations and interoperability for AI-enabled analytics

AI-enabled analytics in healthcare is only as reliable as the data infrastructure that sustains it. Although algorithmic innovation often captures attention, the foundational determinants of real-world success remain data quality, harmonization, and interoperability. Healthcare data is inherently heterogeneous, distributed across silos, and generated in multiple formats—from structured laboratory values and medication codes to unstructured clinical notes, imaging, genomics, and streaming data from connected devices. This heterogeneity creates systematic barriers to scalable AI, particularly when AI models must operate across different hospitals, regions, and regulatory environments.

A persistent limitation is the fragmentation of patient information across EHRs, imaging systems, pharmacy systems, laboratory systems, and payer datasets. The absence of consistent coding practices and semantic alignment makes it difficult to train models that generalize across sites. Furthermore, missing values and inconsistent documentation practices reduce the reliability of predictive performance. These challenges are amplified in real-time analytics scenarios (e.g., early warning systems), where delayed or incomplete data streams can lead to false alarms or missed deterioration signals.

Interoperability standards and structured clinical vocabularies are, therefore, strategic enablers of AI analytics. Standardization allows models to learn from consistent representations of clinical concepts and supports cross-institutional deployment. Importantly, interoperability does not only improve technical performance—it also strengthens governance and auditability, since standardized data pipelines make it easier to validate inputs, track transformations, and explain outputs. In a patient-centric care model, interoperability further supports continuity of care by enabling AI systems to integrate longitudinal histories that span institutions and care settings.

From a policy and implementation perspective, healthcare organizations adopting AI analytics should treat data readiness as a precondition for responsible AI. This involves (a) establishing systematic data quality controls, (b) implementing governance models for data access and stewardship, (c) improving semantic harmonization across datasets, and (d) designing architectures that accommodate both historical datasets and streaming sensor-based information. Without these foundations, advanced analytics may demonstrate impressive performance in controlled settings but fail under real-world clinical complexity.

3.3 New tools, ethics, and the future of patient-centric care

3.3.1 The AI-driven ecosystem: emerging tools and startups

The transformation of healthcare depends on a dynamic ecosystem where specialized analytical tools and groundbreaking startup companies play a central role, extending beyond broad AI applications (Ratti et al., 2025). The value of these tools lies in their ability to provide targeted solutions that enhance particular stages of the value chain, ranging from research to operational management. The incorporation of AI into clinical workflows and the healthcare value chain happens via specialized methods, often driven by innovative startup approaches:

- *Accelerated drug discovery:* Startups leverage generative AI and reinforcement learning in the R&D field to speed up the design and predictive assessment of new molecules. This approach is essential for reducing the high historical failure rates linked to conventional drug development.
- *Advanced imaging diagnostics:* Computer vision models are utilized in pathology and radiology. These advanced systems identify slight irregularities (e.g., early-stage neoplasms) with high accuracy, enhancing diagnostic speed, boosting overall efficiency, and reducing physician workload.
- *Personalized predictive risk stratification:* AI capitalizes on the convergence of multiomics data to forecast disease advancement and treatment response. This detailed analysis forms the basis for personalized therapeutic approaches, fundamentally transforming biomedical research.
- *Operational optimization via digital twins:* Apart from immediate clinical use, startup innovations emphasize the commercialization and streamlined functioning of the healthcare ecosystem. This involves using digital twins to optimize the pharmaceutical supply chain, manage hospital logistics, and forecast equipment requirements.

3.3.2 Ethical, trust, and regulatory challenges

The clinical implementation of AI relies not solely on its analytical accuracy but also on its ability to operate within a structure of ethical governance and trust. The incorporation of AI in patient care presents essential ethical, social, and legal challenges that need to be addressed prior to its extensive implementation.

3.3.2.1 Core ethical corners: the opacity problem

The lack of transparency in advanced AI models poses threats in three key domains:

- *Algorithmic bias and fairness:* Models are trained on historical data, which often mirrors and intensifies current health inequalities. Biased diagnostic recommendations for specific demographic groups can result from training on nonrepresentative datasets.
- *Privacy and data governance:* The significant demand for confidential personal health data (EHRs, imaging) to train algorithms necessitates the existence of strict legal and regulatory frameworks. Methods like Federated Learning are crucial for safeguarding patient privacy and meeting compliance requirements.
- *Opacity and accountability:* The most critical barrier. When a deep learning model generates a diagnosis without providing its rationale (the "Black Box" phenomenon), the clinician cannot entirely assume complete legal and ethical responsibility. The resulting lack of accountability compromises the fundamental trust in the relationship between doctors and patients.

3.3.2.2 Explainable artificial intelligence: the path of responsible adoption

To overcome the "Black Box" impasse, XAI is acknowledged as the essential tool that connects computational capability with clinical insight. XAI is now a regulatory and ethical imperative for the safe integration of AI in healthcare. The significance of XAI is supported by three fundamental pillars:

- *Ensuring clinical safety and error detection:* XAI grants physicians insight into the specific inputs the algorithm used to make the decision. The level of transparency is indispensable for detecting flawed model logic or errors arising from corrupted training data. The physician can thus responsibly challenge the AI, maintaining human oversight as the final safety net.
- *Regulatory compliance and establishing audit trails:* Explainable artificial intelligence transforms the "Black Box" into a "Glass Box" by making the basis of algorithmic decisions more transparent and interpretable. Regulatory compliance and the establishment of audit trails are essential for ensuring traceable decision-making, documented accountability, and auditable processes in healthcare AI systems.
- *Enhancing trust and patient empowerment:* The ability to provide a clear justification ("Diagnosis X was made because the AI identified pattern Y") enhances patient confidence in the process. This transparency empowers the individual to comprehend the basis of their diagnosis, increasing their participation in their treatment journey.

From "Black Box" to "Glass Box": Why Explainable AI Is Nonnegotiable in Healthcare

The challenge: Advanced AI models—particularly deep learning systems—often operate as black boxes, producing accurate predictions without revealing the reasoning behind them. In healthcare, this opacity directly conflicts with clinical accountability, patient safety, and regulatory expectations.

Why it matters

Clinical risk: Clinicians cannot responsibly act on recommendations they cannot interpret.

Legal accountability: Responsibility for decisions cannot be assigned without traceable reasoning.

Trust deficit: Patients are unlikely to accept AI-assisted diagnoses without understandable explanations.

The XAI shift: XAI transforms opaque models into glass boxes by revealing:

Key input features influencing predictions

Relative importance of clinical variables

Model confidence and uncertainty levels

Executive takeaway XAI is not an optional enhancement—it is a regulatory, ethical, and clinical requirement. Without explainability, AI systems cannot be safely scaled in patient-centric healthcare environments.

3.3.3 Operationalizing artificial intelligence analytics: model lifecycle governance and MLOps in healthcare

While AI models can generate value in controlled development environments, sustainable impact in healthcare requires structured operationalization. Clinical and pharmaceutical contexts are high-stakes, dynamic, and regulation-sensitive; as a result, AI-enabled analytics must be managed as "living systems" rather than one-time technical deployments. This necessitates a lifecycle governance approach that spans design, validation, deployment, monitoring, updating, and retirement.

A central challenge is model drift. Patient populations evolve, clinical protocols change, diagnostic technologies advance, and data collection workflows shift over time. These shifts can degrade model performance even if the model was initially accurate. Drift is not merely a technical issue; it directly affects patient safety and accountability. For example, a risk prediction model trained on historical practice patterns may become unreliable after a guideline update or after new diagnostic coding practices are introduced.

To manage such realities, healthcare organizations increasingly adopt "MLOps" principles—structured workflows for reliable and auditable ML operations. In healthcare, MLOps must be strengthened into "Responsible MLOps," incorporating governance requirements such as traceability, explainability, bias monitoring, and compliance documentation. This includes maintaining version control for models and datasets, documenting preprocessing pipelines, and generating audit trails that show how a prediction was produced at a specific point in time.

Equally important is the governance of human oversight. Operationalizing AI in patient care demands an explicit definition of clinical responsibility: who can act on an AI recommendation, when escalation is needed, when a clinician must override, and how disagreements between model output and clinician judgment are resolved. These governance policies should be embedded into clinical workflows and complemented by training programs that build AI literacy, enabling clinicians to interpret outputs, understand limitations, and detect unsafe recommendations. In this way, operationalization becomes a socio-technical process where reliable AI performance and trustworthy clinical integration are inseparable.

3.3.4 Measuring value and safety: clinical validity, utility, and return on investment for AI-enabled analytics

To move from innovation to adoption, AI-enabled analytics must demonstrate measurable value across clinical outcomes, operational performance, and system sustainability. However, healthcare organizations often struggle to evaluate AI because traditional performance metrics (e.g., accuracy, AUC) do not directly translate into clinical utility, patient safety, or economic impact. A model can be statistically strong yet clinically irrelevant, or clinically useful yet unacceptable due to explainability and governance limitations.

A robust evaluation approach should therefore distinguish three complementary layers:

(1) **Technical performance** evaluates predictive capability in controlled settings, using metrics such as sensitivity, specificity, calibration, false alarm burden, and subgroup robustness.

(2) **Clinical validity and utility** evaluate whether AI improves decision-making and patient outcomes in practice. This includes metrics such as earlier detection of deterioration, reduced adverse events, improved time-to-treatment, reduced readmissions, and enhanced precision in diagnostic pathways.

(3) **Organizational and economic value** evaluate the impact on system performance. Key indicators include reduced length of stay, reduced unnecessary testing, improved resource allocation, better patient flow, increased staff productivity, reduced documentation burden, and improved supply chain reliability. In pharma R&D, value indicators include reduced cycle time in discovery and preclinical stages, improved PoS, earlier toxicity detection, and reduced late-stage failure risk.

In parallel, safety must be evaluated as a first-class objective, not a secondary constraint. This requires continuous monitoring for bias, performance decay, explainability quality, and unintended consequences (e.g., automation bias, alert fatigue, inequitable outcomes). Importantly, safety evaluation must be aligned with clinical accountability: evaluation frameworks should specify acceptable risk thresholds, escalation triggers, and post-deployment surveillance mechanisms.

Taken together, these evaluation layers enable responsible scaling. They shift AI adoption from "technology enthusiasm" to evidence-based integration, ensuring that AI-enabled analytics advances patient-centric care while meeting regulatory expectations, ethical obligations, and resource sustainability constraints.

Responsible AI Analytics in Healthcare: An Executive Readiness Checklist

Before deploying AI-enabled analytics in clinical or pharmaceutical settings, organizations should be able to answer "yes" to the following questions:

Clinical and ethical readiness

☐ Can clinicians understand why the AI made a specific recommendation? ☐ Is human oversight explicitly defined and preserved at decision points? ☐ Have bias risks been evaluated across demographic and clinical subgroups?

Data and privacy governance

☐ Are data sources standardized, interoperable, and quality-controlled? ☐ Are privacy-preserving methods (e.g., federated learning) implemented where required? ☐ Is patient consent aligned with AI usage and secondary analytics?

Regulatory and operational readiness

☐ Is there a documented audit trail for every AI-supported decision? ☐ Are model updates, drift detection, and version control formally governed? ☐ Can the system demonstrate compliance with high-risk medical AI regulations?

Value and sustainability

☐ Does the AI deliver measurable clinical, operational, or R&D value? ☐ Are safety and performance continuously monitored post-deployment? ☐ Is the organization prepared to retire or recalibrate models when risk emerges?

Executive takeaway: Responsible AI adoption is not a technical milestone—it is a governance capability. Organizations that treat AI as a managed clinical asset, rather than a standalone tool, are best positioned to scale safely and sustainably.

3.3.5 Regulatory landscape for AI-enabled analytics: from innovation to approved use

AI-enabled analytics in healthcare is increasingly shaped by a risk-based regulatory logic. In practice, AI systems that influence diagnosis, triage, treatment decisions, or clinical trial conduct are treated as high-impact tools, requiring stronger evidence, traceability, and lifecycle oversight than low-risk administrative automation. For healthcare providers and pharmaceutical firms, regulatory readiness is now inseparable from technical readiness.

A practical way to position compliance is through three layers of regulation. First, medical product regulation applies when AI functions as a medical device or influences diagnostic pathways (e.g., under medical device or in vitro diagnostic regimes). Second, data protection and governance regulations apply whenever personal health data is used for training, validation, or deployment monitoring, requiring strict controls on lawful processing, minimization, and access management. Third, quality and clinical research compliance applies in pharmaceutical environments where AI touches trial design, data management, safety monitoring, or manufacturing processes (e.g., GxP environments), requiring validation, change control, and auditability.

From an executive viewpoint, the key shift is clear: healthcare AI must be treated as a regulated clinical asset with documented performance, explainability, drift monitoring, and controlled updates. This aligns directly with your "Glass Box" argument: without explainability and audit trails, compliance becomes fragile, and scaling across institutions becomes impossible.

3.3.6 Limitations and boundary conditions: when artificial intelligence analytics fails in real clinical settings

Despite rapid progress, AI-enabled analytics can fail when deployed outside controlled environments. First, models trained on historical datasets may underperform in new populations due to dataset shift, local clinical practice differences, and incomplete capture of social and behavioral determinants. Second, healthcare environments are susceptible to automation bias, where clinicians may over-trust model outputs, especially under time pressure, increasing risk when the model is wrong. Third, operational realities such as alert fatigue, workflow friction, and data latency can reduce adoption even when model accuracy is high.

A further limitation is that explainability does not automatically equal correctness. XAI can improve transparency and accountability, but explanations can be misleading if the underlying model is unstable or biased. Therefore responsible adoption requires pairing XAI with continuous monitoring, subgroup evaluation, and clearly defined human oversight rules. These boundary conditions reinforce the central argument of this chapter: AI analytics delivers value only when embedded in governance, interoperability, and clinical accountability.

3.4 Discussion

3.4.1 Key conclusions

The comprehensive analysis of AI incorporation into healthcare results in three clear key conclusions. First, AI is confirmed as the primary catalyst for the shift from a reactive to a predictive and personalized care approach. This is clearly demonstrated by its ability to synthesize multiomics data for precise prognosis, exceeding traditional analytical capabilities and establishing the foundation of precision medicine. Second, AI constitutes a critical tool for the holistic optimization of the value chain outside of the clinical setting. Its use in R&D, through generative AI and digital twins, significantly lowers the risk and cost of developing new therapies, accelerating the process from laboratory to patient. Third, technological advancement is intrinsically connected to legal and ethical documentation. Universal acceptance of AI is contingent upon resolving the issues of accountability and opacity.

3.4.2 Critical challenges for the future

The challenges to the full and responsible adoption of AI focus on three critical areas that require immediate attention:

1. *The ethical dilemma of opacity and accountability (the opacity barrier):* The "Black Box" phenomenon remains the most significant regulatory challenge. The clinician's inability to fully understand the reasoning behind a diagnostic recommendation weakens legal accountability and undermines patient trust. XAI serves as the only pathway to resolution, as it transforms the model into a "Glass Box" providing the necessary audit trail for regulatory compliance and safety guarantees.
2. *Bias and privacy management:* Algorithmic bias directly threatens health equity because AI-based decisions reflect and amplify the biases present in historical training data. Addressing this bias must be seamlessly integrated with strict data protection. Technologies like Federated Learning are essential for achieving this balance, allowing collaborative model training without exposing sensitive personal data.
3. *Educational and institutional readiness:* The ultimate success of AI hinges on the human factor. There is an urgent need to reform medical curricula. Healthcare professionals must be trained in the critical evaluation of AI systems and the principles of XAI, guaranteeing that the ultimate decision remains human-centric and that human oversight serves as the final safety net against failure. Without this robust training, the benefits of AI cannot be completely and securely achieved.

3.4.3 Recommendations for future research and adoption

The successful integration of AI into healthcare necessitates coordinated action across three main pillars:

1. *Regulatory harmonization:* There is an urgent need to create globally consistent, stringent standards for the documentation and validation of AI algorithms, with particular emphasis on high-risk diagnostic applications. This will speed up the secure market entry of cutting-edge solutions.
2. *Privacy-preserving technologies:* Research must amplify the development and adoption of methodologies like federated learning. These methods enable the training of models on decentralized data, ensuring privacy while maintaining data representativeness to reduce bias.
3. *Training and human augmentation:* Technology must enhance, not replace, the clinician. Healthcare providers must undergo training programs focused on the critical assessment of XAI explanations, ensuring that the final decision remains human-centric and that human oversight is maintained as the final safety net.

In conclusion, AI is set to guide medicine into a new era. However, realizing this promise hinges on successfully addressing the ethical challenges and implementing a responsible adoption strategy.

Editor's note

This chapter delivers a rigorous and forward-looking analysis of how AI-enabled analytics are reshaping healthcare systems across the full value chain—from pharmaceutical R&D and precision diagnostics to smart hospital operations and mental healthcare. A key strength lies in its clear articulation of the transition from reactive healthcare models to predictive, proactive, and personalized care architectures powered by advanced analytics.

The chapter succeeds in integrating technical innovation with governance considerations. By foregrounding XAI as a prerequisite rather than an optional enhancement, it positions transparency, accountability, and regulatory compliance at the core of responsible AI adoption. This framing is particularly valuable in high-risk clinical and pharmaceutical contexts, where algorithmic opacity directly intersects with patient safety, legal responsibility, and institutional trust.

Equally important is the chapter's emphasis on human oversight and institutional readiness. By recognizing that the success of AI-enabled healthcare systems depends as much on clinician education and organizational capability as on technical performance, the chapter offers a balanced and realistic roadmap for sustainable implementation. As such, it provides both conceptual clarity and practical relevance for researchers, healthcare leaders, and policymakers navigating the next phase of data-driven medicine.

Key takeaways

AI-enabled analytics are the primary driver of the shift toward predictive and personalized healthcare, enabling real-time, data-informed clinical and operational decision-making.

In pharmaceutical R&D, AI reduces cost and failure rates by enabling predictive modeling, toxicogenomics analysis, and digital twin–based simulation across the drug lifecycle.

Precision diagnostics are fundamentally transformed through AI, particularly via multiomics integration and rapid detection of high-risk conditions such as multidrug-resistant infections.

Smart hospital operations benefit from AI-driven optimization, including resource allocation, patient flow management, and automated clinical documentation.

Mental and behavioral health represents a high-impact domain for AI, where voice, text, and behavioral analytics enable early detection, risk prediction, and scalable intervention.

Ethical, legal, and trust challenges—especially model opacity—remain the central barrier to adoption, making XAI a regulatory and clinical necessity.

The future of AI in healthcare is human-centered, requiring clinician training, institutional readiness, and governance frameworks that preserve human oversight.

Mini case study vignette (anonymized)

From black box to glass box: implementing explainable artificial intelligence in clinical decision support

A large tertiary hospital network deployed AI-enabled analytics to support diagnostic decision-making in oncology and infectious disease units. Initial pilot results demonstrated strong predictive performance, particularly in early risk stratification and treatment response forecasting.

However, clinicians expressed growing concern over the opacity of the system. While recommendations were accurate, the lack of interpretable explanations limited clinical confidence and raised legal accountability concerns. Regulatory reviewers also flagged insufficient documentation for auditability.

In response, the hospital integrated XAI mechanisms into the platform. Feature attribution models and visual explanation layers were introduced, allowing clinicians to see which clinical variables and biomarkers influenced each recommendation. This transparency enabled physicians to challenge, validate, or override AI outputs when appropriate.

Following implementation, clinician adoption increased significantly, regulatory review processes accelerated, and patient communication improved, as clinicians could clearly explain diagnostic rationales. The case demonstrated that trust and accountability—not raw accuracy—ultimately determine the clinical viability of AI systems.

Reflection prompt: Should explainability be mandatory for all clinical AI systems, even if it reduces model complexity or marginally impacts predictive performance?

Learning activities

Learning activity 1: mapping artificial intelligence analytics across the healthcare value chain

Format: Individual or pair work. **Time:** 30–40 minutes

Objective: Understand how AI-enabled analytics create value at different stages of healthcare delivery.

Instructions: Map AI applications across the following domains:
Pharmaceutical R&D
Precision diagnostics
Hospital operations
Mental and behavioral health
For each domain, identify:
One core AI analytics technique

One key benefit
One ethical or operational challenge

Deliverable: A one-page value chain map with short explanatory notes.
Learning activity 2: designing a responsible artificial intelligence analytics framework

Format: Team-based (3–5 participants). **Time:** 45–60 minutes

Objective: Develop a governance-aware AI adoption strategy.

Instructions: Design a conceptual framework for deploying AI analytics in a healthcare organization. Your framework should address:
Target clinical or operational use case
Data sources and analytics methods
Explainability and auditability mechanisms
Privacy and bias mitigation strategies
Role of human oversight

Deliverable: A structured framework summary (1 page).
Learning activity 3: executive reflection exercise

Format: Individual. **Time:** 15–20 minutes

Objective: Encourage strategic thinking on AI accountability.

Prompt: Is Explainable AI sufficient to resolve accountability and trust issues in healthcare, or are additional institutional safeguards required?

Deliverable: A reflective response (200–250 words).

References

Alshehade, S. A., Al Zarzour, R. H., Bitar, A. N., Alshehadeh, A. R., Tamilwanan, S., & Safni, S. (2025). Ethical considerations in the application of artificial intelligence in the pharmaceutical industry. In *Conference on Sustainability and Cutting-Edge Business Technologies*. Cham: Springer Nature Switzerland, 326–335.

Bergen, V., Kodella, K., Srikrishnan, S., Barrandon, O., Anderson, S., Rogers-Grazado, M., & Zamanighomi, M. (2025). A large-scale human toxicogenomics resource for drug-induced liver injury prediction. *Nature Communications, 16*(1), 9860.

Bhimani, A., Bhatt, T. C., Ibrahim, M., Detroja, A., Koradiya, J., Mandaliya, V. B., Maharshi, A., Sanghvi, G., & Bishoyi, A. K. (2026). Multidrug-resistant pathogens in UTIs: A concise review of epidemiology, diagnostics, and patent landscaping for precision healthcare. *Diagnostic Microbiology and Infectious Disease, 114*(2). https://doi.org/10.1016/j.diagmicrobio.2025.117125, https://www.sciencedirect.com/science/journal/07328893.

Cherradi, O., Ziti, S., Kharmoum, N., & El Harraj, A. (2025). Artificial intelligence and connected devices in healthcare: Exploring their potential and limitations. In *International Conference on the Global Summit of Digital Health*. Cham: Springer Nature Switzerland, 136–146.

Chin, W. J., Lim, W. Y., Khor, S. M., Ramakrishnan, N., Chee, P. S., & Goh, C. H. (2025). Advancement of machine learning algorithms in biosensors. *Clinica Chimica Acta,* 120677.

Choi, M. Y., Fritzler, M. J., & Mahler, M. (2021). Development of multi-omics approach in autoimmune diseases. In *Precision Medicine and Artificial Intelligence*. Academic Press, 189–201.

El-Jlaidi, K., Ziti, S., & Kharmoum, N. (2025). Artificial intelligence in healthcare: AI-driven diagnostics, tailored medicine, predictive analytics, and robotic surgery. In *International Conference on the Global Summit of Digital Health*. Cham: Springer Nature Switzerland, 355–368.

Georgilas, V. (2025). Automatic speech recognition for greek medical dictation [Bachelor's thesis]. Athens University of Economics and Business.

Hay, M., Thomas, D. W., Craighead, J. L., Economides, C., & Rosenthal, J. (2014). Clinical development success rates for investigational drugs. *Nature Biotechnology, 32*(1), 40–51. https://doi.org/10.1038/nbt.2786.

Maharjan, R., Kim, N. A., Kim, K. H., & Jeong, S. H. (2025). Transformative roles of digital twins from drug discovery to continuous manufacturing: Pharmaceutical and biopharmaceutical perspectives. *International Journal of Pharmaceutics: X,* 100409.

Mohammad, A. A. S., Mohammad, S. I. S., Al Oraini, B., Vasudevan, A., Hindieh, A., Altarawneh, A., & Ali, I. (2025). Strategies for applying interpretable and explainable AI in real world IoT applications. *Discover Internet of Things, 5*(1), 71.

Ratti, E., Morrison, M., & Jakab, I. (2025). Ethical and social considerations of applying artificial intelligence in healthcare—A two-pronged scoping review. *BMC Medical Ethics, 26*(1), 68.

Somara, S., Joshi, A. M., Mitra, K., Desai, S., Lundberg, M. S., Bhasin, S., & Hunsberger, J. (2025). Artificial intelligence in biotechnology and pharmaceuticals: Evolution, applications, and regulatory frontiers. *Current Stem Cell Reports, 11*(1), 1–10.

Further reading

Ali, S., Khan, S.S. A., Khan, B.F., & Ali, A.S. H. (2025). Digital twins and AI for end-to-end sustainable pharmaceutical supply chain management.

Antoniadi, A. M., Du, Y., Guendouz, Y., Wei, L., Mazo, C., Becker, B. A., & Mooney, C. (2021). Current challenges and future opportunities for XAI in machine learning-based clinical decision support systems: A systematic review. *Applied Sciences, 11*(11), 5088.

Deshpande, D., Sharma, K., & Gupta, S. K. (2025). Machine learning models in mental health:: A literature review on voice-based depression. *Screening. SGS-Engineering & Sciences, 1*(1).

Federico, C. A., & Trotsyuk, A. A. (2024). Biomedical data science, artificial intelligence, and ethics: navigating challenges in the face of explosive growth. *Annual Review of Biomedical Data Science, 7*(1), 1–14.

Kalusivalingam, A. K., Sharma, A., Patel, N., & Singh, V. (2021). Leveraging federated learning and explainable AI for advancing health equity: A comprehensive approach to reducing disparities in healthcare access and outcomes. *International Journal of AI and ML, 2*(3).

Labkoff, S., Oladimeji, B., Kannry, J., Solomonides, A., Leftwich, R., Koski, E., & Quintana, Y. (2024). Toward a responsible future: Recommendations for AI-enabled clinical decision support. *Journal of the American Medical Informatics Association, 31*(11), 2730–2739.

Vitorino, R., & Ghavami, S. (2025). Convergence: Multi-omics and AI are reshaping the landscape biomedical research. *Biochimica et Biophysica Acta (BBA)-Molecular Basis of Disease,* 168027.

Zheng, L., Wang, O., Hao, S., Ye, C., Liu, M., Xia, M., & Ling, X. B. (2020). Development of an early-warning system for high-risk patients for suicide attempt using deep learning and electronic health records. *Translational psychiatry, 10*(1), 72.

CHAPTER 4

Artificial intelligence in the pharmaceutical industry: applications, challenges, and future directions

Hani Alhashmi[1], Mohammed Alhefzi[2,3], and Luluh Aldhubayi[4,5]

[1]Medical Affairs, Pfizer Biopharmaceuticals, Riyadh, Saudi Arabia, [2]College of Medicine, Alfaisal University, Riyadh, Saudi Arabia, [3]Saudi Association for Health Informatics (SAHI), Riyadh, Saudi Arabia, [4]College of Computer and Information Sciences, King Saud University, Riyadh, Saudi Arabia, [5]AI Center of Advanced Studies (Thakaa), King Saud University, Riyadh, Saudi Arabia

Summary

Artificial intelligence (AI) is fundamentally transforming the pharmaceutical industry, delivering measurable improvements across the entire value chain—from molecular discovery to patient outcome management. This chapter examines how AI enhances efficiency, accuracy, and clinical relevance in drug development, trial optimization, safety surveillance, manufacturing, and digital health integration. Contemporary AI applications extend beyond traditional pharmaceutical boundaries, enabling patient support programs (PSPs), digital therapeutics, and continuous real-world evidence generation that bridges controlled trial environments with population health outcomes.

Large language models (LLMs), such as GPT-3, GPT-4, GPT-5, and their derivatives, represent a particularly transformative subset of AI technologies. Using transformer architectures to process and generate natural language with remarkable fluency, LLMs are rapidly reshaping drug discovery by accelerating tasks across the pharmaceutical pipeline, processing vast biomedical datasets, generating hypotheses, and interacting with molecular data.

This chapter synthesizes peer-reviewed evidence and validated case studies demonstrating AI's quantifiable impact, including accelerated molecule generation, predictive trial recruitment, automated pharmacovigilance, adaptive manufacturing, and integrated drug-digital therapy approaches. Critical examination of ethical considerations, regulatory frameworks, and convergence with emerging technologies provides a comprehensive understanding of AI's current capabilities and limitations. The analysis concludes with evidence-based

The Future of Pharma Across All Sectors in the Artificial Intelligence Era. DOI: https://doi.org/10.1016/B978-0-443-40572-3.00014-9

projections for the pharmaceutical industry's evolution toward patient-centric, data-driven healthcare delivery models utilizing AI to advance equitable and sustainable global health outcomes.

4.1 Introduction

The pharmaceutical industry confronts persistent challenges that threaten its sustainability and societal impact: development cycles exceeding 10–15 years, costs reaching $2.6 billion per approved drug, and clinical failure rates approaching 90% in late-stage trials (DiMasi et al., 2016). This productivity crisis represents a fundamental challenge requiring transformation in how drugs are discovered, developed, and delivered (Scannell et al., 2012).

Artificial intelligence (AI)—computational systems capable of learning from data, recognizing patterns, and making predictive decisions—offers unprecedented solutions to these challenges. Machine learning (ML) applications in drug discovery demonstrate 80%–90% success rates in Phase I trials, substantially higher than historic industry averages of 40%–65% (Jayatunga et al., 2024), while AI-assisted clinical trials show 10%–20% improvements in enrollment and average timeline reductions of 6 months per asset (ZS Associates, 2025). COVID-19 pandemic exemplified AI's transformative potential, with AI algorithms reducing vaccine development timelines from years to months through accelerated target identification, sequence optimization, and manufacturing scale-up, as demonstrated by companies like Moderna which increased messenger RNA (mRNA) production from 30 to over 1000 molecules per month using AI-driven automation (Evaluating the Impact of Artificial Intelligence on Vaccine Development: Lessons Learned from the COVID-19 Pandemic, 2024).

Contemporary AI integrates diverse data modalities—genomics, proteomics, electronic health records (EHR), medical imaging, and real-world evidence (RWE)—to uncover biological insights previously inaccessible through conventional methods. Advanced ML architectures, including transformer networks, graph neural networks, and generative adversarial networks (GANs), enable sophisticated molecular design, patient stratification, and outcome prediction capabilities. The convergence of these technologies with regulatory frameworks—particularly the Food and Drug Administration's (FDA) guidance on AI/ML-based medical devices and European Medicines Agency's reflection paper on AI throughout medicinal product lifecycles—creates unprecedented opportunities for evidence-based pharmaceutical innovation (European Medicines Agency, 2023; Food and Drug Administration, 2024).

The expansion of the digital health ecosystem further amplifies AI's impact, enabling pharmaceutical companies to evolve from molecule-centric organizations to comprehensive health solution providers. This transformation leverages continuous patient monitoring, personalized intervention delivery, and real-world effectiveness measurement to optimize therapeutic outcomes beyond traditional drug efficacy metrics. The integration of AI across pharmaceutical value chains represents not merely technological advancement but a fundamental reimagining of how medicines are created, tested, and delivered to improve global health outcomes.

To illustrate the comprehensive scope of AI's impact across pharmaceutical operations, Table 4.1 provides a systematic overview of AI applications, technologies, benefits, and performance metrics across the entire pharmaceutical value chain. This framework serves as a roadmap for understanding how AI transforms each stage of pharmaceutical development and commercialization, from initial target discovery through post-market surveillance.

The subsequent sections of this chapter examine each stage of the pharmaceutical value chain in detail, exploring how specific AI technologies deliver the benefits and performance improvements outlined in Table 4.1. Each section provides in-depth analysis of implementation strategies, challenges, and real-world applications that demonstrate AI's transformative impact on pharmaceutical innovation and patient care.

4.2 Large language models in the pharmaceutical industry

Large language models (LLMs) have rapidly transformed the landscape of AI, enabling machines to generate human-like text, code, images, and more. These algorithms and models are revolutionizing fields from healthcare and education to business and creative industries, while also raising new ethical, technical, and societal challenges (Hagos et al., 2024).

LLMs and generative AI refer to algorithms that learn patterns from vast datasets to create new, similar content. LLMs, such as GPT-3, GPT-4, GPT-5, and their derivatives, use transformer architectures to process and generate natural language with remarkable fluency and versatility (Vaswani et al., 2017). These models are trained on massive corpora, allowing them to perform tasks like answering questions, summarizing information, generating code, and even passing professional exams at near-human levels.

In terms of the pharmaceutical industry, AI has a fundamental impact on transforming drug discovery by accelerating timelines, reducing costs, and enabling new approaches to molecule design and optimization. However, LLMs, in particular, are rapidly reshaping drug discovery by accelerating tasks across the pharmaceutical pipeline. The architecture of LLMs shows an ability to derive new research paradigms in the field by processing vast biomedical datasets, generating hypotheses, and interacting with molecular data (Hersh, 2025).

On the other hand, recent publications have shown that the rapid integration of LLMs into chemical science and drug discovery brings significant risks (He et al., 2023; Ramos et al., 2024). The main risks involve dual-use potential, where LLMs can be misused for harmful

Table 4.1 Artificial intelligence (AI) applications across the pharmaceutical value chain.

Value chain stage	AI applications	Technologies used	Key benefits	Performance metrics
Preclinical development	Toxicity prediction, Pharmacokinetic modeling, Safety assessment, Efficacy prediction, Formulation optimization	Predictive modeling, Machine learning algorithms, Computer vision, Multimodal AI, Deep learning	Reduced animal testing, Earlier safety signal detection, Cost reduction, Faster progression decisions, Enhanced predictive accuracy	Reduced preclinical failures, Accelerated development timelines, Enhanced safety prediction, Cost optimization
Clinical trial design	Protocol optimization, Patient stratification strategies, Endpoint selection, Adaptive trial design, Sample size optimization	Bayesian optimization, Predictive analytics, Statistical machine learning, Clinical data mining, Simulation models	Optimized trial protocols, Reduced sample sizes, Enhanced statistical power, Improved success probability, Faster regulatory approval	Significant sample size reduction, Improved statistical validity, Enhanced regulatory acceptance, Reduced development risk
Patient recruitment and enrollment	Patient identification, Eligibility screening, Site selection optimization, Enrollment prediction, Diversity enhancement	Natural language processing, Electronic health record mining, Predictive modeling, Machine learning algorithms, Data integration platforms	Accelerated recruitment, Improved patient matching, Reduced screen failures, Enhanced diversity, Optimized site performance	10%–20% enrollment boost, Reduced recruitment timelines, Decreased screen failure rates, Improved patient diversity
Clinical trial execution	Real-time data monitoring, Protocol deviation detection, Data quality assurance, Patient adherence monitoring, Safety signal detection	Internet of Things integration, Wearable device analytics, Real-time machine learning, Mobile health applications, Continuous monitoring AI	Enhanced data quality, Proactive interventions, Improved patient retention, Faster data processing, Real-time decision making	6-month timeline reduction, Improved data integrity, Enhanced patient retention, Reduced protocol deviations
Regulatory submission	Document automation, Submission optimization, Compliance monitoring, Regulatory intelligence, Risk assessment	Natural language processing, Document generation AI, Regulatory machine learning, Compliance analytics, Risk assessment models	Accelerated submissions, Enhanced compliance, Reduced regulatory risk, Improved documentation quality, Streamlined processes	Faster submission timelines, Enhanced compliance scores, Reduced regulatory delays, Improved approval rates

Manufacturing and quality control	Process optimization, Quality control automation, Predictive maintenance, Yield optimization, Real-time monitoring	Computer vision, Predictive analytics, Internet of Things, Machine learning, Process control AI	Consistent product quality, Reduced manufacturing costs, Minimized downtime, Enhanced compliance, Optimized yields	Nearly 10% COGM reduction, 50% maintenance cost reduction, 25% capacity increase, Improved quality consistency
Supply chain and distribution	Demand forecasting, Inventory optimization, Supply risk management, Cold chain monitoring, Distribution optimization	Forecasting algorithms, optimization models, Internet of Things analytics, Risk assessment ML, Logistics AI	Reduced inventory costs, Minimized stockouts, Enhanced supply security, Optimized distribution, Risk mitigation	Substantial inventory optimization, Reduced stockout occurrences, Enhanced forecast accuracy, Improved supply reliability
Pharmacovigilance	Automated case processing, Safety signal detection, Literature surveillance, Social media monitoring, Adverse event prediction	Natural language processing, Machine learning, Social media analytics, Predictive safety models, Text mining	Earlier signal detection, Comprehensive surveillance, Reduced false positives, Proactive safety monitoring, Enhanced patient safety	Months earlier detection, Enhanced coverage versus 1%–10% traditional, Reduced manual workload, Improved signal accuracy
Medical affairs	Medical information management, Scientific communication, Literature synthesis, Healthcare professional engagement, Evidence generation	Natural language processing, Knowledge synthesis AI, Personalization algorithms, Content generation AI, Analytics platforms	Rapid information delivery, Personalized communications, Enhanced scientific accuracy, Improved engagement, Streamlined processes	Minutes versus days response time, High expert concordance, Improved satisfaction scores, Enhanced engagement rates
Market access and commercialization	Health economics modeling, Market analysis, Pricing optimization, Launch strategy, Competitive intelligence	Health economics AI, Market intelligence, Pricing algorithms, Forecasting models, Competitive analytics	Optimized market access, Enhanced pricing strategies, Improved launch success, Better market positioning, Competitive advantage	Improved market penetration, Optimized pricing outcomes, Enhanced launch performance, Better ROI achievement

(Continued)

Table 4.1 (Continued)

Value chain stage	AI applications	Technologies used	Key benefits	Performance metrics
Patient support and engagement	Adherence monitoring, Risk stratification, Personalized interventions, Outcome tracking, Care coordination	Behavioral analytics, Predictive modeling, Personalization AI, Mobile health platforms, Patient engagement AI	Improved medication adherence, Better patient outcomes, Reduced healthcare costs, Enhanced patient satisfaction, Proactive care management	Meaningful adherence improvements, Reduced healthcare utilization, Enhanced patient satisfaction, Better outcome achievement
Digital therapeutics integration	Behavioral interventions, Therapy combination, Outcome optimization, Adaptive algorithms, Real-world monitoring	Behavioral AI, Adaptive algorithms, Mobile analytics, Integration platforms, Outcome tracking AI	Enhanced therapeutic efficacy, Comprehensive patient care, Improved treatment adherence, Better clinical outcomes, Personalized interventions	Superior outcomes vs monotherapy, Enhanced medication adherence, Improved clinical metrics outcomes, Better patient engagement
Post-market surveillance	Real-world evidence generation, Effectiveness studies, Long-term safety monitoring, Population health analysis, Comparative effectiveness	Real-world data analytics, Epidemiological AI, Outcomes research ML, Population health models, Comparative analytics	Continuous safety monitoring, Real-world validation, Population-level insights, Evidence-based optimization, Regulatory support	RCT-comparable evidence quality, Reduced study costs, Accelerated evidence generation, Enhanced regulatory acceptance

purposes, and the generation of inaccurate or unsafe outputs. Therefore an effective risk control requires technical, regulatory, and collaborative strategies.

Although LLMs have only recently begun to make a significant impact on the pharmaceutical industry, their adoption is rooted in decades of progress in artificial intelligence, natural language processing (NLP), and computational drug discovery. In this section, we will discuss both the transformative opportunities, challenges, and risks of adopting LLMs in the pharmaceutical industry and drug discovery.

4.2.1 From machine learning to large language models

Over the past few decades, drug discovery has undergone a profound transformation, driven largely by rapid advancements in AI. Earlier, tasks such as molecular modeling and virtual screening primarily relied on traditional ML models (Liu et al., 2024). As data availability expanded, these approaches laid the foundation for today's integration of more advanced, language-based models, further enabled by growing computational power (Nuthakki, 2023).

Before the advent of LLMs, AI in drug discovery was primarily driven by ML, deep learning (DL), and traditional NLP techniques. These approaches brought significant advances to drug discovery, especially in property prediction, virtual screening, and early generative design. For example, early applications relied on algorithms such as random forests, support vector machines, deep neural networks, and convolutional neural networks, which were employed in quantitative structure–activity relationship modeling to predict toxicity, bioactivity, and physicochemical properties, while also supporting virtual screening and de novo molecular design (Chen, Liu, et al., 2023; Hessler & Baringhaus, 2018; Rehman et al., 2024). These models required explicit molecular representations—including SMILES strings, molecular fingerprints, and graph-based encodings—and often depended on manual feature engineering to convert chemical structures into machine-readable inputs (Hessler & Baringhaus, 2018).

Moreover, AI methods facilitated the analysis of large-scale datasets for target identification and compound library screening, thereby accelerating hit discovery and lead optimization (Vora et al., 2023). DL approaches also began to show considerable promise in protein structure prediction, with early iterations of AlphaFold demonstrating their potential to support rational drug design (Han et al., 2023; Jumper et al., 2021). In parallel, traditional NLP techniques, such as word2vec (Church, 2017), BioBERT (Lee et al., 2020), and ClinicalBERT (Huang et al., 2019), were employed for literature mining to extract associations between drugs, targets, and diseases from scientific texts. However, these models lacked the generative capacity and multitasking versatility that characterize current LLM-based systems (Liu et al., 2021). While these earlier methods significantly advanced the field of drug discovery, their scope and flexibility remained more constrained compared to the transformative potential of modern LLM-driven approaches.

4.2.2 The adoption of large language models in the pharmaceutical industry and drug discovery

The drug discovery pipeline is a complex, multistage process that translates a scientific concept into a marketable therapeutic product. It involves iterative cycles of design, testing, and optimization across several phases, with decision-making and refinement occurring at multiple points (Rao & Srinivas, 2011). Despite advances, the process typically spans more than a decade, requires investments of billions of dollars, and is characterized by a high attrition rate, particularly during late-stage clinical trials. Increasingly, AI, ML, and other computational approaches are being integrated into modern pipelines to accelerate discovery, enhance predictive accuracy, and support more informed decision-making at each stage. While recent innovations and interdisciplinary collaboration have helped streamline this process, drug discovery remains a lengthy, costly, resource-intensive, and highly complex endeavor (Khanna, 2012). Notably, AI is reshaping this landscape by shortening development timelines, reducing overall costs, and enabling innovative strategies for molecule design, target identification, and lead optimization.

Since 2017, the integration of LLMs into pharmaceutical research began with the development of transformer-based models. These models, trained on vast biomedical and chemical datasets, enabled new capabilities in understanding, generating, and extracting information from unstructured scientific text (Liu et al., 2024). LLMs are applied to achieve certain tasks in the drug discovery lifecycle, such as target identification and target validation. Protein language models and tools like QuoteTarget (Chen, Gu et al., 2023) or TransDTI (Kalakoti et al., 2022) predict druggable protein targets and drug-target interactions, which contribute to the drug discovery lifecycle by identifying a biological target (protein, gene, pathway) linked to a disease.

The second important task in the drug discovery lifecycle is lead optimization or hit-to-design optimization. As part of the lead optimization or hit-to-design optimization process, the molecular design can be generated using transformer-based models, which generate novel molecules with desired properties. The structure-based design, such as SMILES strings and molecular graphs, can enable ligand and scaffold generation (e.g., Transmol, MolGPT, and DrugLLM). In addition, the de novo drug design can be achieved by models like cMolGPT and FSM-DDTR, which create entirely new drug-like molecules optimized for efficacy and safety.

An example of a transformer-based model that uses SMILES strings to represent molecules is ChemBERTa (Chithrananda et al., 2020). This model was developed in 2020 and applies techniques from NLP to predict chemical properties and drug interactions. Its architecture is based on BERT-style transformers, pretrained on massive chemical datasets (up to 77 million compounds), enabling strong performance on property prediction, drug-drug interaction, and drug-target interaction tasks. ChemBERTa consistently matches or outperforms traditional

Table 4.2 Transformer-based models across drug discovery stages.

LLM model	Drug discovery stage(s)	Key application/focus
ChemBERTa (Chithrananda et al., 2020), GraphormerDTI (Gao et al., 2024)	Drug-target interaction (DTI) prediction, Lead optimization	Predicting DTIs, molecular property prediction, prioritizing candidates
DeepMGT-DTI (Zhang et al., 2022)	DTI prediction, Drug repositioning	Integrating molecular structure and sequence for DTI, drug repositioning
DrugGPT (Li et al., 2023), DrugGen (Sheikholeslami et al., 2024)	De novo drug design, Lead generation, Drug repositioning	Generative models for novel molecule creation, binding affinity optimization
Chemformer (Irwin et al., 2022), Molecular transformer (Schwaller et al., 2019)	Retrosynthesis, Chemical synthesis planning	Multistep retrosynthesis, reaction prediction, synthesis planning
TransDTI (Kalakoti et al., 2022)	DTI prediction, Drug recommendation	Multiclass DTI prediction, workflow for drug recommendation
DeepTTA (Jiang et al., 2022)	Drug response prediction, Cancer drug design	Predicting anticancer drug response using transcriptomics

models, achieving high accuracy (e.g., AUROC up to 0.97 for drug-drug interaction prediction), and its embeddings improve downstream tasks in drug discovery and safety screening. The model's impact lies in its scalability, data efficiency, and ability to accelerate early-stage drug development by providing robust molecular representations. However, its main limitations include reduced generalizability to external or heterogeneous datasets, as performance can drop significantly outside the training domain (e.g., AUROC falling from 76% to 44% in some cases), and a strong dependence on the size and diversity of training data (Ahmad et al., 2022; Gromova & Maida, 2025; Kang et al., 2022). More examples of transformer-based models and their primary applications or stages within the drug discovery pipeline, as reported in recent literature, are shown in Table 4.2

4.3 Transforming drug discovery through computational intelligence

Traditional drug discovery confronts the overwhelming complexity of chemical space—-estimated at 10^{60} possible drug-like molecules—while operating under severe experimental throughput constraints. As outlined in Table 4.1, AI addresses these fundamental limitations through sophisticated computational methods that predict molecular properties, design novel compounds, and prioritize candidates with an enhanced probability of clinical success, achieving remarkable 80%–90% Phase I success rates compared to traditional averages of 40%–65%.

Contemporary AI drug discovery integrates molecular property prediction, synthetic accessibility scoring, and toxicity forecasting within unified platforms (Chen et al., 2018; Pu et al., 2019). Graph convolutional networks predict blood-brain barrier permeability with high accuracy, while transformer-based models generate novel scaffolds with improved selectivity profiles (IQVIA, 2024; Zhou et al., 2023). These advances address the historical challenge of optimizing multiple drug properties simultaneously—potency, selectivity, pharmacokinetics, and safety—through multiobjective optimization algorithms that explore chemical space more efficiently than traditional high-throughput screening.

Target identification and validation benefit significantly from AI's ability to integrate multiomics datasets and identify disease-relevant biological pathways. ML models analyze genomic, transcriptomic, and proteomic data to discover novel therapeutic targets while predicting drug-target interactions and potential off-target effects. GANs and reinforcement learning algorithms enable de novo molecular design, creating chemical entities with optimized pharmacokinetic and safety profiles before synthesis and testing (Jagatheesaperumal et al., 2024; Zhavoronkov et al., 2020). Recent advances in protein structure prediction, exemplified by AlphaFold's ability to determine three-dimensional (3D) structures from amino acid sequences, accelerate structure-based drug design by eliminating time-intensive crystallography requirements (Jumper et al., 2021).

Multitarget drug discovery using graph neural networks represents a paradigm shift toward addressing complex diseases through polypharmacology approaches. AI models predict synergistic drug combinations and design molecules capable of modulating multiple targets simultaneously, potentially improving efficacy while reducing side effects. Proteolysis-targeting chimera design benefits from AI-guided molecular generation, enabling targeted protein degradation strategies for previously "undruggable" targets (Gharbi et al., 2024).

The integration of pharmacogenomics with AI-driven drug design enables precision medicine applications from early development stages. ML algorithms identify genetic variants influencing drug response, enabling stratified drug development strategies that improve efficacy while reducing adverse events in specific patient populations. This approach transforms traditional "one-size-fits-all" paradigms toward personalized therapeutic strategies grounded in individual genetic profiles and biomarker status.

These pharmacogenomics advances, combined with AI-driven discovery platforms, have produced measurable improvements in drug development efficiency. For instance, BenevolentAI's, a London-based AI drug discovery company founded in 2013, demonstrated AI's rapid repurposing capabilities during the COVID-19 pandemic by identifying Baricitinib as a therapeutic candidate within weeks rather than years, proceeding rapidly to clinical validation and emergency use authorization (Richardson et al., 2020). Another example is Insilico Medicine, which has demonstrated AI's ability to compress drug development timelines through its INS018_055 program, which progressed from target discovery to Phase I trials in 30 months compared to traditional 4–6 year preclinical phases, with the compound becoming the first AI-discovered and AI-designed drug to advance to Phase II trials (Insilico Medicine, 2023). These validated examples illustrate AI's potential to compress discovery timelines while maintaining rigorous safety and efficacy standards essential for regulatory approval and patient safety.

4.4 Revolutionizing clinical development and trial design

Clinical trials represent the most resource-intensive and failure-prone phases of drug development, with patient recruitment delays, protocol design inefficiencies, and inadequate endpoint selection contributing to extended timelines and escalating costs. As demonstrated in Table 4.1, AI transforms trial operations through sophisticated data integration, predictive modeling, and adaptive design methodologies that optimize recruitment, execution, and outcome measurement, delivering 10%–20% enrollment improvements and 6-month average timeline reductions (Fleming et al., 2020; Terranova et al., 2024).

Predictive recruitment algorithms analyze EHR, claims databases, and genomic repositories to identify eligible patients with unprecedented precision and speed. NLP systems parse structured and unstructured clinical data, enabling rapid patient matching while reducing screen failure rates in oncology trials (Steinhubl et al., 2019). ML models predict patient adherence likelihood, protocol deviation risk, and dropout probability, enabling proactive interventions that maintain trial integrity and statistical power (Bartlett et al., 2019; Khalate et al., 2024).

Decentralized clinical trial (DCT) implementation accelerated dramatically during COVID-19, with AI-powered platforms enabling remote patient monitoring while maintaining data quality and regulatory compliance. Integrated systems combining wearable sensors, smartphone applications, and predictive analytics detect protocol deviations in real-time, enable immediate interventions, and maintain trial integrity across distributed sites. Systematic analysis of DCT implementations demonstrated significant reductions in trial duration, improvements in patient retention, and increases in diverse population enrollment compared to traditional site-based designs (Ghosh et al., 2021; Liu et al., 2020).

Analysis of operational AI/ML data from leading biopharma companies demonstrates that these techniques can boost trial enrollment by 10%–20% and compress development timelines by an average of 6 months per asset across therapeutic areas (Fleming et al., 2020). AI-enabled site selection drives superior trial outcomes by identifying and predicting top-enrolling sites, with top-quartile sites typically outperforming median sites by two to four times (Terranova et al., 2024).

Adaptive trial designs powered by ML algorithms continuously adjust randomization ratios, sample sizes, and endpoint definitions based on accumulating efficacy and safety data.

Bayesian optimization methods enable real-time protocol modifications while preserving statistical validity and regulatory acceptance. Metaanalysis of adaptive trials demonstrated significant reductions in required sample sizes while maintaining statistical power, with particular benefit in rare disease studies where traditional fixed designs prove impractical (Singh et al., 2020; Yang et al., 2022).

Synthetic control arms represent a revolutionary advancement in clinical trial methodology, utilizing AI to create virtual control groups from historical trial data and RWE. These approaches potentially reduce placebo group requirements in diseases with high unmet medical need while addressing ethical concerns regarding treatment withholding. FDA's guidance on external controls and EMA's qualification opinions provide a regulatory framework for synthetic control implementation, supported by validation studies demonstrating equivalence to traditional randomized controlled trials in specific clinical settings (European Medicines Agency, 2023; Food and Drug Administration, 2024).

AI-assisted endpoint selection optimizes trial design by identifying biomarkers and clinical outcomes most predictive of long-term therapeutic benefit. ML models analyze historical trial databases to predict which endpoints offer the greatest statistical power and clinical relevance, thereby reducing trial duration and improving the probability of regulatory approval. Digital biomarker development enables continuous outcome monitoring through wearable devices and smartphone applications, providing objective, quantitative measures of treatment response that complement traditional clinical assessments.

RWE integration during trial conduct enables external validation of efficacy and safety findings while trials progress. AI algorithms harmonize trial data with EHR, insurance claims, and patient registries to assess treatment effectiveness in broader populations than trial participants represent. This integration provides early indicators of real-world performance and identifies potential safety signals that require protocol modifications or enhanced monitoring procedures.

4.5 Pharmacovigilance and post-marketing surveillance

Post-marketing safety surveillance faces fundamental challenges, including underreporting of adverse events, delayed signal detection, and limited ability to establish causal relationships between drugs and rare adverse outcomes. Traditional pharmacovigilance (PV) relies heavily on spontaneous reporting systems that capture only 1%–10% of actual adverse events, as acknowledged by regulatory authorities including the FDA, creating substantial gaps in safety knowledge that persist throughout product lifecycles (FDA Adverse Event Reporting System (FAERS), Underreporting; Chen, Allot, et al., 2023). As shown in Table 4.1, AI revolutionizes PV through automated case processing, literature mining, and RWE analysis, achieving months earlier signal detection compared to traditional methods.

AI revolutionizes PV through automated case processing, literature mining, and RWE analysis, enhancing both the efficiency and sensitivity of safety signal detection. ML algorithms process millions of adverse event reports simultaneously, identifying patterns and associations that human reviewers cannot detect due to volume limitations and cognitive biases. NLP facilitates rapid extraction of adverse event information from unstructured clinical notes, regulatory submissions, biomedical literature, and social media platforms, expanding surveillance beyond traditional reporting channels (Alowais et al., 2023; Yang et al., 2023).

Predictive safety modeling represents a paradigm shift from reactive to proactive PV. AI can analyze molecular structures, mechanisms of action, and population health data to predict potential adverse events before they manifest in spontaneous reporting systems. These models integrate chemical structure–activity relationships, known toxicology pathways, and patient-specific risk factors to generate personalized safety profiles that guide prescribing decisions and monitoring strategies.

RWE integration enhances continuous safety monitoring through EHRs, insurance claims databases, and patient support programs (PSPs). AI algorithms continuously analyze these data streams to detect safety signals, quantify risk-benefit profiles, and identify patient subpopulations at increased adverse event risk. Validation studies demonstrate that AI-powered safety surveillance systems can detect signals significantly earlier than traditional methods while reducing false-positive rates (Li et al., 2020; Obermeyer et al., 2019).

Automated literature surveillance eliminates manual review bottlenecks by continuously scanning biomedical databases, regulatory websites, and scientific publications for safety-relevant information. ML models extract adverse event reports, identify new safety signals, and prioritize findings based on clinical significance and regulatory impact. These systems process volumes of literature that are impossible for human reviewers to process while maintaining high sensitivity in detecting novel safety concerns.

Social media monitoring expands PV reach by analyzing patient-generated content across digital platforms. AI-powered tools identify adverse event mentions in social media posts, online forums, and patient communities, often detecting previously unreported side effects before formal regulatory submissions. Studies demonstrate that social listening can identify substantial numbers of additional adverse events compared to traditional reporting systems while providing real-time insights into patient safety experiences (Council for International Organizations of Medical Sciences CIOMS, 2024; World Health Organization, 2021).

Regulatory authorities increasingly recognize AI's value in PV optimization. FDA's guidance on AI in post-market surveillance provides a framework for algorithm validation, continuous learning implementation, and regulatory submission requirements. EMA's PV risk assessment committee actively evaluates AI-generated safety signals, establishing precedent for algorithm-assisted regulatory decision-making in drug safety evaluation (European Medicines Agency, 2023; Food and Drug Administration, 2024; Yu et al., 2018).

4.6 Autonomous manufacturing and intelligent supply networks

Pharmaceutical manufacturing operates under stringent quality, safety, and regulatory compliance requirements while managing complex global supply chains susceptible to disruption and demand variability. Traditional manufacturing approaches rely on reactive quality control, scheduled maintenance, and linear forecasting methods that inadequately address modern pharmaceutical complexity and regulatory expectations (Patterson et al., 2024; Vora et al., 2023).

AI enables transformation toward predictive, adaptive manufacturing ecosystems that optimize quality, efficiency, and compliance simultaneously. ML algorithms analyze real-time sensor data to identify process anomalies, predict equipment failures, and optimize batch parameters before quality issues manifest. Computer vision systems detect tablet defects, coating irregularities, and packaging errors with exceptional accuracy, surpassing human inspection capabilities while providing objective, consistent quality assessment (Blanco-González et al., 2023; International Council for Harmonisation of Technical Requirements for Pharmaceuticals for Human Use, 2019).

As detailed in Table 4.1, multiple analyses of biopharmaceutical manufacturing performance demonstrate that AI-driven optimization can reduce cost of goods manufactured by 5%–10%, primarily through yield improvement and process control enhancements (McKinsey & Company, 2022). Predictive maintenance implementations have achieved up to 50% reductions in maintenance-related costs, significant reductions in capital expenditure, and 20%–30% increases in available production capacity across benchmarked sites (McKinsey & Company, 2022).

Predictive maintenance algorithms forecast equipment failures by analyzing historical performance data, vibration patterns, temperature fluctuations, and operational parameters. These models generate maintenance schedules tailored to individual asset conditions rather than arbitrary time intervals, reducing unplanned downtime while optimizing maintenance resource allocation. Predictive maintenance particularly benefits complex manufacturing equipment where unexpected failures result in significant production delays and batch losses.

Process optimization utilizes ML to continuously adjust manufacturing parameters—temperature, pressure, mixing speeds, and reaction times—based on real-time quality indicators and historical batch performance. These systems identify optimal operating conditions for each product while adapting to raw material variability, environmental conditions, and equipment status. Advanced process control algorithms significantly reduce batch-to-batch variability while improving yield and reducing waste generation.

From a commercial angle, supply chain forecasting integrates sales history, prescription trends, epidemiological data, and external factors to predict demand and optimize distribution networks. AI models account for seasonal variations, disease outbreaks, and healthcare access patterns to prevent shortages while minimizing inventory costs. Implementations demonstrate substantial improvements in inventory optimization and reductions in stockout occurrences through enhanced demand prediction accuracy (McKinsey & Company, 2022).

Regulatory compliance automation represents a critical advancement in pharmaceutical manufacturing quality assurance. AI systems continuously monitor manufacturing data against FDA, EMA, and International Council for Harmonisation guidelines, automatically generating compliance reports and identifying potential deviations before regulatory impact occurs. ML algorithms analyze manufacturing records, batch documentation, and quality control results to predict inspection outcomes and recommend corrective actions (European Medicines Agency, 2023; Food and Drug Administration, 2024; International Council for Harmonisation of Technical Requirements for Pharmaceuticals for Human Use, 2019).

Quality by design (QbD) implementation benefits from AI's ability to model complex relationships between material attributes, process parameters, and critical quality attributes. ML algorithms identify design space boundaries, predict process robustness, and optimize control strategies based on a comprehensive understanding of manufacturing processes. These capabilities enable a science-based approach to manufacturing that satisfies regulatory expectations while improving operational efficiency.

4.7 Artificial intelligence in medical affairs and commercial strategy

Medical affairs and commercial operations increasingly depend on evidence-based insights to engage healthcare professionals effectively while supporting optimal patient outcomes. As outlined in Table 4.1, AI enhances scientific communication, personalization, and stakeholder engagement through sophisticated data analysis and automated content generation capabilities, reducing medical information response times from days to minutes while maintaining high expert concordance (IQVIA, 2024; Zhou et al., 2023).

NLP transforms medical information management by automatically scanning vast literature volumes, clinical guidelines, and RWE to provide evidence-based responses to healthcare professional inquiries. AI systems synthesize complex scientific information into concise, clinically relevant summaries while maintaining accuracy and regulatory compliance. Studies demonstrate that AI-generated medical information responses achieve high concordance with expert physician reviews while reducing response times from days to minutes (IQVIA, 2024; Zhou et al., 2023).

Healthcare professional engagement utilizes ML algorithms to segment audiences based on specialty, prescribing patterns, communication preferences, and scientific interests. Predictive models identify optimal content, timing, and communication channels for individual physicians while avoiding information overload and ensuring compliance with promotional regulations. Personalized engagement strategies improve healthcare professional satisfaction scores while increasing meaningful scientific interaction rates (IQVIA, 2024; Khalate et al., 2024).

RWE generation leverages AI to analyze EHR, claims databases, and patient registries for post-market effectiveness studies, comparative effectiveness research, and health economic evaluations. ML algorithms identify treatment patterns, predict outcomes, and quantify real-world effectiveness while controlling for confounding variables and selection bias. These capabilities enable pharmaceutical companies to demonstrate value beyond clinical trial efficacy, supporting market access and reimbursement decisions.

Medical writing automation utilizes generative AI to draft regulatory documents, clinical study reports, and scientific publications while maintaining accuracy and compliance with regulatory guidelines. Advanced language models generate initial document drafts that human experts review and refine, reducing authoring time substantially while improving consistency and quality. AI-assisted writing particularly benefits high-volume document production requirements while ensuring adherence to regulatory submission standards.

Scientific platform development integrates AI-powered tools to support healthcare professionals' clinical decision-making through evidence synthesis, guideline recommendations, and patient-specific treatment suggestions. These platforms combine drug information, clinical guidelines, and patient data to provide personalized treatment recommendations that improve prescribing accuracy while supporting evidence-based medicine principles.

On the other hand, DTx codevelopment represents an emerging frontier where pharmaceutical companies integrate AI-powered digital interventions with traditional pharmacotherapy. These solutions provide behavioral modifications, adherence support, and outcome monitoring that enhance drug effectiveness while addressing psychosocial factors influencing treatment success. Validated DTx applications demonstrate significant improvements in medication adherence and clinical outcomes compared to drug therapy alone (Alowais et al., 2023; Obermeyer et al., 2019; Yang et al., 2023).

PSPs utilize AI to predict nonadherence risk, personalize educational content, and deliver timely interventions that improve treatment persistence. ML models analyze patient characteristics, prescription patterns, and engagement behaviors to identify individuals requiring additional support while tailoring intervention strategies to individual preferences and barriers. Such programs demonstrate meaningful improvements in therapy persistence rates across chronic disease populations while reducing healthcare utilization costs.

4.8 Convergence of digital health and pharmaceutical innovation

The convergence of pharmaceutical innovation with digital health technologies creates unprecedented opportunities for comprehensive patient care while raising complex regulatory, ethical, and implementation challenges. Table 4.1 shows how AI serves as the enabling technology that integrates disparate data sources, personalizes interventions, and measures real-world outcomes across traditional healthcare boundaries, with DTx combinations showing superior outcomes compared to monotherapy approaches (European Medicines Agency, 2023; Food and Drug Administration, 2024).

AI-powered data integration harmonizes information streams from EHRs, wearable devices, mobile applications, genomic databases, and national health registries to create comprehensive patient profiles that inform treatment decisions and outcome predictions. Interoperability—which is the ability of different technology systems to communicate–algorithms resolve data format inconsistencies, terminology differences, and temporal misalignments that historically prevented effective healthcare data integration. This unified view enables RWE generation, early disease detection, and treatment personalization based on continuous patient monitoring rather than episodic clinical encounters.

Drug-digital therapy combinations represent a paradigm shift toward holistic treatment approaches where medications are paired with AI-powered digital tools that provide behavioral interventions, biomarker monitoring, and adaptive treatment recommendations. These integrated solutions improve treatment adherence, detect early signs of disease progression, and enable precision medicine delivery that extends beyond pharmacological mechanisms. A recent systematic review of drug-DTx combinations demonstrated superior clinical outcomes compared to pharmacotherapy alone, with particular benefit in chronic diseases requiring long-term management (Alowais et al., 2023; Obermeyer et al., 2019; Yang et al., 2023).

Continuous patient monitoring through wearable sensors, smartphone applications, and home/remote diagnostic devices generates real-time physiological and behavioral data that AI algorithms analyze to detect treatment response, predict adverse events, and recommend intervention adjustments. ML models identify subtle patterns in heart rate variability, activity levels, sleep quality, and medication timing that correlate with clinical outcomes, enabling proactive care management that prevents hospitalizations and improves quality of life.

Regulatory frameworks for AI in pharmaceutical applications continue evolving as agencies develop guidance for algorithm validation, continuous learning systems, and post-market surveillance requirements. FDA's guidance on AI/ML-based medical devices, sometimes referred to as software-as-medical-device establishes a framework for continuous learning algorithms in pharmaceutical applications, emphasizing the need for algorithmic transparency, bias mitigation, and human oversight in AI-assisted healthcare decisions. EMA's reflection paper on AI use throughout the medicinal product lifecycle provides a European perspective on AI validation requirements, post-market monitoring obligations, and quality management system integration (European Medicines Agency, 2023; Food and Drug Administration, 2024).

RWE integration enables pharmaceutical companies to demonstrate effectiveness and safety in diverse patient populations while supporting regulatory submissions, label expansions, and health technology assessments. AI algorithms analyze observational data to generate evidence comparable to traditional clinical studies while reducing costs and accelerating evidence generation. Regulatory authorities increasingly accept high-quality RWE for specific regulatory decisions, particularly in rare diseases where traditional randomized controlled trials prove impractical (European Medicines Agency, 2023; Food and Drug Administration, 2024; Yu et al., 2018).

However, algorithmic bias mitigation requires comprehensive attention to training data diversity, model validation across demographic subgroups, and continuous monitoring for disparate outcomes. AI solutions can perpetuate historical healthcare disparities if training datasets inadequately represent minority populations, socioeconomic diversity, or geographic variations in disease presentation and treatment response. Fairness audits, diverse dataset curation, and algorithmic transparency measures help ensure equitable AI implementation that reduces rather than exacerbates healthcare disparities (Fleming et al., 2020; Obermeyer et al., 2019; Terranova et al., 2024).

Data privacy and security considerations intensify as pharmaceutical AI applications integrate clinical, genetic, and behavioral data across multiple platforms and stakeholders. Federated learning enables model development without centralizing sensitive patient data, while differential privacy techniques protect individual privacy during algorithm training. Blockchain technologies can also provide secure, auditable data sharing mechanisms that maintain patient privacy while enabling multiinstitutional collaboration essential for AI model development and validation.

4.9 Ethical considerations and governance frameworks

Widespread AI adoption in pharmaceutical applications raises fundamental ethical questions regarding fairness, transparency, accountability, and societal impact that require comprehensive governance frameworks and ongoing stakeholder engagement. The potential for AI to improve healthcare outcomes must be balanced against risks of algorithmic bias, privacy violations, and decision-making opacity that could undermine public trust and health equity (Obermeyer et al., 2019; World Health Organization, 2021).

Algorithmic bias represents a critical concern as AI models trained on historical healthcare data may perpetuate existing disparities in care access, treatment effectiveness, and health outcomes. ML algorithms can systematically underperform for racial minorities, women, elderly patients, and socioeconomically disadvantaged populations if training datasets inadequately represent these groups or reflect historical treatment biases. Recent analysis of FDA-approved AI medical devices revealed significant gaps in diversity specifications for training data, highlighting the urgent need for bias mitigation strategies (Obermeyer et al., 2019).

Explainable AI (XAI) techniques address transparency requirements by translating complex algorithmic decisions into clinically interpretable rationales that healthcare professionals and patients can understand and evaluate. Regulatory agencies increasingly demand clear explanations of AI decisions, particularly in safety-critical applications where algorithmic recommendations influence treatment selection, dose adjustment, or safety monitoring. XAI implementation challenges include balancing model performance with interpretability while maintaining user trust and clinical utility (Jagatheesaperumal et al., 2024; Jumper et al., 2021).

Governance frameworks established by leading pharmaceutical companies include AI ethics boards, mandatory bias audits, algorithmic impact assessments, and continuous monitoring protocols that ensure responsible AI development and deployment. These frameworks emphasize human oversight, accountability structures, and clear escalation procedures for addressing algorithmic failures or unintended consequences. The Council for International Organizations of Medical Sciences and regulatory agencies provide guidance on responsible AI use, emphasizing transparency, validation, and patient safety as fundamental requirements (Council for International Organizations of Medical Sciences CIOMS, 2024; World Health Organization, 2021).

Data ownership and consent management become increasingly complex as AI applications integrate information from multiple sources, including EHRs, wearable devices, social media platforms, and genetic databases. Traditional informed consent models prove inadequate for dynamic AI systems that continuously learn and evolve, requiring new approaches to patient engagement and consent management that balance individual autonomy with societal benefits of AI-enabled healthcare improvement.

International collaboration and standardization efforts aim to harmonize AI governance approaches across regulatory jurisdictions while maintaining flexibility for local implementation requirements. Organizations like ICH, the World Health Organization, and the International Medical Device Regulators Forum develop guidance documents that facilitate AI adoption while ensuring patient safety and product quality standards.

Stakeholder engagement processes involve patients, healthcare professionals, advocacy groups, and civil society organizations in AI development and deployment decisions to ensure that technological capabilities align with societal values and patient needs. These participatory approaches help identify potential concerns early in development while building public trust and acceptance of AI-enabled healthcare innovations.

4.10 Future perspectives and industry transformation

AI-driven pharmaceutical industry transformation extends beyond current applications toward fundamental reimagining of how medicines are discovered, developed, manufactured, and delivered to patients. Convergence with emerging technologies, including quantum computing, synthetic biology, and advanced robotics, will create unprecedented capabilities for addressing global health challenges while raising new questions about industry structure, regulatory oversight, and equitable access (Insilico Medicine, 2023; Jagatheesaperumal et al., 2024; Zhavoronkov et al., 2020).

Quantum computing applications in pharmaceutical research promise exponential acceleration of molecular simulation, protein-folding prediction, and drug-target interaction modeling that current classical computers cannot achieve. Early proof-of-concept studies demonstrate quantum advantage for specific pharmaceutical computations, with practical applications expected within 5–10 years as quantum hardware matures and error correction improves. Quantum-enhanced drug discovery could identify novel therapeutic targets, predict drug interactions, and optimize treatment combinations with precision impossible through conventional computational methods (Blanco-González et al., 2023). These may seem to be coming sooner than later with the current pace of overall AI development and unparalleled investments in big and small companies.

Digital twin technologies create virtual patient models that integrate genomic, physiological, behavioral, and environmental data to simulate individual treatment responses and predict optimal therapeutic strategies. These computational models enable in-silico clinical trials that reduce reliance on traditional human studies while providing personalized medicine recommendations based on patient-specific characteristics. Recent validation studies demonstrate significant concordance between digital twin predictions and clinical outcomes in oncology applications, suggesting broad potential for treatment optimization (Khalate et al., 2024).

Synthetic biology integration with AI enables programmable medicine development where therapeutic agents are designed and produced using engineered biological systems guided by ML algorithms. This convergence facilitates personalized drug manufacturing, living therapeutics that adapt to patient conditions, and novel treatment modalities, including engineered immune cells and programmable drug delivery systems.

The pharmaceutical industry structure is evolving toward platform-based organizations that leverage AI to orchestrate comprehensive health solutions rather than focusing solely on molecule development. This transformation requires new business and go-to-market models, partnership strategies, and value demonstration approaches that emphasize health outcomes and real-world effectiveness rather than traditional product-centric metrics. Companies increasingly invest in digital health capabilities, data analytics platforms, and patient engagement technologies that complement pharmaceutical portfolios.

Regulatory science advancement adapts oversight frameworks to accommodate AI-enabled drug development while maintaining safety and efficacy standards. Adaptive regulatory pathways, accelerated approval mechanisms, and RWE integration enable faster access to innovative therapies while ensuring appropriate safety monitoring and post-market surveillance are in place. International harmonization efforts develop consistent AI validation requirements across regulatory jurisdictions while maintaining flexibility for emerging technology applications. Despite how optimistic that is, innovations are often light-years faster than regulations, where such regulations need guiding principles instead of comprehensive legislation.

Global health equity considerations ensure that AI-enabled pharmaceutical innovations address unmet medical needs in low- and middle-income countries (LMIC) rather than exacerbating existing healthcare disparities. Initiatives, including neglected disease drug discovery, affordable manufacturing optimization, and technology transfer programs, utilize AI to develop treatments for diseases affecting global populations while ensuring sustainable access and local capacity building. These are already evident in many, if not all, leading pharmaceutical companies worldwide, with their unique current access models for LMIC.

Healthcare ecosystem integration positions pharmaceutical companies as health solution providers that coordinate care across multiple stakeholders, including healthcare systems, technology companies, payers, and patient organizations. This ecosystem approach leverages AI to optimize treatment pathways, reduce healthcare costs, and improve population health outcomes through comprehensive intervention strategies that extend beyond pharmaceutical products. Where this integration shapes the first version of how future companies will work as in-market health solution partners rather than a commercially driven industry.

4.11 Conclusion

Artificial Intelligence has emerged as a fundamental driver of pharmaceutical industry transformation, delivering quantifiable improvements in drug discovery efficiency, clinical trial optimization, safety surveillance, manufacturing quality, and patient engagement. As comprehensively illustrated in Table 4.1, evidence demonstrates that AI applications reduce development timelines by 20%–40%, improve clinical trial success rates by 30%, and enhance PV sensitivity while reducing costs across the pharmaceutical value chain.

The integration of AI with digital health technologies enables pharmaceutical companies to evolve beyond traditional molecule-centric business models toward comprehensive health solution providers that deliver personalized, evidence-based care throughout patient journeys. This transformation leverages continuous patient monitoring, RWE generation, and adaptive treatment strategies that optimize therapeutic outcomes while addressing individual patient needs and preferences.

Successful AI implementation requires careful attention to ethical considerations, regulatory compliance, and stakeholder engagement to ensure that technological capabilities serve societal needs while maintaining patient safety and public trust. Governance frameworks emphasizing transparency, accountability, and equity help maximize AI benefits while mitigating risks associated with algorithmic bias, privacy violations, and decision-making opacity.

The future pharmaceutical ecosystem will integrate AI across all operational aspects while leveraging convergence with quantum computing, synthetic biology, and digital health technologies to address complex global health challenges. This transformation demands huge interdisciplinary collaboration, regulatory innovation, and commitment to equitable access that ensures AI-enabled pharmaceutical advances benefit all populations regardless of geographic location or socioeconomic status.

As AI capabilities continue advancing, pharmaceutical organizations must balance technological innovation with human oversight, ethical responsibility, and patient-centered care delivery that maintains the fundamental mission of improving human health and alleviating suffering. The successful integration of AI into pharmaceutical practice will ultimately be measured not by technological sophistication alone but by meaningful improvements in patient outcomes, healthcare accessibility, and global health equity.

LLMs represent a transformative force in the pharmaceutical industry, offering unprecedented opportunities to accelerate drug discovery, optimize molecular design, and streamline research processes. The evolution from traditional ML approaches to sophisticated LLMs has enabled researchers to process vast biomedical datasets, generate novel hypotheses, and interact with molecular data at near-human levels of comprehension.

However, realizing the full potential of these technologies requires careful navigation of significant challenges. The dual-use nature of LLMs, the risk of generating inaccurate outputs, and the potential for misuse necessitate robust technical, regulatory, and collaborative frameworks. As the pharmaceutical industry continues to integrate these powerful tools, stakeholders must balance innovation with responsibility—ensuring that AI-driven advances enhance drug discovery while maintaining scientific rigor and ethical standards.

Looking forward, the successful adoption of LLMs in pharmaceutical research will depend on continued collaboration between AI developers, pharmaceutical scientists, and regulatory bodies. By addressing current limitations and establishing best practices for validation and oversight, the industry can harness generative AI to bring safer, more effective therapeutics to patients faster than ever before.

Disclaimer

The views and opinions expressed in this chapter are solely those of the authors and do not necessarily reflect the official positions or policies of their affiliated institutions.

Abbreviations

AI	artificial intelligence
ADMET	absorption, distribution, metabolism, excretion, toxicity
AUROC	area under the receiver operating characteristic curve
BERT	bidirectional encoder representations from transformers
CIOMS	Council for International Organizations of Medical Sciences
COGM	cost of goods manufacturing
COVID-19	Coronavirus Disease 2019
DCT	decentralized clinical trials
DL	deep learning
DTI	drug-target interaction
DTx	digital therapeutics
EHR	electronic health records
EMA	European Medicines Agency
FDA	Food and Drug Administration
GANs	generative adversarial networks
GPT	generative pretrained transformer
ICH	International Council for Harmonisation
IMDRF	International Medical Device Regulators Forum
IoT	Internet of Things
LLMs	large language models
LMIC	low- and middle-income countries
ML	machine learning
mRNA	messenger RNA
NLP	natural language processing
PLMs	protein language models
PROTAC	proteolysis-targeting chimera
PSPs	patient support programs
PV	pharmacovigilance
QbD	quality by design
QSAR	quantitative structure–activity relationship
RWE	real-world evidence
SaMD	software as medical device
SMILES	simplified molecular input line entry system
WHO	World Health Organization
XAI	explainable artificial intelligence

References

Ahmad, W., Simon, E., Chithrananda, S., Grand, G., & Ramsundar, B. (2022). ChemBERTa-2: Towards chemical foundation models. ArXiv, abs/2209.01712. doi: 10.48550/arXiv.2209.01712

Alowais, S. A., Alghamdi, S. S., Alsuhebany, N., et al. (2023). Revolutionizing healthcare: The role of artificial intelligence in clinical practice. *BMC Medical Education, 23*(1), 689. https://doi.org/10.1186/s12909-023-04698-z.

Bartlett, V. L., Dhruva, S. S., Shah, N. D., Ryan, P., & Ross, J. S. (2019). Feasibility of using real-world data to replicate clinical trial evidence. *JAMA Netw Open, 2*(10), e1912869. https://doi.org/10.1001/jamanetworkopen.2019.12869.

Blanco-González, A., Cabezón, A., Seco-González, A., et al. (2023). The role of AI in drug discovery: Challenges, opportunities, and strategies. *Pharmaceuticals (Basel), 16*(6), 891. https://doi.org/10.3390/ph16060891.

Chen, H., Engkvist, O., Wang, Y., Olivecrona, M., & Blaschke, T. (2018). The rise of deep learning in drug discovery. *Drug Discovery Today, 23*(6), 1241–1250. https://doi.org/10.1016/j.drudis.2018.01.039.

Chen, Q., Allot, A., & Lu, Z. (2023). LitCovid: An open database of COVID-19 literature. *Nucleic Acids Research, 51*(D1), D1534–D1540. https://doi.org/10.1093/nar/gkac1005.

Chen, J., Gu, Z., Xu, Y., Deng, M., Lai, L., & Pei, J. (2023). QuoteTarget: A sequence-based transformer protein language model to identify potentially druggable protein targets. *Protein Science, 32*(2).

Chen, W., Liu, X., Zhang, S., & Chen, S. (2023). Artificial intelligence for drug discovery: Resources, methods, and applications. *Molecular Therapy Nucleic Acids, 31*, 691–702. https://doi.org/10.1016/j.omtn.2023.02.019.

Chithrananda, S., Grand, G., & Ramsundar, B. (2020). ChemBERTa: Large-scale self-supervised pretraining for molecular property prediction. arXiv preprint arXiv:2010.09885.

Church, K. W. (2017). Word2Vec. *Natural Language Engineering, 23*(1), 155–162.

Council for International Organizations of Medical Sciences (CIOMS). (2024). Artificial intelligence in pharmacovigilance: Report of CIOMS working group XIV. CIOMS.

DiMasi, J. A., Grabowski, H. G., & Hansen, R. W. (2016). Innovation in the pharmaceutical industry: New estimates of R&D costs. *Journal of Health Economics, 47*, 20–33. https://doi.org/10.1016/j.jhealeco.2016.01.012.

European Medicines Agency. (2023). *Reflection paper on the use of artificial intelligence (AI) in the lifecycle of medicines*. Amsterdam: EMA EMA/CHMP/ICH/44083/2023.

Evaluating the impact of artificial intelligence on vaccine development: Lessons learned from the COVID-19 pandemic. medRxiv. 2024 Oct 23. doi: 10.1101/2024.10.23.24315991

FDA Adverse Event Reporting System (FAERS). Underreporting limitations. Available at: https://www.fda.gov/drugs/fdas-adverse-event-reporting-system-faers

Fleming, T. R., Labriola, D., & Wittes, J. (2020). Conducting clinical trials during the coronavirus pandemic. *Annals of Internal Medicine, 173*(3), 373–379. https://doi.org/10.1001/jama.2020.9286.

Food and Drug Administration. (2024). *Artificial Intelligence and machine learning (AI/ML)-based software as a medical device (SaMD) action plan.* Silver Spring, MD: FDA.

Gao, M., Zhang, D., Chen, Y., Zhang, Y., Wang, Z., Wang, X., & Song, J. (2024). GraphormerDTI: A graph transformer-based approach for drug-target interaction prediction. *Computers in Biology and Medicine, 173*, 108339.

Gharbi, Y., Zhao, Y., Yang, Y., & Mercado, R. (2024). A comprehensive review of emerging approaches in machine learning for de novo PROTAC design. *Drug Discovery Today, 29*(9), 104125. https://doi.org/10.1016/j.drudis.2024.104125.

Ghosh, R., Lewis, D., Wadhwa, B., & Koopmans, I. (2021). Artificial intelligence and machine learning in pharmacovigilance: A systematic review. *Drug safety: An International Journal of Medical Toxicology and Drug Experience, 44*(8), 815–841. https://doi.org/10.1007/s40264-021-01076-1.

Gromova, A., & Maida, A. (2025). ChemBERTaDDI: Transformer driven molecular structures and clinical data for predicting drug-drug interactions. *bioRxiv*. https://doi.org/10.1101/2025.01.22.634309.

Hagos, D., Battle, R., & Rawat, D. (2024). Recent advances in generative AI and large language models: Current status, challenges, and perspectives. *IEEE Transactions on Artificial Intelligence, 5*, 5873–5893. https://doi.org/10.1109/TAI.2024.3444742.

Han, R., Yoon, H., Kim, G., Lee, H., & Lee, Y. (2023). Revolutionizing medicinal chemistry: The application of artificial intelligence (AI) in early drug discovery. *Pharmaceuticals, 16*. https://doi.org/10.3390/ph16091259.

He, J., Feng, W., Min, Y., Yi, J., Tang, K., Li, S., Zhang, J., Chen, K., Zhou, W., Xie, X., Zhang, W., Yu, N., & Zheng, S. (2023). Control risk for potential misuse of artificial intelligence in science. ArXiv, abs/2312.06632. doi: 10.48550/arXiv.2312.06632

Hersh, W. (2025). Generative artificial intelligence: Implications for biomedical and health professions education. Annual Review of Biomedical Data Science. doi: 10.48550/arXiv.2501.10186

Hessler, G., & Baringhaus, K. (2018). Artificial intelligence in drug design. *Molecules (Basel, Switzerland), 23*. https://doi.org/10.3390/molecules23102520.

Huang, K., Altosaar, J., & Ranganath, R. (2019). ClinicalBERT: Modeling clinical notes and predicting hospital readmission. arXiv preprint arXiv:1904.05342.

Insilico Medicine. (2023). First generative AI drug begins phase II trials with patients. Available at: https://insilico.com/blog/first_phase2

International Council for Harmonisation of Technical Requirements for Pharmaceuticals for Human Use. (2019). *ICH E9(R1) statistical principles for clinical trials: Addendum on estimands and sensitivity analysis in clinical trials*. ICH.

IQVIA. (2024). The crucial role of real-time data use in pharma marketing: AI-powered analytics for enhanced decision-making. IQVIA Blog

Irwin, R., Dimitriadis, S., He, J., & Bjerrum, E. J. (2022). Chemformer: A pre-trained transformer for computational chemistry. *Machine Learning: Science and Technology, 3*(1), 015022.

Jagatheesaperumal, S. K., Rahouti, M., Ahmad, K., Al-Fuqaha, A., & Guizani, M. (2024). Explainable artificial intelligence for drug discovery and development: A comprehensive survey. *IEEE Access, 12*, 40112–40137. https://doi.org/10.1109/ACCESS.2024.3373195.

Jayatunga, M. K. P., Ayers, M., Bruens, L., Jayanth, D., & Meier, C. (2024). How successful are AI-discovered drugs in clinical trials? A first analysis and emerging lessons. *Drug Discovery Today, 29*(6), 104009. https://doi.org/10.1016/j.drudis.2024.104009.

Jiang, L., Jiang, C., Yu, X., Fu, R., Jin, S., & Liu, X. (2022). DeepTTA: A transformer-based model for predicting cancer drug response. *Briefings in Bioinformatics, 23*(3).

Jumper, J., Evans, R., Pritzel, A., Green, T., Figurnov, M., Ronneberger, O., Hassabis, D., et al. (2021). Highly accurate protein structure prediction with AlphaFold. *Nature, 596*(7873), 583–589. https://doi.org/10.1038/s41586-021-03819-2.

Kalakoti, Y., Yadav, S., & Sundar, D. (2022). TransDTI: Transformer-based language models for estimating DTIs and building a drug recommendation workflow. *ACS Omega, 7*(3), 2706–2717.

Kang, H., Goo, S., Lee, H., Chae, J., Yun, H., & Jung, S. (2022). Fine-tuning of BERT model to accurately predict drug–target interactions. *Pharmaceutics, 14*. https://doi.org/10.3390/pharmaceutics14081710.

Khalate, P., Gite, S., Pradhan, B., & Lee, C. W. (2024). Advancements and gaps in natural language processing and machine learning applications in healthcare: A comprehensive review of electronic medical records and medical imaging. *Frontiers in Physics, 12*, 1445204. https://doi.org/10.3389/fphy.2024.1445204.

Khanna, I. (2012). Drug discovery in pharmaceutical industry: Productivity challenges and trends. *Drug Discovery Today, 17*(19-20), 1088–1102.

Lee, J., Yoon, W., Kim, S., Kim, D., Kim, S., So, C. H., & Kang, J. (2020). BioBERT: A pre-trained biomedical language representation model for biomedical text mining. *Bioinformatics (Oxford, England), 36*(4), 1234–1240.

Li, T., Sahu, A. K., Talwalkar, A., & Smith, V. (2020). Federated learning: Challenges, methods, and future directions. *IEEE Signal Processing Magazine, 37*(3), 50–60. https://doi.org/10.1109/MSP.2020.2975749.

Li, Y., Gao, C., Song, X., Wang, X., Xu, Y., & Han, S. (2023). DrugGPT: A GPT-based strategy for designing potential ligands targeting specific proteins. *bioRxiv*.

Liu, S., Wang, Y., Thijssen, B., et al. (2020). Mining adverse drug events from social media for pharmacovigilance. *npj Digital Medicine, 3*, 137. https://doi.org/10.1038/s41746-020-00354-4.

Liu, X., Lu, Z., Wang, T., & Liu, F. (2024). Large language models facilitating modern molecular biology and novel drug development. *Frontiers in Pharmacology, 15.* https://doi.org/10.3389/fphar.2024.1458739.

Liu, Z., Roberts, R., Lal-Nag, M., Chen, X., Huang, R., & Tong, W. (2021). AI-based language models powering drug discovery and development. *Drug Discovery Today, 26*, 2593–2607. https://doi.org/10.1016/j.drudis.2021.06.009.

McKinsey & Company. (2022). Human-machine harmonization to upgrade biopharma production.

Nuthakki, S. (2023). AI and the future of medicine: Pioneering drug discovery with language models. *International Journal of Science and Research (IJSR).* https://doi.org/10.21275/sr24304173757.

Obermeyer, Z., Powers, B., Vogeli, C., & Mullainathan, S. (2019). Dissecting racial bias in an algorithm used to manage the health of populations. *Science (New York, N.Y.), 366*(6464), 447–453. https://doi.org/10.1126/science.aax2342.

Patterson, J. D., Lee, K. M., & Wright, N. (2024). Automated compliance monitoring in pharmaceutical manufacturing using machine learning. *Pharmaceutical Technology, 48*(4), 36–42.

Pu, L., Govindaraj, R. G., Lemoine, J. M., Wu, H. C., & Brylinski, M. (2019). DeepDrug3D: Classification of ligand-binding pockets in proteins with a convolutional neural network. *PLoS Computational Biology, 15*(2), e1006718. https://doi.org/10.1371/journal.pcbi.1006718.

Ramos, M., Collison, C., & White, A. (2024). A review of large language models and autonomous agents in chemistry. *Chemical Science, 16*, 2514–2572. https://doi.org/10.48550/arXiv.2407.01603.

Rao, V. S., & Srinivas, K. (2011). Modern drug discovery process: An in silico approach. *Journal of Bioinformatics and Sequence Analysis, 2*(5), 89–94.

Rehman, A., Li, M., Wu, B., Ali, Y., Rasheed, S., Shaheen, S., Liu, X., Luo, R., & Zhang, J. (2024). Role of artificial intelligence in revolutionizing drug discovery. *Fundamental Research.* https://doi.org/10.1016/j.fmre.2024.04.021.

Richardson, P., Griffin, I., Tucker, C., et al. (2020). Baricitinib as potential treatment for 2019-nCoV acute respiratory disease. *Lancet, 395*(10223), e30–e31. https://doi.org/10.1016/S0140-6736(20)30304-4.

Scannell, J. W., Blanckley, A., Boldon, H., & Warrington, B. (2012). Diagnosing the decline in pharmaceutical R&D efficiency. *Nature Reviews Drug Discovery, 11*(3), 191–200. https://doi.org/10.1038/nrd3681.

Schwaller, P., Laino, T., Gaudin, T., Bolgar, P., Hunter, C. A., Bekas, C., & Lee, A. A. (2019). Molecular transformer: A model for uncertainty-calibrated chemical reaction prediction. *ACS Central Science, 5*(9), 1572–1583.

Sheikholeslami, M., Mazrouei, N., Gheisari, Y., Fasihi, A., Irajpour, M., & Motahharynia, A. (2024). DrugGen: Advancing drug discovery with large language models and reinforcement learning feedback. arXiv preprint arXiv:2411.14157.

Singh, R., Dwivedi, A. D., & Srivastava, G. (2020). Internet of things based blockchain for temperature monitoring and counterfeit pharmaceutical prevention. *Sensors, 20*(14), 3951. https://doi.org/10.3390/s20143951.

Steinhubl, S. R., Waalen, J., & Edwards, A. M. (2019). Digital clinical trials: Creating a vision for the future. *npj Digital Medicine, 2*, 38. https://doi.org/10.1038/s41746-019-0109-6.

Terranova, N., Giraud, S., Ouwerkerk-Mahadevan, S., et al. (2024). Artificial intelligence for quantitative modeling in drug discovery and development: An innovation and quality consortium perspective on use cases and best practices. *Clinical Pharmacology and Therapeutics, 115*(4), 758–767. https://doi.org/10.1002/cpt.3053.

Vaswani, A., et al. (2017). Attention is all you need. *Advances in Neural Information Processing Systems, 30.*

Vora, L., Gholap, A., Jetha, K., Thakur, R., Solanki, H., & Chavda, V. (2023). Artificial intelligence in pharmaceutical technology and drug delivery design. *Pharmaceutics, 15.* https://doi.org/10.3390/pharmaceutics15071916.

World Health Organization. (2021). *Ethics and governance of artificial intelligence for health: WHO guidance.* WHO.

Yang, Y., Adelstein, S. J., & Kassis, A. I. (2023). Digital therapeutics in pharmaceutical care: Current landscape and future prospects. *Digital Medicine, 6*, 78. https://doi.org/10.1038/s41746-023-00823-6.

Yang, Y., Adelstein, S. J., & Kassis, A. I. (2022). Target discovery from data mining approaches. *Drug Discovery Today, 27*(6), 103200. https://doi.org/10.1016/j.drudis.2022.01.006.

Yu, K. H., Beam, A. L., & Kohane, I. S. (2018). Artificial intelligence in healthcare. *Nature Biomedical Engineering, 2*(10), 719–731. https://doi.org/10.1038/s41551-018-0305-z.

Zhang, P., Wei, Z., Che, C., & Jin, B. (2022). DeepMGT-DTI: Transformer network incorporating multilayer graph information for drug–target interaction prediction. *Computers in Biology and Medicine, 142*, 105214.

Zhavoronkov, A., Vanhaelen, Q., & Oprea, T. I. (2020). Will artificial intelligence for drug discovery impact clinical pharmacology? *Clinical Pharmacology and Therapeutics, 108*(4), 780–785. https://doi.org/10.1002/cpt.1795.

Zhou, B., Yang, G., Shi, Z., & Ma, S. (2023). Natural language processing for smart healthcare. *IEEE Reviews in Biomedical Engineering, 16*, 337–360. https://doi.org/10.1109/RBME.2022.3210270.

ZS Associates. (2025). Pharmaceutical industry trends 2025: Outlook on AI, supply chain resilience and digital transformation strategies. Available at: https://www.zs.com/insights/pharmaceutical-trends-2025-outlook-ai-supplychain-and-beyond

CHAPTER 5

Trends shaping the future of the pharmaceutical industry

Lamyaa Munahi AlQahtani
Faculty of Pharmaceutical Sciences graduate, Monash University, Melbourne, VIC, Australia

5.1 Drug development in the era of artificial intelligence

5.1.1 Artificial intelligence in pharma: from tool to infrastructure

Artificial intelligence (AI) is no longer a future-facing supplement to pharmaceutical innovation; it has become a core infrastructural element in how drug discovery, development, and deployment are imagined. AI, particularly its subsets machine learning (ML) and deep learning (DL), is reshaping pharmaceutical drug discovery by addressing long-standing inefficiencies and limitations. AI refers to computational systems designed to replicate tasks that typically require human intelligence, including pattern recognition, decision-making, and language understanding (Kühl et al., 2020). ML enables these systems to learn from data and make predictions, improving accuracy over time without explicitly programmed instructions. DL, a more advanced subset, uses multilayered neural networks to uncover complex patterns in vast, high-dimensional biomedical datasets.

The integration of AI into drug discovery gained momentum in the early 2000s, with DL breakthroughs in the 2010s enabling more refined insights into molecular interactions and disease biology (Abbas et al., 2024). These technologies evolved alongside advances in computational capacity and data availability, particularly from high-throughput screening and genomic platforms. This digital shift has revolutionized pharmaceutical R&D, moving beyond trial-and-error approaches to data-driven decision-making (Blanco-González et al., 2022).

AI applications are driving value across multiple domains of drug development (Deng et al., 2021). Increased efficiency and speed are evident as ML algorithms rapidly screen compound libraries and predict pharmacokinetic profiles, accelerating early-stage discovery. Enhanced predictive accuracy, especially in genomics and toxicology, stems from DL's capacity to identify nonobvious biological correlations (Hughes et al., 2015). Optimizing clinical trial design through AI-driven patient stratification improves recruitment and response prediction, potentially raising success rates while lowering costs (Liu et al., 2021a, 2021b). Furthermore, cost reduction is realized by minimizing unnecessary laboratory experiments through virtual

The Future of Pharma Across All Sectors in the Artificial Intelligence Era. DOI: https://doi.org/10.1016/B978-0-443-40572-3.00009-5

simulations and compound prioritization (Maharao et al., 2020). Finally, AI facilitates personalized medicine, enabling tailored therapeutic strategies based on individual genetic and phenotypic data (Alum & Ugwu, 2025).

In summary, AI is no longer a supplementary tool but a central pillar in modern drug discovery. By enhancing precision, accelerating timelines, and reducing costs, AI-enabled technologies are redefining how medicines are discovered and developed. Continued innovation in this domain holds immense promise for addressing unmet clinical needs and transforming global healthcare.

5.1.2 Rebuilding the pipeline: artificial intelligence's expanding role from target to trial

The integration of AI, ML, and DL into pharmaceutical pipelines is now influencing every stage of drug development, from target identification to clinical trials. This integration has reshaped every stage of drug discovery and development. These technologies enhance decision-making, streamline processes, and improve outcomes across target identification, hit-to-lead optimization, preclinical modeling, and clinical trials.

Target identification in early-phase discovery: AI has proven instrumental in uncovering novel therapeutic targets. ML algorithms, including generative adversarial networks, can mine vast biological datasets to reveal nonobvious targets with high therapeutic potential. For instance, successfully employed AI to identify and validate endometriosis targets, accelerating early-stage research efforts (Balica et al., 2023). Demonstrated how AI-driven screening approaches contributed to the identification of glioblastoma-related targets, highlighting AI's ability to augment traditional discovery with scalable, data-intensive methods (Xu et al., 2020).

Hit-to-lead optimization: The progression from hit compounds to optimized leads is a critical bottleneck in drug development. AI addresses this by enabling efficient structure–activity relationship analysis and predicting compound-target interactions. Deep reinforcement learning and other generative techniques allow the design of molecules with improved pharmacological profiles. Predictive modeling using AI led to higher success rates in lead selection by uncovering relationships not apparent through manual methods (Potanin et al., 2023), further emphasizing AI's potential in automating this optimization and accelerating compound refinement cycles (Xia et al., 2024).

Preclinical in silico modeling: In the preclinical phase, AI-powered in silico models are redefining how researchers evaluate compound safety and efficacy. DL-based models simulate complex pharmacokinetic and pharmacodynamic (PK/PD) profiles, enabling predictions of absorption, distribution, metabolism, and excretion characteristics. It has been shown that AI plays a role in predicting toxicity and drug interactions, reducing reliance on extensive animal testing (Vo et al., 2019). Likewise, the use of computational models to validate therapeutic targets supports informed transitions to in vivo testing (Chelliah and van der Graaf, 2022).

Clinical trials: AI is playing an increasingly prominent role in optimizing clinical trial design and execution (Liu et al., 2021a, 2021b). One major application is patient stratification—AI analyzes clinical, genetic, and demographic data to match patients to appropriate trials, improving recruitment and trial efficiency. AI tools also enable the prediction of patient responses using historical datasets, allowing for adaptive trial designs. Such enhancements can significantly reduce trial durations and costs, accelerating the time to market for new therapeutics (DiMasi, 2002).

Benefits across the pipeline: The overarching advantages of AI integration in drug development are multifold:

Increased efficiency: Automated data analysis accelerates lead identification and decision-making (Ocana et al., 2025).

Cost reduction: By replacing labor-intensive processes with scalable computation, AI reduces R&D expenditures (Grisoni et al., 2021).

Improved predictive capabilities: AI enhances the accuracy of drug candidate screening and patient outcome forecasting (Mao et al., 2025).

Optimized resource allocation: Through early identification of promising candidates, AI minimizes resource waste and enhances pipeline productivity (Ocana et al., 2025).

In conclusion, AI is no longer an experimental add-on but a foundational tool across all phases of drug development. From discovering targets to running clinical trials, its capacity to extract insights from complex datasets is revolutionizing pharmaceutical research. As algorithms grow more sophisticated and datasets expand, the impact of AI on drug development is expected to deepen, offering scalable, cost-effective, and personalized solutions to enduring challenges in the field.

5.1.3 When artificial intelligence delivers: case studies and cautionary lessons

The growing influence of AI in pharmaceutical research is often illustrated through a series of high-profile success stories. AI has emerged as a pivotal force in drug discovery, with several real-world applications illustrating its profound impact on pharmaceutical research and development. A notable example is AlphaFold, the AI system developed by DeepMind, which has dramatically advanced protein structure prediction, an essential step in rational drug design. By accurately modeling the three-dimensional structures of proteins, AlphaFold has accelerated target discovery and deepened our understanding of complex biological systems. Its use in exploring proteins linked to neglected tropical diseases, such as Trypanosoma cruzi, facilitated the identification of new drug targets for Chagas disease, underscoring its potential to drive innovation in underfunded therapeutic areas (Osorio-Méndez et al., 2025). Another groundbreaking application comes from In Silico Medicine, a biotechnology company that employs

DL across multiple stages of the drug development pipeline. Their AI-driven approach enabled the discovery of a novel fibrosis drug candidate in under 46 days, an unprecedented timeline in pharmaceutical R&D (Ren et al., 2022). This achievement reflects how AI can overcome traditional barriers like high costs and lengthy development cycles by automating and accelerating hit identification and lead optimization processes. Similarly, BioNTech has integrated AI technologies to refine its vaccine design strategies, particularly in the context of mRNA platforms. During the COVID-19 pandemic, the company's AI-enhanced tools were instrumental in selecting optimal mRNA sequences capable of generating strong and specific immune responses, which contributed significantly to the rapid development of an effective vaccine. Beyond pandemic response, BioNTech's AI framework supports ongoing efforts in personalized cancer immunotherapy, demonstrating how AI can be leveraged to tailor treatments to individual patient profiles (Alum & Ugwu, 2025).

Collectively, these case studies illustrate the versatility and scalability of AI across all stages of drug development. AI enables faster identification of viable drug candidates, more accurate predictions of efficacy and toxicity, and more efficient design and execution of clinical trials. By automating complex processes and extracting actionable insights from high-dimensional data, AI helps pharmaceutical companies reduce time-to-market and improve success rates in both preclinical and clinical settings. These real-world examples not only validate the practical utility of AI but also signal a broader paradigm shift within the pharmaceutical industry. As these technologies continue to mature, they are expected to yield even more success stories, reinforcing the role of AI as a cornerstone of future drug discovery and a critical enabler of innovation in modern medicine.

5.1.4 Ethical, regulatory, and technical challenges

While AI continues to reshape pharmaceutical research, its integration into drug development presents several complex ethical, regulatory, and technical challenges that must be addressed to ensure responsible and equitable innovation. From an ethical perspective, one of the most pressing concerns is algorithmic bias. AI models trained on skewed or nonrepresentative datasets risk reinforcing health disparities, as predictions may be less accurate for underrepresented populations (Marko et al., 2025). Ensuring the inclusion of diverse, high-quality datasets is critical to mitigating this issue. Compounding this problem is the "black box" nature of many AI systems, which lack transparency in how decisions are made. This opacity complicates accountability, particularly in clinical or regulatory settings where understanding the rationale behind a prediction is essential for trust and compliance (Marey et al., 2024). Moreover, the use of extensive health data to train AI models introduces serious concerns regarding data ownership, informed consent, and privacy. Clear data governance frameworks and ethical oversight are urgently needed to protect patient rights while supporting scientific advancement (Larson et al., 2020).

In parallel, the regulatory environment has struggled to keep pace with the rapid evolution of AI-driven technologies. Traditional frameworks, such as those overseen by the U.S. Food and Drug Administration (FDA), are not yet fully adapted to assess the dynamic and iterative nature of AI systems. Key regulatory concerns include validating AI models, ensuring reproducibility, and establishing criteria for safety and efficacy in AI-supported drug development (Blanco-González et al., 2022). These issues are further complicated by the need for algorithmic transparency and explainability, which are difficult to achieve in many high-performance DL models. As a result, AI-based drug development often faces prolonged approval timelines, which may hinder the introduction of urgently needed therapies into the market.

From a technical standpoint, the success of AI applications is heavily dependent on data availability, quality, and consistency. Many pharmaceutical datasets are fragmented, incomplete, or siloed, posing challenges for developing robust and generalizable models (Huang et al., 2021). Moreover, integrating AI tools into existing pharmaceutical workflows demands significant infrastructural and cultural adaptation (Terranova et al., 2023). Collaboration between computational scientists and domain experts is essential to ensure that AI tools are both technically sound and practically usable. A persistent technical hurdle lies in the interpretability of complex AI models, particularly those based on DL, which often fail to provide clear explanations for their outputs (Mandala, 2023). To bridge this gap, the development of explainable AI (xAI) is gaining traction as a means to increase transparency and foster greater acceptance of AI in clinical and research settings.

Although AI presents transformative opportunities in drug development, its implementation must be guided by rigorous ethical standards, adaptive regulatory strategies, and technical innovation. Proactively addressing these challenges through multidisciplinary collaboration and thoughtful policymaking will be critical to ensuring that AI technologies deliver on their promise to improve therapeutic outcomes while maintaining public trust and scientific integrity.

Strategic synthesis: key trends reshaping the pharmaceutical industry

The future pharmaceutical industry is undergoing a structural transformation driven by three converging forces:

Artificial intelligence as infrastructure: AI is no longer a tool but a foundational system embedded across discovery, trials, manufacturing, and post-market surveillance.

From scale to precision: Therapies are increasingly individualized, data-driven, and adaptive—reshaping clinical, regulatory, and commercial models.

Innovation with responsibility: Sustainability, ethics, and global equity are emerging as core strategic imperatives rather than peripheral concerns.

Together, these shifts redefine pharma as a digitally intelligent, socially accountable, and sustainability-oriented ecosystem.

5.2 New and disruptive technologies in pharma

5.2.1 Digital therapies and wearables: hype, promise, and patient realities

As digital health technologies mature, their integration into therapeutic contexts, especially chronic disease and mental health management, has sparked both excitement and skepticism. Digital therapeutics, powered by AI, wearables, and smart health applications, are increasingly being recognized as transformative tools in the management of chronic diseases and mental health conditions. As digital health technologies evolve, they offer new opportunities for personalized, data-driven interventions, while also introducing important challenges related to adoption, ethics, and integration into clinical practice.

One of the most impactful uses of AI within digital therapeutics lies in the mental health sector, where intelligent applications such as chatbots and mobile health platforms are being developed to deliver interventions based on established psychological frameworks like cognitive-behavioral therapy (Jovanovic et al., 2021). These AI-enabled tools dynamically assess user input, behavior, and feedback to adapt therapeutic content in real time. Such personalization enhances user engagement and therapeutic compliance, particularly for individuals managing anxiety, depression, and stress-related conditions (Wang et al., 2023). Additionally, AI facilitates early detection of mental health deterioration by identifying behavioral changes and linguistic patterns in data sources such as electronic health records and social media, allowing for timely interventions that could prevent crisis escalation (Poudel et al., 2025).

The proliferation of wearable technologies has further expanded the scope of digital therapeutics. These devices enable continuous, real-time monitoring of physiological and behavioral metrics, such as heart rate, sleep quality, physical activity, and even mood fluctuations. When integrated with AI algorithms, wearable data becomes a powerful tool for both patients and clinicians, offering deeper insights into individual health patterns (Zheng et al., 2021). For example, AI-powered wearables can alert healthcare providers to abnormal fluctuations in blood pressure or glucose levels, enhancing chronic disease management and potentially preventing hospitalizations. In the context of mental health, wearables are being used to track indicators of emotional well-being, thereby supporting early, unobtrusive interventions tailored to individual needs (Asif et al., 2024).

Despite the promising advancements, the adoption of digital therapeutics remains hindered by several practical and ethical concerns. Patient engagement continues to be a significant challenge, with studies reporting low long-term adherence to digital health tools (O'Connor et al., 2016). Contributing factors include technological complexity, limited user customization, and skepticism regarding the efficacy of digital therapies compared to face-to-face care. Moreover, the vast amounts of personal health data collected by these tools raise serious privacy and security issues. Ensuring data protection and compliance with regulations such as the Health Insurance Portability and Accountability Act is crucial for maintaining user trust and safeguarding patient rights (Martínez-Pérez et al., 2014).

Beyond individual concerns, integrating digital therapeutics into existing healthcare infrastructures presents logistical hurdles. Clinicians require appropriate training to interpret and act upon data generated by AI and wearable systems, and healthcare organizations must address digital literacy and access disparities to avoid exacerbating existing health inequalities (Lee et al., 2022). Without deliberate strategies to bridge these gaps, the benefits of digital therapeutics may remain inaccessible to vulnerable populations.

In summary, AI-driven digital therapeutics and wearable technologies are reshaping the future of chronic disease and mental health management by enabling personalized care, real-time monitoring, and data-informed decision-making. However, their successful integration into mainstream healthcare requires concerted efforts to overcome challenges related to engagement, privacy, equity, and infrastructure. As the field matures, interdisciplinary collaboration between technologists, clinicians, regulators, and patients will be essential to ensure these innovations deliver on their promise of more accessible, effective, and personalized care.

5.2.2 Drug discovery innovations

Advances in drug discovery technologies are reshaping the pharmaceutical landscape by enhancing precision, accelerating timelines, and expanding the therapeutic frontier. Among the most promising innovations are DNA-encoded libraries (DELs), CRISPR-Cas9 gene editing, and messenger RNA (mRNA) technologies beyond vaccines. These emerging tools are not only improving the efficiency of drug development but also unlocking new modalities for treating complex diseases.

DELs have emerged as a highly efficient platform for high-throughput compound screening. By attaching unique DNA barcodes to small molecules, researchers can synthesize and screen millions of compounds simultaneously within a single reaction vessel (Song & Hwang, 2020). This approach drastically reduces the time and cost traditionally associated with drug discovery. DELs have proven instrumental in identifying potent inhibitors for various protein targets, with multiple pharmaceutical companies incorporating the technology into their early-stage pipelines. The ability to conduct iterative screening campaigns using expansive chemical space makes DELs a valuable tool in the pursuit of novel therapeutics.

Complementing chemical screening innovations, CRISPR-Cas9 has transformed the way researchers approach gene function and target validation (Campenhout et al., 2019). As a highly precise gene-editing tool, CRISPR enables the targeted modification or knockout of genes implicated in disease, allowing scientists to assess their functional roles within cellular systems. In drug discovery, this capability is crucial for confirming the relevance of potential therapeutic targets. When combined with high-throughput screening technologies,

CRISPR platforms allow for genome-wide analyses that elucidate key genetic drivers of disease and identify novel intervention points (Xue et al., 2020). This intersection of genomics and pharmacology enhances target selection strategies and paves the way for mechanism-based drug development.

Beyond their initial use in COVID-19 vaccines, mRNA technologies are expanding into broader therapeutic domains, including protein replacement therapies, cancer immunotherapy, and gene editing (Li et al., 2023). By delivering synthetic mRNA into cells, these therapies can induce the production of therapeutic proteins in vivo, offering promising avenues for treating genetic disorders and chronic illnesses. The flexibility and rapid adaptability of mRNA platforms also enable tailored interventions, such as the engineering of T-cells to enhance immune responses against tumors. These applications signal a paradigm shift in how genetic information is used to influence cellular function, highlighting mRNA as a versatile and scalable therapeutic modality.

The convergence of these technologies is driving new frontiers in drug design. Integrating DELs with CRISPR enables researchers to screen vast compound libraries against genetically modified models, streamlining both target validation and hit identification (Lee et al., 2022). Simultaneously, the incorporation of AI and ML enhances these platforms by enabling predictive modeling, structural optimization, and real-time analysis of biological interactions (Jena et al., 2024). This systems-level approach to drug discovery facilitates the design of more effective, safer, and personalized therapies.

In summary, DELs, CRISPR-Cas9, and mRNA technologies represent transformative innovations in drug discovery. Their ability to improve specificity, efficiency, and scalability addresses long-standing challenges in pharmaceutical research. As these platforms continue to evolve and integrate with digital and computational tools, they will not only accelerate the development of new drugs but also reshape the future of medicine toward more individualized and mechanism-driven care.

5.2.3 Next-gen manufacturing and automation

Next-generation pharmaceutical manufacturing is undergoing a radical transformation driven by digitalization, automation, and advanced analytics. These technologies are reshaping traditional production models, shifting the focus from batch-based manufacturing to continuous, real-time, and highly integrated systems. The adoption of smart manufacturing practices not only improves production efficiency and scalability but also enhances quality assurance, sustainability, and regulatory compliance.

At the core of this shift is continuous manufacturing, which replaces discrete production steps with an end-to-end, uninterrupted process. Unlike traditional batch production, which involves multiple start-stop stages, manual handling, and quality control delays, continuous manufacturing allows for real-time monitoring and control, significantly reducing cycle times and minimizing variability (Burcham et al., 2018). This model has proven particularly valuable during public health emergencies, such as the COVID-19 pandemic, where the rapid and flexible production of mRNA vaccines required scalable and agile platforms. Regulatory bodies like the U.S. FDA and EMA have endorsed continuous manufacturing approaches, citing their potential to enhance product quality and reduce risks associated with supply chain disruptions.

Automation technologies, including robotics, process analytical technologies, and industrial Internet of Things (IIoT), are also playing a pivotal role. These systems enable real-time data capture and automated process adjustments, reducing the need for manual intervention and lowering the risk of human error (Silva et al., 2021). For instance, automated aseptic filling lines and robotic arms in sterile manufacturing environments have improved both safety and throughput, especially for biologics and advanced therapy medicinal products (ATMPs). Meanwhile, digital twins, virtual replicas of physical manufacturing systems, are being used to simulate, optimize, and predict manufacturing outcomes before changes are implemented in the real world, saving time and resources.

Furthermore, artificial intelligence and ML are enhancing the intelligence of manufacturing systems. AI algorithms can analyze vast datasets from production lines to detect anomalies, predict equipment failures, and optimize process parameters. These capabilities not only reduce downtime and waste but also support adaptive control systems that respond dynamically to process changes (Plathottam et al., 2023). For quality control, AI-enabled vision systems and predictive models are being deployed to detect deviations with higher precision than conventional sampling methods. In doing so, AI supports the move toward real-time release testing, where finished products are evaluated and approved based on continuous in-process monitoring rather than postproduction testing.

The implementation of next-gen manufacturing also supports broader sustainability goals. Automated systems reduce energy consumption and raw material waste, while continuous manufacturing lowers the environmental footprint by requiring less equipment, space, and water usage. As global attention shifts toward green pharmaceutical production, these digital and automated solutions provide a viable path to meeting both regulatory and environmental standards.

In summary, next-generation manufacturing and automation are redefining the pharmaceutical production paradigm by enhancing flexibility, quality, and responsiveness. These innovations not only meet the growing demand for personalized and complex therapies but also build resilience in the face of global health challenges. As automation technologies mature and become more integrated with AI and digital infrastructure, the pharmaceutical industry stands to benefit from unprecedented levels of efficiency, scalability, and sustainability.

5.2.4 Chimeric antigen receptor T-cell therapy and artificial intelligence: precision for whom?

The integration of AI into personalized therapies marks a critical frontier in oncology, particularly in the context of chimeric antigen receptor (CAR) T-cell therapy. Artificial intelligence is playing a transformative role in advancing precision medicine, particularly in the development and refinement of CAR T-cell therapy. These therapies, which involve reprogramming a patient's T-cells to target and destroy cancer cells, represent a highly personalized form of immunotherapy. Integrating AI into this framework has significantly enhanced the precision, safety, and efficacy of treatment by enabling clinicians to make informed, real-time decisions based on complex biological data.

At the core of AI-guided precision medicine is the ability to analyze massive, multi-dimensional datasets to uncover clinically relevant biomarkers that inform individualized treatment plans. By leveraging genomic, transcriptomic, and proteomic data, AI algorithms can predict how a patient is likely to respond to CAR T-cell therapy, thereby enabling the personalization of dosing strategies and patient selection (Beider et al., 2021). This approach minimizes the risk of toxicity while improving therapeutic outcomes, especially in cases where tumor burden, immune environment, and genetic heterogeneity present substantial variability across patients. Through this lens, AI acts as a powerful decision-support system, guiding clinicians toward optimal treatment pathways tailored to each patient's unique disease profile.

Real-time monitoring of CAR T-cells is equally vital in ensuring the safety and responsiveness of therapy. Advanced imaging technologies, including ferumoxytol-enhanced MRI and PET-based techniques, have enabled clinicians to track CAR T-cell trafficking in vivo, providing critical insights into their distribution across target and off-target tissues. Continuous monitoring allows for the early detection of immune-related complications such as cytokine release syndrome and neurotoxicity, two of the most significant risks associated with CAR T-cell therapies (Du et al., 2020). For example, as demonstrated, real-time data on CAR T-cell expansion can inform the timely adjustment of immunosuppressive support or modification of dosing, enhancing both safety and efficacy.

Personalized dosing strategies represent another critical component of AI-guided CAR T-cell therapy. Traditional dosing models often rely on population-based pharmacokinetic assumptions, which may not reflect an individual's immune dynamics or tumor responsiveness. ML models are now being used to analyze patient-specific parameters, including tumor size, immune markers, and T-cell proliferation rates, to generate tailored dosing schedules. Techniques such as quantitative PCR and digital cell tracking enable clinicians to dynamically assess CAR T-cell levels, informing decisions on whether additional infusions or alternative interventions are required (Sarikonda et al., 2020).

The integration of cutting-edge technologies further amplifies these advancements (Wang et al., 2020). Nanoparticle labeling of CAR T-cells, for example, enables high-resolution visualization of cell activity in real time, improving the precision of targeting and reducing the likelihood of off-target effects. When combined with AI-powered analytics, these imaging and monitoring technologies provide a comprehensive view of the therapeutic landscape, allowing clinicians to adapt treatment plans with unprecedented accuracy and confidence.

In conclusion, the convergence of AI, real-time cellular monitoring, and personalized dosing is redefining the paradigm of CAR T-cell therapy. These innovations not only enhance the safety and effectiveness of treatments for cancer patients but also exemplify the broader potential of AI-guided precision medicine. As these technologies mature, they are likely to extend beyond oncology, setting the stage for a new era of individualized therapies across diverse disease areas.

Precision for whom? AI, access, and global health equity

While AI-driven pharmaceutical innovation promises unprecedented precision and efficiency, it also raises critical questions of access and justice. Advanced therapies such as CAR T-cell treatments and AI-powered diagnostics risk reinforcing global and socioeconomic disparities if infrastructure, affordability, and governance are not addressed.

Ensuring that AI delivers precision with inclusion requires:

Ethical-by-design AI systems

Context-aware deployment in low-resource settings

Policy frameworks that prioritize public value over technological exclusivity

The true success of AI in pharma will be measured not only by innovation speed—but by who benefits.

5.3 Sustainability and the future of pharmacy

5.3.1 Environmental impact of pharma

The pharmaceutical industry is undergoing a transformative shift toward more sustainable and efficient manufacturing practices, largely driven by the adoption of continuous manufacturing, smart pharmaceutical factories, the Internet of Things (IoT), and robotics. These advancements reflect the sector's transition into the era of Industry 4.0, characterized by interconnected, data-driven, and environmentally conscious production systems. Together, they are redefining how medicines are developed, produced, and delivered while also addressing pressing environmental concerns such as energy consumption, waste generation, and resource inefficiencies.

Continuous manufacturing is at the forefront of this transformation, offering a more sustainable alternative to traditional batch processing. Unlike batch methods, which often involve lengthy production cycles and higher material waste, continuous systems support uninterrupted operations with real-time monitoring and control. This approach enables consistent product quality and significantly reduces production times and energy use. Recent developments, such as the implementation of digital twins, virtual simulations of physical manufacturing processes, have further optimized system performance, allowing manufacturers to detect inefficiencies and fine-tune operations with precision (Sarikonda et al., 2020). Moreover, continuous manufacturing aligns with green chemistry principles by minimizing waste and improving resource utilization, thus contributing to broader environmental and regulatory goals (Poechlauer et al., 2012).

Smart pharmaceutical factories enhance these benefits by incorporating AI, IoT, and robotics into fully integrated manufacturing environments. These intelligent systems leverage data from embedded sensors and connected devices to continuously monitor critical quality attributes, such as dosage uniformity and temperature control, in real time (Bordawekar et al., 2015). Techniques like near-infrared spectroscopy, for instance, enable noninvasive quality assessments during production, helping ensure batch consistency without halting operations. Beyond quality control, smart factories also facilitate agile production scaling, allowing manufacturers to quickly adapt to market demand fluctuations and reduce excess inventory or overproduction, key contributors to pharmaceutical waste.

IoT plays a critical enabling role in this ecosystem by connecting machinery, sensors, and control systems into cohesive digital networks. These networks enhance process visibility and traceability, allowing for improved oversight of environmental variables essential to pharmaceutical stability, such as humidity, air purity, and temperature (Sharma et al., 2020). By embedding IoT-enabled devices across the supply chain, companies can maintain optimal conditions, preemptively identify risks, and reduce deviations that might otherwise lead to product recalls or discarded materials.

Robotics is another integral component driving both operational efficiency and sustainability. Robotic systems ranging from traditional industrial robots to collaborative robots (cobots) are increasingly used for tasks such as aseptic filling, packaging, sorting, and visual inspection. Their precision reduces material loss and minimizes the risk of contamination, while their speed and consistency boost throughput. Importantly, automation through robotics also reduces reliance on energy-intensive manual labor and helps maintain high productivity with minimal environmental footprint, particularly in continuous manufacturing environments.

Despite these advances, challenges remain. The high capital costs associated with transitioning to smart manufacturing platforms can be prohibitive for small and mid-sized enterprises (Mittal et al., 2019). Furthermore, a workforce skilled in digital technologies, automation, and data analytics is essential to operate and maintain these systems effectively. This creates an urgent need for educational initiatives and industry-academic partnerships focused on upskilling professionals in the pharmaceutical manufacturing sector (Lim & Teng, 2021). Data security and regulatory compliance are also critical concerns, as the increasing interconnectedness of systems raises vulnerability to cyber threats and adds complexity to audit and validation processes.

In conclusion, the integration of continuous manufacturing, smart factories, IoT, and robotics represents a paradigm shift in pharmaceutical production. These innovations not only enhance operational performance and product quality but also contribute meaningfully to environmental sustainability. As the pharmaceutical industry navigates increasing pressures to meet global health demands while reducing its ecological footprint, the continued evolution of these technologies will be essential in shaping a more resilient and responsible manufacturing future.

5.3.2 Sustainable drug manufacturing and distribution

The pharmaceutical industry is rapidly evolving through the adoption of sustainable manufacturing practices, driven by technologies that enhance both environmental stewardship and operational efficiency. Among the most promising innovations are AI-based resource optimization and 3D printing, both of which are transforming traditional production and distribution models. These technologies not only reduce the environmental footprint of pharmaceutical operations but also support more agile, personalized, and resilient systems of care delivery.

AI has emerged as a powerful tool for optimizing resource use across the pharmaceutical manufacturing value chain through advanced data analytics and ML algorithms. AI can identify inefficiencies in production workflows, forecast demand fluctuations, and refine inventory management strategies (Plathottam et al., 2023). These capabilities contribute to a significant reduction in waste, energy usage, and raw material consumption, key factors in lowering carbon emissions associated with drug production. For example, AI systems can adjust energy inputs in real-time based on process requirements, maintaining quality standards while minimizing resource depletion. Additionally, the integration of AI into logistics and supply chain operations allows companies to dynamically reallocate materials and workforce in response to shifting demands, enhancing both environmental and economic sustainability (Helo & Hao, 2021).

In parallel, 3D printing, or additive manufacturing, is redefining how pharmaceuticals are formulated and delivered. Unlike traditional batch manufacturing, which often results in surplus production and material waste, 3D printing operates on a just-in-time basis, producing only what is needed, when it is needed. This approach significantly reduces excess inventory and environmental burden (Pawar & Pawar, 2022). Beyond waste reduction, 3D printing enables the creation of complex and customizable drug formulations, offering precise control over dose, release profile, and ingredient combinations (Bagheri et al., 2023). Such flexibility accelerates the prototyping and approval of new therapies, shortening time to market while also enabling a higher degree of personalization for patients with unique therapeutic needs.

The convergence of AI and 3D printing technologies introduces a novel paradigm in sustainable pharmaceutical manufacturing. AI can guide the 3D printing process by analyzing patient data to determine optimal drug formulations, ensuring that medications are tailored to individual biological profiles. Simultaneously, AI systems can monitor the printing process in real time to adjust variables such as temperature, print speed, and material deposition, ensuring consistency and compliance with quality standards. This dynamic feedback loop not only improves production accuracy but also supports adaptive manufacturing environments capable of responding rapidly to emerging clinical demands.

From an environmental perspective, the integration of these technologies supports broader sustainability goals within the pharmaceutical sector by reducing energy consumption, minimizing raw material usage, and streamlining distribution logistics. Companies can lower their ecological impact and contribute to global climate targets (Bade et al., 2023). Moreover, the rise of green chemistry, in tandem with AI-optimized processes and additive manufacturing, reflects an industry-wide shift toward more responsible innovation (Kar et al., 2021). These advancements help pharmaceutical firms meet stringent environmental regulations while aligning with growing consumer expectations for environmentally conscious healthcare solutions.

The intersection of AI and 3D printing is redefining sustainable drug manufacturing and distribution. These technologies enable a shift from centralized, high-waste production models to adaptive, personalized, and resource-efficient systems. As the pharmaceutical industry continues to face pressures to expand therapeutic access while minimizing its environmental impact, embracing these innovations will be essential in achieving a balance between technological progress and ecological responsibility.

5.3.3 Access versus extraction: can artificial intelligence deliver global health justice?

AI is frequently hailed as a leveling force in global healthcare, a tool that can democratize access to innovation, reduce clinical trial disparities, and expand health service delivery in low- and middle-income countries (LMICs). AI, when integrated with mobile health (mHealth) platforms and innovative clinical trial models, offers a transformative opportunity to address persistent disparities in healthcare access and quality, particularly in LMICs. These technologies collectively hold the potential to democratize access to medical innovations, expand clinical research to underrepresented populations, and improve public health outcomes in regions traditionally excluded from mainstream pharmaceutical development.

AI-driven enhancements in clinical trials are a key area of advancement. Traditionally, the cost, complexity, and time required to conduct clinical research have limited trial implementation in LMICs. However, AI can help streamline these processes by optimizing trial design, accelerating patient recruitment, and improving data management (Mourya et al., 2024). For instance, AI algorithms can rapidly analyze electronic health records to identify suitable trial participants, ensuring not only quicker enrollment but also greater diversity among study populations. This inclusivity is critical for generating evidence that is generalizable and applicable across different demographic and genetic backgrounds. Moreover, integrating AI into trial protocols can standardize methodologies, improve the accuracy of outcome measurements, and reduce administrative burden, all of which help lower trial costs and make research in resource-constrained settings more viable.

In parallel, mobile health technologies are expanding the reach of healthcare delivery to underserved communities. The widespread penetration of mobile phones in LMICs provides a powerful platform for disseminating health information, monitoring treatment adherence, and facilitating patient-provider communication. mHealth applications offer a cost-effective and scalable solution to bridge access gaps, particularly in rural or remote regions (Kahn et al., 2010). Mobile reminders have shown notable success in improving medication adherence, an essential factor in chronic disease management, where noncompliance can significantly compromise outcomes. Furthermore, mHealth platforms support patient education and telemedicine capabilities, empowering individuals to actively manage their health even in the absence of formal healthcare infrastructure.

However, the implementation of AI and mHealth in LMICs is not without challenges. Technological limitations such as inadequate internet access, unreliable power supply, and lack of digital literacy can hinder adoption and effectiveness (Alami et al., 2020). These barriers underscore the importance of infrastructure development and the deployment of context-specific technological solutions. Additionally, health literacy plays a crucial role in the success of digital interventions. If patients cannot comprehend or effectively use these tools, their impact may be significantly diminished. Tailoring content to local languages, cultures, and levels of understanding is essential to ensure engagement and long-term sustainability.

To fully harness the benefits of AI and mHealth in promoting global health equity, a holistic and inclusive approach is needed. This involves not only investing in technological solutions but also addressing the social, cultural, and infrastructural determinants that affect access to and engagement with these tools. Policymakers, industry stakeholders, and global health organizations must collaborate to build systems that are resilient, adaptable, and equitable.

The convergence of AI-powered clinical trials and mobile health innovations presents a significant opportunity to improve access to healthcare and research in LMICs. These technologies can help dismantle long-standing barriers by making clinical development more inclusive and healthcare delivery more efficient. However, realizing this potential requires deliberate efforts to address the unique challenges of low-resource settings and to embed equity considerations at every stage of innovation deployment. When implemented thoughtfully, these digital health strategies can serve as powerful catalysts for global health equity.

5.3.4 A new compact: rethinking progress through equity and sustainability

The pharmaceutical industry stands at a pivotal juncture, technologically sophisticated, globally interdependent, and under growing pressure to respond to both planetary and social crises. The future of the pharmaceutical industry is increasingly being shaped by the convergence of AI, sustainability, and global access. This multidimensional vision aims not only to accelerate drug innovation and improve therapeutic outcomes but also to ensure equitable distribution of medicines and reduce the environmental footprint of pharmaceutical practices. Together, these shifts signal a transition toward a smarter, more inclusive, and environmentally responsible healthcare ecosystem (Fig. 5.1).

AI continues to play a pivotal role in the evolution of personalized medicine. By analyzing vast and complex datasets, including genomic profiles, electronic health records, and real-time biomarker data, AI systems are capable of identifying clinically relevant patterns that inform the development of individualized treatment plans (Alum & Ugwu, 2025). This approach enhances therapeutic efficacy and minimizes adverse effects, ultimately improving patient outcomes and treatment adherence. Moreover, AI is transforming the clinical trial landscape by streamlining participant selection, identifying responsive subpopulations, and accelerating trial execution. These capabilities support the broader aim of reducing time-to-market while improving access to innovative therapies. AI also facilitates drug repurposing by uncovering

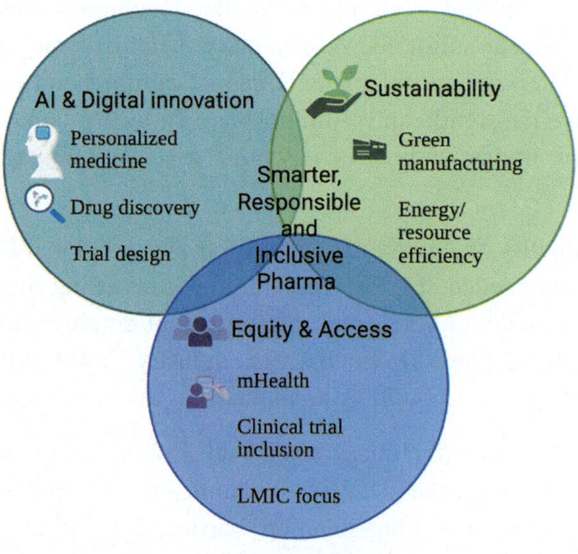

Figure 5.1
New compact: rethinking progress through equity and sustainability.
Convergence of key pillars shaping the future of the pharmaceutical industry: technological innovation (AI and digital tools), environmental sustainability, and equitable access intersect to define a smarter, more responsible, and inclusive pharma landscape.

new indications for existing molecules, thereby enhancing the cost-effectiveness and sustainability of pharmaceutical R&D pipelines (Wan et al., 2025).

Sustainability is becoming an equally integral pillar of the future pharmaceutical landscape. Faced with mounting environmental pressures, pharmaceutical companies are increasingly adopting green chemistry principles and digital tools to reduce waste, energy consumption, and carbon emissions. AI plays a central role in optimizing resource allocation within manufacturing processes, improving production efficiency, and identifying opportunities for process improvements that align with environmental objectives (Plathottam et al., 2023). Leading firms such as Novartis and Johnson & Johnson have embedded sustainability into their corporate strategies, aligning business operations with the UN Sustainable Development Goals while committing to broader health equity agendas (Eang et al., 2022). These efforts not only reflect corporate responsibility but also respond to growing consumer and regulatory expectations for ethical and sustainable practices in healthcare.

Equitable global access to medicines remains a defining challenge in contemporary healthcare. The COVID 19 pandemic exposed and amplified disparities in the availability of vaccines and treatments, prompting urgent calls for reform in global health governance (Abu El Kheir-Mataria et al., 2023). In response, collaborative frameworks involving governments, industry stakeholders, and nongovernmental organizations are being developed to ensure more inclusive access to essential medicines. Technologies such as mobile health (mHealth) applications are also playing a critical role in extending pharmaceutical services to underserved populations, offering education, diagnostics, and treatment support in real time. When coupled with AI-driven analytics, these platforms can inform healthcare planning by identifying emerging needs, optimizing distribution routes, and ensuring that innovations reach the communities that need them most.

Despite these promising trends, several challenges regulatory systems must evolve to accommodate the unique complexities introduced by AI and digital technologies, particularly regarding patient safety, data privacy, and algorithmic transparency. Many LMICs still face barriers such as inadequate digital infrastructure, limited health data availability, and workforce gaps in technical capacity, all of which can limit the impact of these technologies (Lamichhane & Neupane, 2022). Establishing robust governance frameworks, investing in capacity-building, and fostering global cooperation will be essential to overcoming these limitations and ensuring that the benefits of innovation are distributed equitably.

In summary, the pharmaceutical industry's future lies at the intersection of technological advancement, environmental responsibility, and equitable access. By aligning innovation with sustainability and social responsibility, the industry can begin to address the most pressing global health challenges. However, the realization of this vision requires more than innovation alone—it demands cross-sector collaboration, ethical foresight, and a sustained commitment to global health equity.

Key Takeaways

AI is becoming infrastructural in pharma—embedded across target discovery, preclinical modeling, clinical trials, manufacturing, and post-market surveillance, rather than acting as an isolated tool.

Next-generation modalities and platforms (e.g., CRISPR, mRNA beyond vaccines, DELs, digital therapeutics, and AI-enabled monitoring) are expanding both therapeutic ambition and operational complexity.

Manufacturing is shifting toward continuous, smart, and automated systems, where real-time monitoring, digital twins, and AI-driven quality control enable higher resilience, scalability, and reduced waste.

Precision therapies (including CAR T-cell approaches) illustrate both promise and constraint: AI improves personalization and safety, yet affordability, infrastructure, and governance determine who can benefit.

Sustainability and equity are no longer peripheral; they are emerging as strategic requirements—demanding responsible data governance, ethical deployment, and context-aware implementation in low-resource settings.

5.3.4.1 Editor's note

This chapter provides a timely and well-grounded synthesis of the forces reshaping the pharmaceutical industry—highlighting how AI, disruptive technologies, and sustainability imperatives are converging into a new operating reality for drug development and delivery. Importantly, it does not treat technological progress as inherently beneficial; rather, it frames innovation as a responsibility that must be governed through ethics, regulatory adaptability, and equity-oriented strategies. As the broader volume argues, the long-term value of AI-enabled pharma will depend not only on scientific acceleration and operational efficiency, but also on the industry's ability to sustain public trust and ensure that the benefits of innovation are distributed fairly across populations and regions.

5.3.4.2 Learning activities: trends shaping the future of the pharmaceutical industry

These learning activities are designed to support graduate students, researchers, and healthcare professionals in critically engaging with the technological, ethical, and sustainability-driven transformations shaping the future pharmaceutical industry. The activities encourage analytical thinking, interdisciplinary reasoning, and strategic foresight.

1. Short essay prompts

Select one of the following topics and write a structured essay (600–800 words), supported by academic and industry sources:

Essay A: Artificial intelligence as infrastructure: How AI is reshaping the pharmaceutical value chain?

Essay B: Balancing precision and equity: Can AI-driven pharma deliver global health justice?

Essay C: Sustainable innovation in pharma: How AI and automation redefine environmental responsibility?

2. Applied case analysis

Case focus: AI-enabled drug development

A pharmaceutical company integrates AI across target identification, clinical trials, and manufacturing while expanding into low- and middle-income markets.

Discussion questions:

Which AI applications generate the greatest strategic value across the pipeline?

What ethical and regulatory risks emerge from large-scale AI deployment?

How can sustainability and equity be embedded into AI-driven innovation strategies?

3. Digital research and critical review

Students are asked to explore **two** of the following resources:

Regulatory bodies (FDA, EMA)

Global health organizations (WHO)

Industry innovation platforms (AI in pharma startups)

Tasks:

Identify one emerging AI-driven pharmaceutical innovation

Assess its ethical, regulatory, and sustainability implications

Propose one policy or governance improvement

4. Bloom's taxonomy–based learning tasks

Cognitive level	Activity
Remember	List key AI applications across drug discovery and manufacturing
Understand	Explain how AI enhances precision medicine
Apply	Design a simple AI-supported patient monitoring workflow
Analyze	Compare AI benefits in CAR T-cell therapy vs. traditional oncology
Evaluate	Assess risks of algorithmic bias in pharma AI systems
Create	Propose an AI-enabled sustainable pharma model for LMICs

5. Team activity: designing the pharma of tomorrow

Working in small teams, design a future-ready pharmaceutical model that integrates:

AI-driven drug development

Sustainable manufacturing

Equitable global access

Ethical governance

Teams present a 5–7 minute strategic pitch outlining priorities, risks, and impact.

References

Abbas, M. K. G., et al. (2024). The role of AI in drug discovery. *Chembiochem: A European Journal of Chemical Biology, 25*(14). https://doi.org/10.1002/cbic.202300816.

Abu El Kheir-Mataria, W., El-Fawal, H., & Chun, S. (2023). Global health governance performance during Covid-19, what needs to be changed? A delphi survey study. *Globalization and Health, 19*(1). https://doi.org/10.1186/s12992-023-00921-0.

Alami, H., et al. (2020). Artificial intelligence in health care: Laying the foundation for responsible, sustainable, and inclusive innovation in low- and middle-income countries. *Globalization and Health, 16*(1). https://doi.org/10.1186/s12992-020-00584-1.

Alum, E. U., & Ugwu, O. P. (2025). Artificial intelligence in personalized medicine: Transforming diagnosis and treatment. *Discover Applied Sciences, 7*(3). https://doi.org/10.1007/s42452-025-06625-x.

Asif, M. et al. (2024). Proactive emotion tracker: AI-driven continuous mood and emotion monitoring. arXiv (Cornell University). https://doi.org/10.48550/arxiv.2401.13722

Bade, C., et al. (2023). Sustainability in the pharmaceutical industry—An assessment of maturity and effects of measure implementation on supply chain security. *Corporate Social Responsibility and Environmental Management, 31*(1), 224–242. https://doi.org/10.1002/csr.2564.

Bagheri, A., et al. (2023). 3D printing of customized drug delivery systems with controlled architecture via reversible addition-fragmentation chain transfer polymerization. *Advanced Engineering Materials, 25*(10). https://doi.org/10.1002/adem.202201785.

Balica, A. et al. (2023). Augmenting endometriosis analysis from ultrasound data with deep learning. arXiv (Cornell University). https://doi.org/10.48550/arxiv.2302.09621

Beider, K., et al. (2021). In vitro analysis predicts clinical response of B cell lymphatic malignancies to Cd19 Car-T cells: Phenotypic, transcriptional and functional study. *Hematological Oncology, 39*(S2). https://doi.org/10.1002/hon.191_2880.

Blanco-González, A. et al. (2022). The role of AI in drug discovery: Challenges, opportunities, and strategies. arXiv (Cornell University). https://doi.org/10.48550/arxiv.2212.08104

Bordawekar, S., et al. (2015). Industry perspectives on process analytical technology: Tools and applications in API manufacturing. *Organic Process Research & Development, 19*(9), 1174–1185. https://doi.org/10.1021/acs.oprd.5b00088.

Burcham, C. L., Florence, A. J., & Johnson, M. D. (2018). Continuous manufacturing in pharmaceutical process development and manufacturing. *Annual Review of Chemical and Biomolecular Engineering, 9*(1), 253–281. https://doi.org/10.1146/annurev-chembioeng-060817-084355.

Campenhout, C. V., et al. (2019). Guidelines for optimized gene knockout using CRISPR/Cas9. *Biotechniques, 66*(6), 295–302. https://doi.org/10.2144/btn-2018-0187.

Chelliah, V., & van der Graaf, P. H. (2022). Model-informed target identification and validation through combining quantitative systems pharmacology with network-based analysis. *CPT: Pharmacometrics & Systems Pharmacology, 11*(4), 399–402. https://doi.org/10.1002/psp4.12766.

Deng, J. et al. (2021). Artificial intelligence in drug discovery: Applications and techniques. arXiv (Cornell University). https://doi.org/10.48550/arxiv.2106.05386

DiMasi, J. A. (2002). The value of improving the productivity of the drug development process. *Pharmacoeconomics, 20*(Supplement 3), 1–10. https://doi.org/10.2165/00019053-200220003-00001.

Du, M., et al. (2020). Biomarkers in individualized management of chimeric antigen receptor T cell therapy. *Biomarker Research, 8*(1). https://doi.org/10.1186/s40364-020-00190-8.

Eang, M., Clarke, A., & Ordonez-Ponce, E. (2022). The roles of multinational enterprises in implementing the United Nations Sustainable Development Goals at the local level. *BRQ Business Research Quarterly, 26*(1), 79–97. https://doi.org/10.1177/23409444221140912.

Grisoni, F., et al. (2021). Combining generative artificial intelligence and on-chip synthesis for de novo drug design. *Science Advances, 7*(24). https://doi.org/10.1126/sciadv.abg3338.

Helo, P., & Hao, Y. (2021). Artificial intelligence in operations management and supply chain management: An exploratory case study. *Production Planning & Control, 33*(16), 1573–1590. https://doi.org/10.1080/09537287.2021.1882690.

Huang, D. Z., Baber, J. C., & Bahmanyar, S. S. (2021). The challenges of generalizability in artificial intelligence for ADME/Tox endpoint and activity prediction. *Expert Opinion on Drug Discovery, 16*(9), 1045–1056. https://doi.org/10.1080/17460441.2021.1901685.

Hughes, T. B., Miller, G. P., & Swamidass, S. J. (2015). Modeling epoxidation of drug-like molecules with a deep machine learning network. *ACS Central Science, 1*(4), 168–180. https://doi.org/10.1021/acscentsci.5b00131.

Jena, G. K., et al. (2024). Artificial intelligence and machine learning implemented drug delivery systems: A paradigm shift in the pharmaceutical industry. *Journal of Bio-X Research, 7.* https://doi.org/10.34133/jbioxresearch.0016.

Jovanovic, M., Jevremović, A., and Pejović-Milovančević, M. (2021). Intelligent interactive technologies for mental health and well-being. arXiv (Cornell University). https://doi.org/10.48550/arxiv.2105.05306

Kahn, J. G., Yang, J. S., & Kahn, J. S. (2010). Mobile' health needs and opportunities in developing countries. *Health Affairs, 29*(2), 252–258. https://doi.org/10.1377/hlthaff.2009.0965.

Kar, S., et al. (2021). Green chemistry in the synthesis of pharmaceuticals. *Chemical Reviews, 122*(3), 3637–3710. https://doi.org/10.1021/acs.chemrev.1c00631.

Kühl, N. et al. (2020). Machine learning in artificial intelligence: Towards a common understanding. arXiv (Cornell University). https://doi.org/10.48550/arxiv.2004.04686

Lamichhane, B., & Neupane, N. (2022). Improved healthcare access in low-resource regions: A review of technological solutions. arXiv (Cornell University). https://doi.org/10.48550/arxiv.2205.10913

Larson, D. B., et al. (2020). Ethics of using and sharing clinical imaging data for artificial intelligence: A proposed framework. *Radiology, 295*(3), 675–682. https://doi.org/10.1148/radiol.2020192536.

Lee, U. et al. (2022). Toward data-driven digital therapeutics analytics: Literature review and research directions. arXiv (Cornell University). https://doi.org/10.48550/arxiv.2205.01851

Li, D., et al. (2023). Messenger RNA-based therapeutics and vaccines: What's beyond COVID-19? *ACS Pharmacology & Translational Science, 6*(7), 943–969. https://doi.org/10.1021/acsptsci.3c00047.

Lim, K. H., & Teng, C. S. (2021). University engagement to improve safety education. *Process Safety Progress, 40*(3), 12–17. https://doi.org/10.1002/prs.12241.

Liu, J. et al. (2021a). A machine learning approach for recruitment prediction in clinical trial design. arXiv (Cornell University). https://doi.org/10.48550/arxiv.2111.07407

Liu, X. et al. (2021b). A scalable AI approach for clinical trial cohort optimization. arXiv (Cornell University). https://doi.org/10.48550/arxiv.2109.02808

Maharao, N., et al. (2020). Entering the era of computationally driven drug development. *Drug Metabolism Reviews, 52*(2), 283–298. https://doi.org/10.1080/03602532.2020.1726944.

Mandala, S.K. (2023). XAI renaissance: Redefining interpretability in medical diagnostic models. arXiv (Cornell University). https://doi.org/10.48550/arxiv.2306.01668

Mao, Y., et al. (2025). Emerging artificial intelligence-driven precision therapies in tumor drug resistance: Recent advances, opportunities, and challenges. *Molecular Cancer, 24*(1). https://doi.org/10.1186/s12943-025-02321-x.

Marey, A., et al. (2024). Explainability, transparency and black box challenges of AI in radiology: Impact on patient care in cardiovascular radiology. *Egyptian Journal of Radiology and Nuclear Medicine, 55*(1). https://doi.org/10.1186/s43055-024-01356-2.

Marko, J. G. O., Neagu, C. D., & Anand, P. B. (2025). Examining inclusivity: The use of AI and diverse populations in health and social care: A systematic review. *BMC Medical Informatics and Decision Making, 25*(1). https://doi.org/10.1186/s12911-025-02884-1.

Martínez-Pérez, B., de la Torre-Díez, I., & López-Coronado, M. (2014). Privacy and security in mobile health apps: A review and recommendations. *Journal of Medical Systems, 39*(1). https://doi.org/10.1007/s10916-014-0181-3.

Mittal, S., et al. (2019). A smart manufacturing adoption framework for SMEs. *International Journal of Production Research, 58*(5), 1555–1573. https://doi.org/10.1080/00207543.2019.1661540.

Mourya, A., Jobanputra, B., & Pai, R. (2024). AI-powered clinical trials and the imperative for regulatory transparency and accountability. *Health and Technology, 14*(6), 1071–1081. https://doi.org/10.1007/s12553-024-00904-0.

O'Connor, S., et al. (2016). Understanding factors affecting patient and public engagement and recruitment to digital health interventions: A systematic review of qualitative studies. *BMC Medical Informatics and Decision Making, 16*(1). https://doi.org/10.1186/s12911-016-0359-3.

Ocana, A., et al. (2025). Integrating artificial intelligence in drug discovery and early drug development: A transformative approach. *Biomarker Research, 13*(1). https://doi.org/10.1186/s40364-025-00758-2.

Osorio-Méndez, J. F., et al. (2025). Exploring the mechanisms of action of the antimicrobial peptide CZS-5 against Trypanosoma cruzi epimastigotes: Insights from metabolomics and molecular dynamics. *Parasites & Vectors, 18*(1). https://doi.org/10.1186/s13071-025-06861-5.

Pawar, R., & Pawar, A. (2022). 3D printing of pharmaceuticals: Approach from bench scale to commercial development. *Future Journal of Pharmaceutical Sciences, 8*(1). https://doi.org/10.1186/s43094-022-00439-z.

Plathottam, S. J., et al. (2023). A review of artificial intelligence applications in manufacturing operations. *Journal of Advanced Manufacturing and Processing, 5*(3). https://doi.org/10.1002/amp2.10159.

Poechlauer, P., et al. (2012). Continuous processing in the manufacture of active pharmaceutical ingredients and finished dosage forms: An industry perspective. *Organic Process Research & Development, 16*(10), 1586–1590. https://doi.org/10.1021/op300159y.

Potanin, M. et al. (2023). Startup success prediction and VC portfolio simulation using CrunchBase data. arXiv (Cornell University). https://doi.org/10.48550/arxiv.2309.15552

Poudel, U., et al. (2025). AI in mental health: A review of technological advancements and ethical issues in psychiatry. *Issues in Mental Health Nursing,* 1–9. https://doi.org/10.1080/01612840.2025.2502943.

Ren, F. et al. (2022). AlphaFold accelerates artificial intelligence powered drug discovery: Efficient discovery of a novel cyclin-dependent kinase 20 (CDK20) small molecule inhibitor. arXiv (Cornell University). https://doi.org/10.48550/arxiv.2201.09647

Sarikonda, G., et al. (2020). Monitoring cell kinetics in clinical trials by multiparametric flow cytometry: Benefits and challenges. *Cytometry Part B: Clinical Cytometry, 100*(1), 72–78. https://doi.org/10.1002/cyto.b.21891.

Sharma, A., Kaur, J., & Singh, I. (2020). Internet of things (IoT) in pharmaceutical manufacturing, warehousing, and supply chain management. *SN Computer Science, 1*(4). https://doi.org/10.1007/s42979-020-00248-2.

Silva, T. C., Eppink, M., & Ottens, M. (2021). Automation and miniaturization: Enabling tools for fast, high-throughput process development in integrated continuous biomanufacturing. *Journal of Chemical Technology & Biotechnology, 97*(9), 2365–2375. https://doi.org/10.1002/jctb.6792.

Song, M., & Hwang, G. T. (2020). DNA-encoded library screening as core platform technology in drug discovery: Its synthetic method development and applications in DEL synthesis. *Journal of Medicinal Chemistry, 63*(13), 6578–6599. https://doi.org/10.1021/acs.jmedchem.9b01782.

Terranova, N., et al. (2023). Artificial intelligence for quantitative modeling in drug discovery and development: An innovation and quality consortium perspective on use cases and best practices. *Clinical Pharmacology & Therapeutics, 115*(4), 658–672. https://doi.org/10.1002/cpt.3053.

Vo, A. H., et al. (2019). An overview of machine learning and big data for drug toxicity evaluation. *Chemical Research in Toxicology, 33*(1), 20–37. https://doi.org/10.1021/acs.chemrestox.9b00227.

Wan, Z., et al. (2025). Applications of artificial intelligence in drug repurposing. *Advanced Science, 12*(14). https://doi.org/10.1002/advs.202411325.

Wang, X., et al. (2020). Nanotechnology-based CAR-T strategies for improving efficacy and safety of tumor immunotherapy. *Advanced Functional Materials, 31*(1). https://doi.org/10.1002/adfm.202004713.

Wang, Z. et al. (2023). Personalized state anxiety detection: An empirical study with linguistic biomarkers and a machine learning pipeline. arXiv (Cornell University). https://doi.org/10.48550/arxiv.2304.09928

Xia, Y., et al. (2024). A comprehensive review of molecular optimization in artificial intelligence-based drug discovery. *Quantitative Biology, 12*(1), 15–29. https://doi.org/10.1002/qub2.30.

Xu, D., et al. (2020). Phenotypic screening of chemical libraries enriched by molecular docking to multiple targets selected from glioblastoma genomic data. *ACS Chemical Biology, 15*(6), 1424–1444. https://doi.org/10.1021/acschembio.0c00078.

Xue, V. W., Wong, S. C. C., & Cho, W. C. S. (2020). Genome-wide CRISPR screens for the identification of therapeutic targets for cancer treatment. *Expert Opinion on Therapeutic Targets, 24*(11), 1147–1158. https://doi.org/10.1080/14728222.2020.1820986.

Zheng, Y., et al. (2021). Smart materials enabled with artificial intelligence for healthcare wearables. *Advanced Functional Materials, 31*(51). https://doi.org/10.1002/adfm.202105482.

CHAPTER 6

AI-driven pharma strategy and operating models: from digital adoption to intelligent transformation

Miltiadis Lytras[1] **and Hani Alhashmi**[2]

[1]Computer Science Department, College of Engineering, Effat University, Jeddah, Saudi Arabia, [2]Senior Medical Director, Pfizer Saudi Arabia, Riyadh, Saudi Arabia

6.1 From digital adoption to intelligent transformation: why strategy must lead artificial intelligence in pharma

The pharmaceutical industry has entered a decisive inflection point in its digital evolution. Over the past decade, most pharmaceutical organizations have invested heavily in digital technologies—advanced analytics platforms, automation tools, real-world data infrastructures, and isolated artificial intelligence (AI) applications. Yet despite this widespread adoption, the strategic impact of AI across the industry remains uneven. Many organizations exhibit high levels of technological sophistication but struggle to translate these capabilities into sustained competitive advantage, faster evidence generation, or more adaptive operating models. This disconnect reveals a fundamental insight: AI transformation in pharma is not primarily a technology problem—it is a strategic and organizational one.

Digital adoption and intelligent transformation are not synonymous. Digital adoption refers to the deployment of tools: machine learning models for prediction, natural language processing for document review, or robotic process automation for operational efficiency. Intelligent transformation, by contrast, reflects a deeper shift in how decisions are made, how evidence is generated, how accountability is assigned, and how value is created across the pharmaceutical value chain. In intelligent organizations, AI does not operate at the margins; it reshapes the logic of strategy, governance, and execution.

6.1.1 The limits of tool-centric artificial intelligence adoption

Most pharmaceutical companies began their AI journey through use-case-driven experimentation. Data science teams were tasked with developing models to optimize clinical trial recruitment, predict manufacturing deviations, or enhance pharmacovigilance signal detection.

The Future of Pharma Across All Sectors in the Artificial Intelligence Era. DOI: https://doi.org/10.1016/B978-0-443-40572-3.00012-5

While many of these initiatives delivered localized benefits, they often remained siloed, disconnected from enterprise strategy and decision-making authority.

This tool-centric approach creates three structural limitations:

First, AI remains operational rather than strategic. Models support individual functions but do not inform portfolio-level trade-offs, investment prioritization, or long-term capability development. As a result, AI becomes a cost center rather than a strategic asset.

Second, decision accountability becomes blurred. When AI outputs are embedded into workflows without clearly defined ownership, it becomes unclear who is responsible for outcomes—particularly when recommendations conflict with human judgment. In a regulated environment such as pharma, this ambiguity undermines trust and slows adoption.

Third, organizational learning is fragmented. Without a unifying strategy, insights generated in one domain (e.g., clinical development) fail to inform others (e.g., regulatory strategy or supply chain planning). The organization learns locally but not systemically.

These limitations explain why many AI initiatives stall at the pilot stage or fail to scale beyond individual departments. Intelligent transformation requires a shift away from isolated optimization toward strategic integration.

6.1.2 Artificial intelligence as a strategic capability, not a functional add-on

To move beyond digital fragmentation, pharmaceutical leaders must reconceptualize AI as a strategic capability—on par with R&D excellence, regulatory expertise, or global manufacturing scale. A strategic capability is not defined by individual tools but by the organization's ability to repeatedly deploy knowledge, coordinate action, and adapt to uncertainty.

In this context, AI's true value lies in its capacity to:

Integrate heterogeneous data across the enterprise (clinical, genomic, operational, regulatory, and market data)

Enable predictive and scenario-based decision-making

Support continuous evidence generation rather than episodic analysis

Enhance organizational learning through feedback loops

When AI is embedded at the strategic level, it influences how portfolios are designed, how risks are assessed, how trials are structured, and how regulatory engagement is planned. Strategy no longer precedes data; instead, strategy and analytics co-evolve.

This shift is particularly critical in pharmaceutical environments characterized by long development cycles, high uncertainty, and irreversible investment decisions. AI-enabled strategic intelligence allows leaders to explore multiple futures, test assumptions, and adjust direction before costs escalate.

AI as a Strategic Capability, Not a Functional Add-on

From "AI Projects" to "AI Capability": The Executive Maturity Model for Pharma

Most pharma organizations are currently stuck between experimentation and transformation. Use this maturity model to benchmark where your organization stands—and what must change to scale.

Level 1—Use-case pilots: AI exists as isolated proofs-of-concept, typically led by data science teams. Value is local and fragile.

Level 2—Functional optimization: AI supports individual functions (e.g., R&D analytics, recruitment, manufacturing monitoring) but remains siloed.

Level 3—Cross-functional integration: AI outputs start influencing adjacent functions. Shared datasets and governance appear, but decision rights remain unclear.

Level 4—Enterprise intelligence operating model: AI informs portfolio strategy, evidence strategy, supply chain resilience, and regulatory planning through coordinated decision architecture.

Level 5—Adaptive intelligence loops (Intelligent Pharma): Continuous learning loops connect trial data, RWE, manufacturing signals, safety surveillance, and market feedback. Governance and accountability are lifecycle-based.

Executive takeaway: AI transformation is achieved when decision-making becomes intelligence-driven—not when more models are deployed.

6.1.3 From linear value chains to adaptive intelligence loops

Traditional pharmaceutical operating models are largely linear. Discovery feeds development; development feeds regulatory submission; approval feeds manufacturing and commercialization. While feedback exists, it is slow and often retrospective.

AI enables a fundamentally different model: adaptive intelligence loops. In these loops, data generated at every stage of the lifecycle continuously informs upstream and downstream decisions. Real-world evidence (RWE) feeds back into clinical strategy. Manufacturing data informs formulation design. Post-market safety signals reshape trial endpoints.

However, such intelligence loops cannot function without strategic orchestration. Without clear governance, AI systems risk generating conflicting signals, reinforcing local optimization at the expense of global performance. Strategy provides the alignment mechanism that determines:

Which decisions should be AI-augmented
Which outcomes matter most
How uncertainty is handled
When human judgment overrides algorithmic recommendations

In intelligent pharma organizations, strategy defines the "decision architecture" within which AI operates.

6.1.4 Leadership, governance, and decision rights in AI-driven pharma

One of the most underappreciated aspects of AI transformation is its impact on decision rights. AI systems introduce new actors into decision-making processes—algorithms that rank options, flag risks, or recommend actions. Without explicit governance, these systems can unintentionally shift power, accountability, and responsibility.

Strategic AI adoption requires leadership to address several critical questions:
Who owns AI-driven decisions?
What level of explainability is required before action?
How are disagreements between human experts and AI systems resolved?
How is performance monitored over time?

In pharmaceutical contexts, where regulatory scrutiny is intense and patient safety paramount, these questions cannot be deferred. Explainable AI becomes not merely a technical requirement but a governance mechanism that enables accountability, auditability, and trust.

Decision Rights in the AI Era: A Practical Governance Blueprint

AI introduces a new actor in decision-making: the algorithm. Without explicit governance, organizations drift into ambiguity—where AI recommendations exist but accountability is unclear.

A workable governance model answers five questions:

What decisions are AI-augmented? Define the list of high-value decisions (e.g., site selection, safety signal triage, batch release risk) where AI is allowed to influence outcomes.

Who is accountable for each decision? Assign a single accountable owner (clinical, quality, regulatory, operations)—not "the AI team."

What evidence must AI provide to be actionable? Specify thresholds for explainability, confidence/uncertainty reporting, and subgroup performance.

What is the override and escalation policy? Codify when clinicians/experts can override, when escalation is mandatory, and what is logged.

How is performance governed over time? Establish drift monitoring, periodic revalidation, version control, and retirement triggers.

Executive takeaway: In pharma, governance is not a barrier to AI. It is the mechanism that makes AI deployable, auditable, and scalable.

Leading organizations establish AI governance frameworks that integrate ethics, compliance, clinical oversight, and data stewardship into a single operating model. These frameworks ensure that AI systems evolve responsibly and remain aligned with both corporate strategy and societal expectations.

6.1.5 Human-centered intelligence: augmentation over automation

A defining principle of intelligent transformation in pharma is human-centered AI. Despite advances in automation, pharmaceutical innovation remains deeply human—dependent on scientific judgment, ethical reasoning, and contextual understanding.

AI excels at processing complexity and scale; humans excel at interpreting meaning, weighing values, and exercising responsibility. Intelligent transformation does not replace human expertise—it amplifies it.

Strategically mature organizations design AI systems to support:
Better scientific hypotheses
Faster learning cycles
More informed regulatory dialogue
Safer, more equitable patient outcomes

This requires investment not only in technology but also in capability building: training leaders, clinicians, and researchers to understand AI outputs, question assumptions, and engage critically with algorithmic insights.

6.1.6 Strategic implications for the pharma enterprise

The transition from digital adoption to intelligent transformation carries profound implications for the pharmaceutical enterprise:
AI strategy must be articulated at the board and executive levels, not delegated solely to IT or data science teams.
Organizational structures must evolve to support cross-functional intelligence rather than functional silos.
Governance models must shift from static compliance to lifecycle accountability.
Talent strategies must prioritize AI literacy alongside scientific excellence.

Ultimately, the organizations that succeed will not be those with the most sophisticated algorithms, but those that align AI with purpose, governance, and strategy.

This chapter builds on this foundation by examining how AI reshapes the pharmaceutical value chain in practice—moving from strategic framing to operational execution, evidence generation, and responsible innovation across the full lifecycle.

6.2 AI-driven operating models across the pharmaceutical value chain

AI reshapes the pharmaceutical industry most profoundly not through isolated innovations, but through the reconfiguration of operating models across the entire value chain. While traditional pharmaceutical models are structured around sequential handovers between discovery, development, manufacturing, and commercialization, AI enables a more integrated, adaptive, and intelligence-driven architecture. In this architecture, data, analytics, and decision-making flow continuously rather than episodically, supporting faster learning and more resilient execution.

An AI-driven operating model is not defined by the presence of advanced algorithms alone. Rather, it reflects how analytics are embedded into core decision points, how insights are translated into action, and how feedback loops are institutionalized. This section examines how AI transforms each major segment of the pharmaceutical value chain and, critically, how these transformations interconnect to form a coherent enterprise intelligence system.

6.2.1 Reconfiguring discovery and early research through predictive intelligence

Drug discovery has traditionally been characterized by high uncertainty, long timelines, and extensive trial-and-error experimentation. AI fundamentally alters this paradigm by enabling predictive intelligence at the earliest stages of research. Machine learning models can analyze vast chemical, biological, and genomic datasets to identify promising targets, predict molecular interactions, and prioritize candidate compounds with higher probabilities of success.

However, the strategic impact of AI in discovery lies not merely in speed, but in decision quality. Predictive models allow organizations to explore alternative research pathways, compare risk profiles across candidate molecules, and make earlier stop–go decisions. This shifts discovery from an exploratory art toward a more disciplined, hypothesis-driven process supported by data.

Importantly, AI-enabled discovery requires integration with downstream considerations. Insights from clinical development, regulatory precedent, and real-world outcomes increasingly inform early research choices. Organizations that treat discovery analytics as an isolated function miss the opportunity to align scientific ambition with translational feasibility.

6.2.2 Transforming clinical development into a learning system

Clinical development represents one of the most resource-intensive and risk-laden phases of the pharmaceutical lifecycle. AI-driven operating models reframe clinical development as a learning system, rather than a sequence of fixed trials.

AI supports this transformation in several ways. Predictive analytics inform protocol design by simulating eligibility criteria against real-world populations, improving feasibility and inclusivity. Natural language processing accelerates patient identification and recruitment by mapping eligibility criteria to structured and unstructured clinical data. Machine learning models forecast enrollment rates, dropout risk, and site performance, enabling proactive intervention.

Beyond operational efficiency, AI enables adaptive trial designs that respond dynamically to emerging data. Interim analyses supported by AI allow modifications to dosing, stratification, or endpoints while preserving scientific integrity. This adaptability is particularly valuable in precision medicine contexts, where patient heterogeneity challenges traditional trial assumptions.

Critically, AI-driven clinical development demands robust governance. Adaptive decisions must be traceable, explainable, and prespecified within regulatory frameworks. Organizations that embed governance into their operating models can leverage AI's flexibility without compromising credibility or compliance.

6.2.3 Intelligent manufacturing and supply chain resilience

Manufacturing and supply chain operations have emerged as strategic priorities for the pharmaceutical industry, particularly in light of recent global disruptions. AI-driven operating models enhance resilience by shifting from reactive management to predictive and prescriptive control.

In manufacturing, AI models analyze process data in real time to detect deviations, predict equipment failures, and optimize yield. Digital twins—virtual representations of production processes—enable scenario testing and continuous optimization without interrupting operations. These capabilities reduce variability, improve quality, and support regulatory compliance through enhanced process understanding.

Across the supply chain, AI integrates demand forecasting, inventory optimization, and logistics planning. Predictive models anticipate shortages, identify bottlenecks, and recommend mitigation strategies before disruptions materialize. Importantly, supply chain intelligence increasingly incorporates external signals, such as epidemiological trends, geopolitical risk, and market dynamics.

From an operating model perspective, AI-enabled manufacturing and supply chains require cross-functional coordination. Quality, operations, regulatory affairs, and IT must align around shared data infrastructures and decision frameworks. Without such alignment, predictive insights remain underutilized.

6.2.4 Artificial intelligence in regulatory strategy and evidence generation

Regulatory engagement has traditionally been treated as a downstream activity—focused on submission preparation and compliance. AI-driven operating models elevate regulatory strategy to a continuous, intelligence-informed function.

AI supports regulatory decision-making by analyzing historical approvals, identifying precedent patterns, and simulating evidence strategies. Machine learning models can assess the likelihood of regulatory success under different trial designs or endpoint selections, informing early development choices.

Moreover, AI enhances evidence generation through the integration of RWE, synthetic controls, and post-market surveillance. These capabilities support more dynamic regulatory dialogues, particularly in contexts where traditional randomized trials are impractical.

However, regulatory acceptance of AI-generated evidence depends on transparency and explainability. Operating models must therefore ensure that analytics outputs are interpretable, auditable, and aligned with evolving regulatory guidance. Regulatory intelligence becomes a strategic capability rather than a compliance afterthought.

6.2.5 Commercialization and market intelligence in the artificial intelligence era

Commercial success in pharmaceuticals increasingly depends on the ability to understand complex stakeholder ecosystems, including patients, providers, payers, and regulators. AI-driven operating models enhance commercialization by enabling granular market intelligence and personalized engagement strategies.

Predictive analytics support launch planning, pricing strategy, and demand forecasting. Natural language processing extracts insights from scientific literature, policy documents, and stakeholder communications. AI-enabled segmentation allows organizations to tailor value propositions to specific patient populations and healthcare contexts.

Crucially, commercialization intelligence feeds back into upstream functions. Market response data informs lifecycle management decisions, label expansion strategies, and future R&D priorities. In intelligent operating models, commercialization is not the end of the value chain but a source of continuous learning.

6.2.6 Integrating the value chain: from functional silos to enterprise intelligence

The defining characteristic of an AI-driven pharmaceutical operating model is **integration**. While individual AI applications can optimize local performance, transformative impact emerges only when insights flow across functions and inform enterprise-level decisions.

Integration requires shared data architectures, interoperable platforms, and aligned governance. It also requires cultural change: incentives must reward collaboration and learning rather than siloed optimization. Leadership plays a critical role in articulating a unifying vision and ensuring that AI investments align with strategic priorities.

In integrated operating models, the pharmaceutical enterprise functions as an adaptive intelligence system. Decisions are informed by data, guided by strategy, and refined through continuous feedback. AI becomes a connective capability that links discovery, development, manufacturing, regulation, and commercialization into a coherent whole.

The "Enterprise Intelligence Loop": How AI Connects the Pharma Value Chain

Traditional pharma operates as a linear chain (discovery → development → approval → manufacturing → commercialization). AI enables a different architecture: an enterprise intelligence loop, where every stage continuously informs the others.

What flows inside the loop

Clinical signals → Discovery: biomarkers, heterogeneity patterns, responder profiles inform target selection.

Manufacturing signals → Development: process variability and quality insights inform formulation and scale-up design.

RWE → Clinical strategy: post-market outcomes reshape endpoints, inclusion criteria, and trial design.

Regulatory interactions → Evidence planning: precedent analytics guide submission strategy and evidence generation choices.

Market response → Portfolio decisions: payer, provider, and patient signals influence lifecycle management and next indications.

What breaks the loop

Siloed data ownership and incompatible standards

AI deployed without shared governance and decision rights

Local optimization incentives that override enterprise goals

Missing interoperability across R&D, quality, regulatory, and commercial systems

Executive takeaway AI's strategic value in pharma is not a better model; it is a better enterprise—one that learns continuously across the lifecycle.

6.2.7 State of the art: AI-driven digital transformation and operating models in pharma

Across the last five years, the state of the art has shifted decisively from asking whether AI can improve isolated pharmaceutical functions to examining how AI restructures operating models, governance, and value creation across the end-to-end pharmaceutical enterprise. Contemporary research converges on one central conclusion: AI's impact is maximized when it is treated as a strategic capability embedded in cross-functional decision systems, rather than as a collection of tools deployed in functional silos (Harrer et al., 2024; Henstock, 2019; Kulkov, 2021).

6.2.8 From digitalization to enterprise transformation

A major strand of the literature emphasizes that "digital transformation" in pharma increasingly means enterprise-scale capability building: internal AI teams, data platforms, partnerships, and acquisitions that expand the organization's data and AI footprint and enable new business models in digital health (Harrer et al., 2024). This transformation extends beyond R&D—spanning clinical development, manufacturing, distribution, and marketing—because the strategic value of AI emerges when insights travel across the lifecycle and reshape decisions systemically (Debnath et al., 2025; Harrer et al., 2024).

This enterprise view is reinforced by work focusing on how organizations actually lead transformation rather than simply deploy technology. A practical example is the articulation of a digital transformation roadmap in global drug development, grounded in data science to generate operational intelligence and actionable insights (Finelli & Narasimhan, 2020). Complementary perspectives argue that AI transformation requires internal investment in data management and AI talent, supported by robust data governance to unlock value from diverse datasets typical of large pharma (Henstock, 2019). Together, this stream aligns directly with your chapter's argument that strategy and governance—not algorithms alone—determine transformation outcomes.

6.2.9 Adoption barriers and operating-model constraints

A second strand focuses on why AI adoption remains uneven and what delays implementation. Empirical work on pharmaceutical manufacturing organizations identifies high ROI areas for AI adoption (operations efficiency, product quality, supply chain integrity, market penetration, and engineering/maintenance) while highlighting delay factors including lack of strategy, talent scarcity, functional silos, insufficient management commitment, and behavioral change barriers (Pazhayattil & Konyu-Fogel, 2023). These findings reinforce the chapter's logic that operating models, incentives, and leadership commitment are structural determinants of scaling.

Related work addresses how organizations structure AI programs and teams, noting a shift toward hybrid organizational models balancing central standardization with application-specific knowledge (Henstock, 2021). This is consistent with the view that scaling AI requires an operating model that manages shared assets (data, platforms, governance) while enabling domain specificity in regulated functions such as quality, clinical, and regulatory affairs.

At the level of business transformation, qualitative evidence suggests that AI affects processes differently depending on organizational size and maturity. Smaller companies may focus on transforming R&D and master data/reporting functions, while larger companies emphasize production, sales, marketing, and analytics-led transformations (Kulkov, 2021). This reinforces the need for contextual operating-model design rather than one-size-fits-all AI strategies.

6.2.10 Pharma 4.0, Industry 4.0, and intelligent manufacturing

Manufacturing transformation appears as one of the most mature "at-scale" domains for AI applications. A prominent Industry 4.0 view argues that IoT, AI, and robotics challenge traditional manufacturing models and enable visions of full digitization and autonomy—leading to end-to-end automation and demand-driven operations (Arden et al., 2021). This perspective is complemented by work on biopharmaceutical manufacturing, highlighting "Bioprocessing 4.0" and pragmatic guidance for digital transformation strategies and operating models, including the evolution of Quality by Design under Industry 4.0 through digital twins and Process Analytical Technology expansions (Isoko et al., 2024).

Recent discussions specifically emphasize AI's contribution to manufacturing efficiency, product quality, and safety, enabled by real-time data, automation, and analytics that support process improvements and reduced waste (Rajesh & Elumalai, 2025). From an operations perspective, reviews further link AI deployment to inventory optimization, predictive maintenance, productivity improvement, and compliance support—again suggesting that AI's manufacturing value is inseparable from operating-model readiness and process integration (Mottaghi-Dastjerdi et al., 2024; Saini et al., 2025).

6.2.11 Digital transformation across R&D, clinical development, and regulatory affairs

Several sources frame AI as a driver compressing drug development cycles through predictive modeling and pipeline-wide integration, spanning virtual screening, target identification, and downstream monitoring and pharmacovigilance (Debnath et al., 2025; Kandhare et al., 2025). Digital transformation in pharma and biotech is also positioned as a convergence of AI/ML with IoT, blockchain, and cloud computing to improve speed, accuracy, and efficiency across drug research, clinical trials, and manufacturing (Subha et al., 2024).

Regulatory affairs and drug development governance emerge as another critical domain. Work on drug development and regulatory affairs highlights favored AI technologies (machine learning, deep learning, natural language processing, robotic process automation) and emphasizes the informational impact of AI tools for decision-making across the lifecycle (Nene et al., 2024). This aligns strongly with your chapter's emphasis on decision rights, explainability, and lifecycle accountability: if AI reshapes evidence and regulatory interactions, it must be governable and auditable as part of the operating model—not treated as an "analytics add-on."

6.2.12 Commercial operations, patient engagement, and digital health expansion

The state of the art also shows a shift from internal optimization to stakeholder-centered digital models. AI is increasingly linked to digital health use cases such as diagnostics, prognostics, personalized treatment, prevention, digital therapeutics, digital diagnostics, telehealth, and patient monitoring (Harrer et al., 2024). In commercial operations, AI is discussed as a driver of next-best-action optimization, behavioral analytics, forecasting, and dynamic pricing, with attention to measurable performance outcomes like time-to-therapy reduction, sales productivity, customer satisfaction, and patient retention (Sabapathy, 2025).

At the broader "pharmacy ecosystem" level, recent discussions outline AI's role across drug safety, quality control, inventory management, and patient counseling, while also acknowledging constraints around privacy, ethics, and regulation (Khan et al., 2023). This strengthens the chapter's argument that pharma transformation must be human-centered and governance-led because commercialization and patient engagement amplify trust and accountability requirements.

6.2.13 The strategic synthesis: operating models, investment, and governance as the differentiator

Taken together, the literature supports a synthesis consistent with your chapter's core thesis: AI is a transformation force across discovery, development, manufacturing, regulatory strategy, and commercialization—but the differentiator is not technical capability alone. Transformation depends on (a) internal investment and talent, (b) strong data governance, (c) operating models that integrate intelligence across functions, and (d) leadership mechanisms that align AI with strategic objectives (Finelli & Narasimhan, 2020; Henstock, 2019; Pazhayattil & Konyu-Fogel, 2023).

Finally, several works explicitly position AI as foundational to new operating paradigms, where predictive analytics and real-time decision systems reshape supply chains, production, and program management—especially when integrated with cloud infrastructure and cybersecurity as enabling conditions (Arden et al., 2021; Stephen, 2025). The state of the art, therefore, reinforces that "AI-driven pharma" is best understood as an enterprise intelligence system: a combination of technology, governance, and organizational design that institutionalizes learning loops across the value chain.

6.3 AI-enabled evidence generation and the transformation of clinical research

Clinical research and evidence generation are undergoing a structural shift driven by AI. This shift is not simply methodological; it redefines how evidence is conceptualized, produced, validated, and translated into clinical and regulatory decisions. AI enables a transition from episodic, trial-centric evidence toward continuous, data-driven, and adaptive evidence ecosystems that better reflect real-world complexity.

Traditional randomized controlled trials (RCTs) remain foundational to clinical science, yet they face increasing pressure. Rising costs, slow timelines, limited population diversity, and challenges in rare diseases and precision medicine expose structural constraints. AI does not replace RCTs; instead, it extends the evidentiary toolkit, allowing clinical research to operate across a broader spectrum of data sources, analytical methods, and temporal horizons.

6.3.1 Reimagining the clinical trial lifecycle with artificial intelligence

AI reshapes the clinical trial lifecycle by embedding intelligence at every decision point. From protocol design to post-trial monitoring, AI transforms trials from static experiments into learning systems.

During protocol development, machine learning models simulate eligibility criteria against real-world patient populations, improving feasibility and inclusivity. Natural language processing enables automated interpretation of complex inclusion and exclusion criteria, aligning them with structured and unstructured clinical data. These capabilities reduce protocol amendments, accelerate startup, and enhance representativeness.

During execution, AI supports dynamic monitoring through predictive analytics. Models anticipate enrollment bottlenecks, dropout risk, and site performance variability, allowing proactive intervention. Safety monitoring evolves from periodic review to continuous signal detection, particularly in decentralized and hybrid trials where data volume and velocity exceed traditional oversight capacity.

Critically, AI-enhanced trials remain governed by scientific rigor. Adaptive decisions must be prespecified, auditable, and aligned with regulatory expectations. When embedded responsibly, AI strengthens—not weakens—the integrity of clinical research.

6.3.2 Real-world evidence as a core evidence pillar

One of the most significant contributions of AI to clinical research is the elevation of RWE from a supplementary input to a core evidentiary pillar. Electronic health records, registries, claims databases, wearable devices, and patient-reported outcomes generate continuous streams of real-world data that reflect routine clinical practice.

AI enables the extraction, harmonization, and analysis of these heterogeneous data sources at scale. Machine learning models identify treatment effects, safety signals, and outcome patterns that may not emerge in controlled trial environments. Natural language processing unlocks insights from unstructured clinical notes, imaging reports, and pathology narratives, expanding the evidentiary surface.

For regulators and payers, AI-enhanced RWE supports post-marketing surveillance, comparative effectiveness research, and long-term outcome assessment. However, its credibility depends on transparent methodologies, bias mitigation, and robust validation. AI-driven RWE must be governed by the same evidentiary discipline as traditional trials to ensure trust and regulatory acceptance.

6.3.3 Synthetic control arms and external comparators

AI has enabled the practical implementation of synthetic control arms—one of the most disruptive innovations in evidence generation. Synthetic controls leverage historical trial data and real-world cohorts to construct comparator groups when randomization is infeasible or ethically problematic.

Using causal inference methods and advanced matching algorithms, AI identifies patients with similar clinical, demographic, and molecular profiles to trial participants. These external comparators reduce reliance on placebo arms, accelerate recruitment, and minimize patient exposure to ineffective treatments—particularly valuable in rare diseases and oncology.

Yet synthetic evidence raises important methodological and ethical questions. Transparency in cohort construction, sensitivity to hidden confounders, and reproducibility across datasets are essential. Regulators increasingly scrutinize not only outcomes, but also how comparability was achieved. Explainability and documentation are, therefore, prerequisites for acceptance.

6.3.4 Digital biomarkers and continuous outcome measurement

AI also expands the definition of clinical endpoints through digital biomarkers derived from continuous data streams. Wearable devices, mobile applications, and connected sensors generate granular physiological and behavioral data that capture disease dynamics beyond episodic clinic visits.

Machine learning algorithms translate raw signals—such as movement patterns, speech characteristics, heart rate variability, or sleep metrics—into clinically meaningful indicators. These digital endpoints enable earlier detection of deterioration, more sensitive measurement of treatment response, and reduced patient burden.

Digital biomarkers are particularly impactful in neurological, cardiovascular, and mental health research, where disease trajectories are dynamic and context-dependent. However, their adoption requires validation, standardization, and regulatory qualification. AI-driven endpoints must demonstrate reliability, clinical relevance, and interpretability to gain acceptance.

6.3.5 Adaptive and pragmatic trial designs

AI enables more flexible and responsive trial designs that align with real-world clinical complexity. Adaptive trials adjust key parameters—such as randomization ratios, dosing strategies, or eligibility criteria—based on interim data. While adaptive designs are not new, AI enhances their precision and scalability.

Pragmatic trials, conducted in routine care settings, benefit from AI's ability to manage heterogeneity and confounding. Machine learning supports patient stratification, outcome adjustment, and real-time analytics without compromising methodological rigor.

These designs shift clinical research toward patient-centricity and efficiency, but they also increase governance demands. Adaptive decisions must be transparent, traceable, and ethically justified. AI-driven flexibility must be balanced with accountability.

6.3.6 Implications for the future of clinical evidence

AI-enabled evidence generation represents a fundamental evolution in clinical research. Evidence is no longer confined to isolated trials but emerges from interconnected data ecosystems spanning development, deployment, and post-market monitoring.

This evolution challenges traditional hierarchies of evidence and demands new evaluation frameworks. Regulators, clinicians, and researchers must collaborate to define standards for AI-generated evidence that preserve scientific rigor while embracing innovation.

Ultimately, AI's value lies not in replacing established methodologies but in augmenting human judgment, accelerating learning, and improving alignment between research findings and patient outcomes. When governed responsibly, AI transforms clinical research into a continuously learning system capable of supporting safer, faster, and more equitable healthcare innovation.

6.4 Governance, ethics, and regulatory readiness in AI-driven clinical research

As AI becomes embedded across the clinical research lifecycle, the question is no longer whether AI can generate value, but whether it can do so responsibly, transparently, and at scale. Governance, ethics, and regulatory readiness are therefore not peripheral considerations; they are structural prerequisites for sustainable adoption. In high-stakes environments such as clinical research, where evidence informs regulatory approval, clinical guidelines, and patient care, failures of governance directly translate into risks to safety, trust, and legitimacy.

AI challenges existing oversight models because it introduces systems that are probabilistic, adaptive, and often opaque. Unlike traditional statistical analyses, AI models may evolve over time, learn from new data streams, and produce outputs that are difficult to interpret without specialized tools. This reality requires a shift from static compliance frameworks toward lifecycle-based governance architectures that treat AI as a regulated clinical asset rather than a one-off analytical method.

6.4.1 The governance gap in AI-enabled clinical research

Clinical research governance has historically relied on well-defined structures such as ethics committees, protocol review boards, good clinical practice standards, and regulatory inspections. These mechanisms were designed for deterministic study designs and relatively stable analytical approaches. AI disrupts this equilibrium.

The core governance gap emerges from three characteristics of AI systems:
Adaptivity—Models may change behavior as data distributions shift.
Opacity—Advanced models may not provide intuitive explanations for outputs.
Scale and automation—Decisions can be generated rapidly and at volume, amplifying the impact of errors or bias.

Without explicit governance frameworks, AI risks being deployed in ways that blur accountability, obscure decision logic, and weaken evidentiary traceability. In clinical research, such ambiguity is unacceptable. Governance must therefore define who is responsible, when oversight applies, and how decisions are documented across the AI lifecycle.

6.4.2 Explainability and accountability as ethical imperatives

Among the ethical challenges associated with AI, explainability is the most consequential for clinical research. The so-called "black box" problem undermines trust at multiple levels: clinicians may hesitate to rely on recommendations they cannot interpret, patients may question consent validity, and regulators may reject evidence that lacks transparency.

Explainable artificial intelligence provides mechanisms to address this challenge by enabling insight into how models generate predictions or classifications. Feature attribution, counterfactual analysis, uncertainty estimation, and model visualization techniques help translate complex computations into interpretable signals.

However, explainability must be understood as an ethical and governance requirement, not merely a technical enhancement. Explanations must be:
Clinically meaningful, not only mathematically accurate
Context-aware, reflecting patient-specific factors
Actionable, supporting validation, challenge, or override by human experts

Accountability in AI-driven research depends on traceability. It must be possible to reconstruct how a model influenced a decision, what data were used, which assumptions were embedded, and where human judgment intervened. Without such traceability, responsibility becomes diffused—undermining both ethical integrity and legal defensibility.

6.4.3 Regulatory alignment and evidence acceptability

Regulatory agencies increasingly acknowledge the potential of AI to improve clinical research efficiency and evidence generation. However, acceptance is conditional and cautious. Regulators emphasize that AI-generated evidence must meet at least the same standards of validity, reliability, and transparency as traditional approaches.

Key regulatory concerns include:
Reproducibility across populations and settings
Bias and fairness, particularly for underrepresented groups
Data provenance and quality
Model lifecycle management, including updates and drift

Unlike static analytical tools, AI models require continuous oversight. Regulatory readiness, therefore, demands documentation practices that include version control, audit trails, validation reports, and performance monitoring plans. Increasingly, regulators are moving toward lifecycle-based oversight, recognizing that approval is not a single event but an ongoing process.

For sponsors and research organizations, this means that regulatory alignment must be designed into AI systems from inception—not retrofitted after deployment.

6.4.4 Human oversight and responsibility allocation

Despite automation advances, AI does not eliminate the need for human judgment in clinical research; it amplifies its importance. AI systems can surface patterns, predictions, and signals, but responsibility for decisions must remain human-centered.

Effective governance frameworks explicitly define:
When AI outputs may inform decisions
When escalation is required
When human judgment must override algorithmic recommendations

These rules should be embedded in protocols, standard operating procedures, and training programs. Human oversight is not symbolic; it is operational. Clinicians, researchers, and regulators must be empowered to interrogate AI outputs, recognize limitations, and intervene when necessary.

Responsibility allocation must also be clear across interdisciplinary teams. Data scientists, clinical investigators, sponsors, and oversight bodies must share a common understanding of roles and accountability. Governance failures often arise not from technical flaws, but from organizational ambiguity.

6.4.5 Data governance, privacy, and trust

AI-driven clinical research depends on access to large volumes of sensitive health data. This reliance intensifies concerns about privacy, consent, and data stewardship. Traditional consent models—designed for narrowly defined data use—are strained by AI systems that derive value from secondary analysis and longitudinal learning.

Robust data governance frameworks must address:
Data access controls and stewardship roles
Consent management and transparency
Anonymization and deidentification practices
Secure data architectures and interoperability

Privacy-preserving technologies, such as federated learning and secure computation, offer promising pathways by enabling collaborative model development without centralized data aggregation. However, these approaches require strong governance and technical maturity to be effective.

Trust is the ultimate currency of clinical research. Patients must trust that their data are used responsibly, clinicians must trust AI-supported insights, and regulators must trust the evidence presented for approval. Governance frameworks that prioritize transparency and ethical integrity are essential to sustaining this trust.

6.4.6 From compliance to responsible innovation

A narrow compliance-focused approach risks reducing governance to a procedural exercise. In contrast, responsible innovation frames governance as an enabler of sustainable impact. This perspective recognizes that AI systems operate in dynamic environments and that not all risks can be anticipated in advance.

Responsible innovation emphasizes:
Continuous monitoring and learning
Stakeholder engagement across disciplines
Ethical reflection alongside technical development
Adaptive governance rather than static rules

Responsible AI in Pharma: The Non-Negotiables Checklist (Executive)

Responsible AI is the condition for scale in pharma. If any of the elements below are missing, adoption may occur—but sustainability will fail.

Clinical and scientific integrity: · The model's intended use is clinically meaningful and properly scoped. · Performance is validated against external data and across relevant subgroups. · The system reports uncertainty, limitations, and failure modes.

(cont'd)

Explainability and accountability: · Explanations are understandable to clinical and regulatory stakeholders. · Decision ownership is explicit and documented. · Override and escalation rules exist and are followed.

Data governance and privacy: · Data provenance, consent alignment, and access controls are documented. · Data quality controls exist for completeness, bias risks, and drift. · Privacy-preserving approaches are used when required (e.g., federated learning)

Operational readiness: · Continuous monitoring exists (drift, bias, performance decay). · Version control and audit trails are maintained for models and datasets. · A formal retirement/recalibration policy exists

Executive takeaway: In pharma, "responsible AI" is not an ethics add-on. It is the operating requirement for regulatory acceptance, patient trust, and enterprise scale.

In this model, governance is not a barrier to progress but a foundation for legitimacy, scalability, and societal acceptance. AI-enabled clinical research succeeds not when models are merely accurate, but when they are trusted, accountable, and aligned with human values.

6.5 Future directions: artificial intelligence as the foundation of next-generation clinical evidence

AI is no longer a peripheral innovation within clinical research; it is rapidly becoming the foundational infrastructure upon which next-generation evidence generation is built. As healthcare systems face escalating complexity, accelerating innovation cycles, and growing expectations for transparency and inclusivity, AI-enabled clinical research offers a pathway to reimagine how evidence is generated, evaluated, and sustained over time.

The future of clinical research will not be defined by isolated technological breakthroughs, but by system-level transformation—where AI reshapes the architecture of evidence itself. This transformation spans methodological design, institutional capability, regulatory models, and the very definition of what constitutes credible and actionable clinical evidence.

6.5.1 From episodic trials to continuous evidence generation

Traditional clinical research has been structured around episodic trials: discrete studies with fixed protocols, predefined endpoints, and finite timelines. While this paradigm has produced robust causal evidence, it struggles to keep pace with rapidly evolving therapies, precision medicine, and real-world clinical complexity.

AI enables a transition toward continuous evidence generation, where clinical trials, real-world data, post-market surveillance, and digital health signals are integrated into a unified learning ecosystem. In this model, evidence does not conclude at publication or regulatory approval; it evolves dynamically as new data emerge.

Continuous evidence generation allows research programs to adapt to emerging safety signals, shifting patient populations, and evolving standards of care. AI serves as the analytical backbone that links these data streams, enabling real-time learning while preserving methodological rigor through governance and validation frameworks.

6.5.2 Personalized and context-aware evidence

One of the most profound implications of AI-driven research is the shift from population-average evidence to personalized and context-aware insights. Traditional trials are designed to estimate average treatment effects, often masking clinically meaningful heterogeneity across patient subgroups.

AI-enabled analytics—particularly when integrating genomics, imaging, digital biomarkers, and longitudinal clinical histories—enable evidence to be stratified by individual characteristics, disease trajectories, and contextual factors. This supports precision medicine by answering not only whether an intervention works, but for whom, under what conditions, and at which stage of disease.

However, personalized evidence also challenges existing regulatory and methodological norms. Regulators must determine how to evaluate evidence that varies across subpopulations, while researchers must guard against algorithmic bias and overfitting. The future of personalized evidence will therefore depend on robust validation strategies and fairness-aware governance models.

6.5.3 Synthetic evidence and virtual trial augmentation

AI is also redefining the structure of clinical trials through the generation of synthetic data and virtual control arms. Synthetic evidence—constructed using historical trials, real-world data, and advanced causal inference techniques—offers opportunities to reduce reliance on placebo groups, accelerate recruitment, and improve patient experience.

These approaches are particularly valuable in rare diseases, oncology, and ethically sensitive contexts where traditional randomization may be impractical. AI-enabled virtual trial augmentation can complement physical trials, enabling hybrid designs that balance scientific rigor with feasibility.

At the same time, synthetic evidence raises critical questions about validity, transparency, and reproducibility. Regulatory acceptance will depend on clear documentation of data sources, modeling assumptions, sensitivity analyses, and performance benchmarking against real-world outcomes. As such, synthetic evidence is not a shortcut—but a new evidentiary modality requiring rigorous governance.

6.5.4 Institutional transformation and skills evolution

The integration of AI into clinical research demands profound institutional transformation. Research organizations must move beyond ad hoc AI adoption toward systematic capability building, encompassing data infrastructure, governance frameworks, and interdisciplinary collaboration.

Clinical researchers will increasingly work alongside data scientists, AI ethicists, informaticians, and regulatory specialists. This shift requires new skill sets: not necessarily coding expertise, but AI literacy—the ability to critically interpret model outputs, understand limitations, and participate in governance decisions.

Education and training will therefore be decisive success factors. Institutions that invest in workforce development, cross disciplinary communication, and ethical competence will be best positioned to scale AI responsibly. Leadership commitment is essential: AI transformation is as much a cultural and organizational challenge as it is a technical one.

6.5.5 Regulatory evolution and global harmonization

As AI reshapes evidence generation, regulatory frameworks must evolve accordingly. Regulators are increasingly exploring adaptive approval pathways, integration of RWE, and lifecycle-based oversight models. AI itself can support these efforts by enabling continuous monitoring, automated signal detection, and dynamic risk assessment.

However, regulatory fragmentation across jurisdictions remains a significant barrier. Divergent standards for AI validation, transparency, and governance complicate global trials and slow innovation. International harmonization of AI governance principles—particularly around explainability, bias mitigation, and lifecycle management—will be essential to unlock the full potential of AI-enabled research.

Proactive engagement between sponsors, researchers, and regulators will be critical. AI systems must be designed with regulatory expectations in mind from the outset, rather than retrofitted for compliance after deployment.

6.5.6 A human-centered vision for AI-driven evidence

Despite its transformative power, AI does not replace the human core of clinical research. Instead, it redefines roles and responsibilities. AI excels at handling complexity, scale, and uncertainty—but humans remain responsible for ethical judgment, accountability, and trust.

A human-centered vision positions AI as a decision-support capability rather than a decision-maker. Clinicians, researchers, and regulators retain authority over interpretation, risk-benefit assessment, and final decisions. This balance is essential to preserving professional integrity and public confidence.

The most successful AI-enabled research systems will therefore be those that augment human expertise, rather than attempt to automate it away.

6.5.7 Strategic implications for the next decade

Looking ahead, several strategic imperatives emerge:

Clinical research will shift from isolated studies to integrated evidence ecosystems.

Explainability and governance will become primary determinants of adoption and regulatory acceptance.

Personalized evidence will challenge traditional evaluation models and demand new methodological standards.

Institutional readiness—not algorithmic sophistication alone—will determine success.

Trust, transparency, and accountability will outweigh raw predictive performance as success metrics.

In conclusion, AI is redefining what clinical evidence means, how it is generated, and how it is trusted. Organizations that embrace AI responsibly—integrating technical innovation with ethical governance and human oversight—will shape the future of clinical research. Those who fail to adapt risk marginalization in an increasingly data-driven and accountability-focused healthcare landscape.

6.5.8 Editor's note

This chapter offers a rigorous and forward-looking analysis of how AI is redefining clinical research and evidence generation. Rather than presenting AI as a collection of isolated tools, the authors frame it as a structural capability that reshapes the entire evidence lifecycle—from protocol design and trial execution to RWE generation and regulatory decision-making.

A key strength of the chapter lies in its balanced integration of innovation and governance. While it clearly demonstrates how AI accelerates feasibility assessment, patient recruitment, monitoring, and adaptive analysis, it also foregrounds the ethical, regulatory, and accountability challenges that must be addressed to ensure legitimacy and trust. The emphasis on explainability, human oversight, and lifecycle governance reflects current regulatory expectations and anticipates future policy developments.

Importantly, the chapter advances a human-centered vision of AI-enabled research. It recognizes that predictive accuracy alone is insufficient; sustainable impact depends on institutional readiness, interdisciplinary collaboration, and transparent responsibility allocation. By positioning AI as an augmentation of clinical and scientific judgment—rather than a replacement—the chapter provides a realistic and responsible roadmap for the next generation of evidence-based medicine.

This contribution will be particularly valuable to researchers, clinical leaders, regulators, and policymakers seeking to understand not only what AI can enable in clinical research but also how it must be governed to deliver safe, credible, and socially acceptable evidence.

6.5.9 Key takeaways

AI is transforming clinical research from a linear, episodic process into a continuous, adaptive evidence generation system.

AI enhances efficiency and feasibility across the full clinical research lifecycle, including protocol design, site selection, recruitment, monitoring, and reporting.

RWE, synthetic controls, and digital biomarkers expand the evidentiary toolkit beyond traditional RCTs.

Personalized and context-aware evidence generation supports precision medicine but challenges population-average evaluation models.

Synthetic data and virtual trial augmentation offer major efficiency gains, particularly in rare and high-risk conditions, but require rigorous validation.

Explainable AI is essential for clinical accountability, regulatory acceptance, and sustained trust.

Effective AI adoption depends more on institutional readiness and governance than on algorithmic sophistication alone.

Human oversight remains indispensable; AI augments scientific judgment but does not replace ethical or professional responsibility.

Regulatory evolution toward lifecycle-based oversight will be critical to scaling AI-enabled clinical research globally.

Trust, transparency, and accountability will ultimately determine the success of AI-driven evidence generation.

6.5.10 Mini case study vignette (anonymized)

6.5.10.1 Transforming evidence generation through AI-enabled adaptive research

A multinational clinical research consortium implemented an AI-enabled platform to support oncology trials across academic hospitals and regional care centers. The platform integrated electronic health records, imaging data, genomic profiles, and real-world outcomes to assist with protocol feasibility assessment, patient eligibility screening, adaptive monitoring, and posttrial evidence generation.

During early deployment, the system significantly reduced recruitment timelines and improved early detection of safety signals compared to historical benchmarks. Investigators reported operational efficiencies, particularly in identifying eligible patients and monitoring protocol deviations across sites.

However, regulatory reviewers and clinicians expressed concern about the system's initial lack of transparency. While predictions were accurate, the rationale behind patient risk stratification and response predictions was not sufficiently interpretable, limiting clinician confidence and slowing regulatory review.

In response, the consortium embedded Explainable AI components, including feature attribution dashboards and uncertainty indicators. These enhancements allowed clinicians to trace AI recommendations back to specific clinical variables and enabled regulators to audit decision pathways.

Following these changes, adoption increased, regulatory engagement improved, and the platform transitioned from an automation tool to a trusted decision-support system.

Key insight: In clinical research, predictive performance alone is insufficient. Explainability, governance, and alignment with clinical accountability are decisive for real-world adoption.

6.5.11 Learning activities

Learning activity 1: mapping artificial intelligence across the clinical research lifecycle (lifecycle blueprint)

Purpose and learning value: This activity helps learners build a structured, end-to-end mental model of where AI creates value in clinical research—while recognizing the governance and ethical constraints that determine whether that value is acceptable and scalable.

Recommended format: Individual (preferred for accountability) or small group (2–3 students for richer discussion)

Estimated time: 30–40 minutes (plus 10 minutes optional sharing)

Learning outcomes: By the end of this activity, learners will be able to:
Identify core clinical research lifecycle phases and the decision points within them
Match AI methods (e.g., NLP, predictive models, anomaly detection) to practical research tasks
Articulate benefits and governance constraints for each AI-enabled capability
Explain how lifecycle integration strengthens evidence quality and operational performance

Instructions (step-by-step)

Create a lifecycle map using a single page (diagram, table, or flowchart). Include the following phases:

Protocol design and feasibility assessment
Patient recruitment and eligibility screening
Trial monitoring and safety surveillance
Analysis, reporting, and interpretation
Post-market evidence generation and RWE

For each phase, add three structured elements: A. AI-enabled capability (what AI does here) B. Value contribution (what improves: speed, quality, equity, cost, compliance, safety) C. Governance/ethical constraint (what must be controlled: bias, transparency, consent, data provenance, model drift, accountability)

Add a "handoff link" between phases (one arrow note per transition) describing:
What data or decision output moves forward (e.g., feasibility estimates → protocol refinement)
What risk must be tracked (e.g., eligibility automation → fairness auditing)

Student prompts (to guide high-quality answers)

Where does AI reduce latency (time delay) versus improve validity (trustworthiness of evidence)?

Which phase is most sensitive to bias, and why?

Where is explainability non-negotiable, and who requires it (patients, regulators, clinicians, sponsors)?

What would "failure" look like at each phase, and how would AI governance detect it early?

Deliverable: A one-page lifecycle blueprint (diagram/table) with concise explanatory notes (2–3 sentences per phase).

Light assessment criteria (instructor rubric)

Completeness (all phases addressed)

Specificity (capabilities are realistic and properly matched to the phase)

Balance (benefits and risks are addressed)

Integration (handoff links show lifecycle thinking, not isolated use cases)

Learning activity 2: designing a responsible artificial intelligence evidence framework (governance-by-design workshop)

Purpose and learning value: This team-based activity moves learners from "AI use cases" to governance-by-design—building an implementable framework that would satisfy both scientific rigor and regulatory expectations.

Recommended format: Team-based (3–5 students). Assign roles for realism:
Clinical investigator
Data science lead
Regulatory/QA lead
Ethics/privacy lead
Program manager (optional)

Estimated time: 45–60 minutes (plus 10 minutes optional peer critique)

Learning outcomes: Learners will be able to:
Translate clinical research objectives into AI-enabled evidence workflows
Define validation, explainability, and monitoring requirements aligned with accountability
Specify human oversight and decision-rights allocation
Propose lifecycle monitoring and change control mechanisms (versioning, drift, escalation)

Scenario options (choose one): Select one context to anchor the framework:
Rare disease trial (small sample, high ethical constraints)
Decentralized trial (high data variability from devices and remote monitoring)
Oncology precision trial (complex heterogeneity, high-stakes endpoints)
Post-market surveillance (continuous monitoring, signal detection, regulatory reporting)

Framework design instructions (what teams must produce): Your framework must address the following components:

Evidence goal and decision context

What decision will the evidence support (approval, label expansion, safety signal, guideline change)?

What constitutes "acceptable evidence" for this decision?

Data strategy and provenance

Data sources (EHR, trial data, wearables, claims, registries)

Data quality controls and documentation of provenance

Consent, privacy, and access governance rules

Model strategy and validation plan

Model type and purpose (prediction, eligibility matching, anomaly detection, causal comparator)

Validation approach (internal, external, prospective, where possible)

Performance metrics and subgroup fairness checks

Explainability mechanisms (what users must understand and why)

Human oversight and decision rights

What decisions are AI-supported versus human-controlled

Escalation rules (when AI flags risk, who reviews, what action follows)

Accountability mapping (who owns outcomes)

Lifecycle monitoring and change control

Monitoring (drift, calibration decay, bias emergence, data shifts)

Version control and auditability

Model updates and revalidation triggers

Documentation practices for regulatory readiness

Student prompts (to move beyond superficial frameworks)

If your model's performance drops in one patient subgroup, what happens next (who is notified, what is paused, what is revalidated)?

What does "explainability" mean for your selected stakeholder—clinician versus regulator versus patient?

Which part of the workflow is your highest-risk point, and what control reduces that risk?

Deliverable A 1–2 page Responsible AI Evidence Framework (structured outline with short paragraphs and a simple diagram if desired).

Light assessment criteria (instructor rubric)

Coherence (framework reads like a real operating model)
Governance completeness (oversight + monitoring + auditability)
Practicality (implementable decisions and controls)
Regulatory realism (evidence acceptability and traceability are addressed)

Learning activity 3: executive reflection exercise (trust, trade-offs, and regulatory reality)

Purpose and learning value: This activity strengthens executive reasoning: learners must take a defensible position on the trade-off between model complexity and accountability—mirroring real regulatory and governance debates.

Recommended format: Individual

Estimated time: 15–20 minutes

Learning outcomes: Learners will be able to:

Formulate a reasoned position on governance versus performance trade-offs

Use stakeholder-based logic (patient safety, regulatory acceptance, operational feasibility)

Identify conditions under which complex AI is acceptable and when it is not

Reflection prompt (expanded and student-friendly): Regulators and healthcare leaders often face a dilemma:

Highly complex AI models may be more accurate, but harder to explain and audit.

More interpretable models may be easier to govern, but less powerful.

Question: Should regulatory approval prioritize explainability and governance even if it limits the use of highly complex AI models? Take a position and justify it.

Required structure (students must follow) Write 200–250 words with the following structure:

Your position (1–2 sentences): Yes / No / Conditional (recommended)

Your reasoning (3–5 sentences): include at least two stakeholder perspectives

Your conditions (2–3 sentences): what safeguards would change your answer? Examples: subgroup fairness testing, audit trails, monitoring, human override, prospective validation

Optional extension (for advanced cohorts): Add one sentence proposing a "compromise policy," such as:

complexity allowed only with stronger lifecycle monitoring and independent auditing

tiered approval where explainability standards vary by risk level and intended use

Deliverable: A 200–250 word reflective memo written in a professional tone.

Light assessment criteria

Clarity of stance

Strength of justification (not opinion-based; uses governance logic)

Stakeholder awareness

Practical safeguards and realism

References

Arden, N. S., Fisher, A. C., Tyner, K., Yu, L. X., & Lee, S. L. (2021). Industry 4.0 for pharmaceutical manufacturing: Preparing for the smart factories of the future. *International Journal of Pharmaceutics*.

Debnath, B., Wilson, S. K., & Basu, S. (2025). The pharmaceutical industry's future: How artificial intelligence is transforming medicine. *Advanced Pharmaceutical Bulletin*. https://pmc.ncbi.nlm.nih.gov.

Finelli, L. A., & Narasimhan, V. (2020). Leading a digital transformation in the pharmaceutical industry: Reimagining the way we work in global drug development. *Clinical Pharmacology & Therapeutics*.

Harrer, S., Menard, J., Rivers, M., & Green, D. V. S. (2024). Artificial intelligence drives the digital transformation of pharma. *Artificial Intelligence in Clinical Practice*.

Henstock, P. V. (2019). Artificial intelligence for pharma: Time for internal investment. In *Trends in pharmacological sciences*. Elsevier.

Henstock, P. (2021). Artificial intelligence in pharma: Positive trends but more investment needed to drive a transformation. *Archives of Pharmacology and Therapeutics*.

Isoko, K., Cordiner, J. L., Kis, Z., & Moghadam, P. Z. (2024). Bioprocessing 4.0: A pragmatic review and future perspectives. *Digital Discovery*. https://pubs.rsc.org.

Kandhare, P., Kurlekar, M., Deshpande, T., et al. (2025). Artificial intelligence in pharmaceutical sciences: A comprehensive review. *Medicine in Novel*.

Khan, O., Parvez, M., Kumari, P., Parvez, S., & Ahmad, S. (2023). The future of pharmacy: How AI is revolutionizing the industry. *Intelligent Pharmacy*.

Kulkov, I. (2021). The role of artificial intelligence in business transformation: A case of pharmaceutical companies. *Technology in Society*.

Mottaghi-Dastjerdi, N., et al. (2024). Advancements and applications of artificial intelligence in pharmaceutical sciences: A comprehensive review. *Iranian Journal of Pharmaceutical Research*. https://pmc.ncbi.nlm.nih.gov.

Nene, L., Flepisi, B. T., Brand, S. J., Basson, C., & Balmith, M. (2024). Evolution of drug development and regulatory affairs: The demonstrated power of artificial intelligence. *Clinical Therapeutics*.

Pazhayattil, A. B., & Konyu-Fogel, G. (2023). An empirical study to accelerate machine learning and artificial intelligence adoption in pharmaceutical manufacturing organizations. *Journal of Generic*. https://journals.sagepub.com.

Rajesh, M. V., & Elumalai, K. (2025). The transformative power of artificial intelligence in pharmaceutical manufacturing: Enhancing efficiency, product quality, and safety. *Journal of Holistic Integrative Pharmacy*.

Sabapathy, G. (2025). Artificial intelligence in pharmaceutical commercial operations: Transforming sales performance and patient engagement in the digital era. *Journal of Computer Science and Technology*. https://al-kindipublishers.org.

Saini, J. P. S., Thakur, A., & Yadav, D. (2025). AI driven Innovations in pharmaceuticals: Optimizing drug discovery and industry operations. *RSC Pharmaceutics*. https://pubs.rsc.org.

Stephen, G. (2025). The future of pharma program management: Integrating AI, cybersecurity, and cloud solutions. *International Journal of AI, BigData, Computational and Management Studies*. https://ijaibdcms.org.

Subha, S., Shanmugathai, M., Prasanth, A., et al. (2024). Digital Transformation in the pharmaceutical and biotech industry: Challenges and research directions. In *Digital twins in industrial production and smart manufacturing: An understanding of principles, enhancers, and obstacles*. Wiley Online Library.

CHAPTER 7

Generic drugs and biosimilars: opportunities for access and affordability

Abdullah Saeed
Ministry of Health, Abha, Asir, Saudi Arabia

7.1 Introduction

As healthcare costs continue to soar, access to pharmaceutical treatments has become a growing concern for patients and healthcare providers alike. This is especially true regarding access to expensive biologics, which have been developed to treat complex diseases such as cancer and rheumatoid arthritis. Unfortunately, although the recent introduction of biosimilars has led to the patent expiration of several innovative biologics, patients still face challenges. Similarly, access to medications is complicated by a plethora of generic drugs, with some countries and patients having difficulty finding the correct formulation. Generic drugs are copies of original pharmaceutical compounds that have lost market exclusivity due to patent expiration. This comprehensive analysis aims to discuss the impact of generics and biosimilars on access and affordability within the pharmaceutical industry. Particular emphasis will be placed on the challenges these two categories of drugs pose for patients and healthcare providers in obtaining the necessary medication (Rahman Kabir et al., 2019).

For generics, the focus will be on oral solid dosage forms, the most widely used drug delivery system worldwide; for biosimilars, the focus will be on injectable drugs. Both categories of drugs are crucial components of modern healthcare systems, and patients are often dependent on them. However, recently, so-called "drug shortages" have arisen regarding both generics and biosimilars. New pharmaceutical discoveries are crucial for treating complex diseases, but considering the developing landscape regarding generics and biosimilars, it is imperative to evaluate pharmaceuticals currently on the market with respect to access and affordability. Therefore this comprehensive analysis will address the questions concerning what generics and biosimilars are and how they impact access and affordability. What are the unique challenges associated with these medications? What must be considered regarding the future evolution of the pharmaceutical landscape? As artificial intelligence (AI) continues to permeate industry and research, special attention will be paid to this new frontier regarding generics and biosimilars (Shaikh et al.2025).

The Future of Pharma Across All Sectors in the Artificial Intelligence Era. DOI: https://doi.org/10.1016/B978-0-443-40572-3.00001-0

7.1.1 Background and significance of generic drugs and biosimilars

In the complex landscape of the pharmaceutical industry, generic drugs and biosimilars have emerged as pivotal players, shaping the rules of the game and challenging the incumbents. The historical backdrop of generics and biosimilars paints a vivid picture of triumph over adversity. From the early days of crude medicines and patent controversies to the establishment of the Drug Price Competition and Patent Term Restoration Act in 1984, generics carved a niche for themselves. The allure of generics lies in their potential to address the critical question of patient access to life-saving medicines. In an ideal world, every patient would have access to the medications deemed vital by the World Health Organization (WHO). However, the reality is starkly different. Millions of lives remain at risk due to the prohibitive costs of essential treatments. Statistically, generics and biosimilars hold the key to financial salvation, despite the naysayers who predict doom and gloom for the pharmaceutical industry (Rahman Kabir et al., 2019). In the United States alone, the average wholesale price of a drug is approximately 276% higher than the manufacturer's list price. This discrepancy speaks volumes about the impact of pharmacy benefit managers and the need for public awareness regarding generic options. There is a compelling case for generics and biosimilars, backed by statistical arguments that could fill volumes. However, the critical focus should remain on the rules and nuances shaping the current landscape. Quid pro quo arrangements, kickbacks, and legal loopholes undermine the efficacy of the Drug Enforcement Administration and the Health Insurance Portability and Accountability Act in safeguarding patient health secrets. At the heart of the issue lie patents and exclusivity periods, which can either break or shape an empire (Lynch, 2017). The overarching desire to "reduce healthcare expenditures" without compromising the efficacy of medications is an uphill battle. Every minutia and corner needs to be meticulously examined to "identify the most critical therapeutic areas" that are either "currently underserved" or "flourishing." With nearly 10 million lives at stake, it is prudent to explore the overlooked therapeutic avenues on the verge of obsolescence. A meticulous examination of the rules of the game governing the market is essential. The objective is to provide a concise account illuminated by personal experiences, particularly during PhD doctoral degree endeavors that regrettably remained unpublished. Based on publicly accessible information, every effort will be made to present a clear depiction of the current scenario as simply as possible.

7.1.2 Scope and objectives of the study

The scope of this study is to conduct a thorough analysis of the impact of generic drugs and biosimilars on access and affordability within the pharmaceutical industry. In accomplishing this task, the scope delineates the specific parameters and focus areas involved in carrying out the study. As a result, the contribution this analysis is intended to make is clearly articulated. Although prior research has looked at various aspects of this issue, comprehensive studies highlighting the overall impact of generics and biosimilars are limited. Therefore, to fill this gap, the objectives of this analysis are to provide a comprehensive understanding of the impact of generic drugs and biosimilars in terms of access and affordability. More specifically, the key targets are to assess the contribution of generics and biosimilars in terms of cost reduction and improved access in healthcare systems, as well as to explore key factors shaping the impact of generics and biosimilars (Wouters et al., 2017).

This study utilizes a qualitative methodology, with a systematic literature review as the main approach in conducting the analysis. A review of peer-reviewed research articles published over the last ten years is conducted to gather relevant data and insights on the impact of generics and biosimilars. This impact is examined from three different angles: the overall assessment of the impact of generics and biosimilars, the analysis of the pharmaceutical market as a determining factor for the impact of generics and biosimilars, and the examination of policy and regulatory frameworks as shaping factors for the impact of generics and biosimilars. By defining the boundaries of the study, it is clarified what will be covered and what will be excluded. In this sense, the focus is limited to an analysis of the impact of generics and biosimilars on access and affordability in developed countries. Therefore, although still highly relevant, the discussion on the impact of generics and biosimilars in low- and middle-income countries is not included (Lynch, 2017). On the one hand, this is justified by the recognition that the developing world has been severely underrepresented in terms of research output. On the other hand, this limitation acknowledges that the pharmaceutical industry has a responsibility toward all countries.

7.2 Understanding generic drugs and biosimilars

7.2.1 What are generic drugs and biosimilars?

Despite rapidly advancing technologies and staggering economic growth, good health remains a luxury for many people around the globe. Access to affordable medicines is a fundamental tenet of global health, but the pharmaceutical industry functions like a market plagued by excessive monopolistic tendencies. Patent protections grant brand-name drugs monopoly rights for a minimum of 20 years postinvention, granting sole control over the drug's market price, which is often exorbitant and beyond the reach of most patients in developing countries—if they can access the drug at all. In response to this ethical dilemma, the World Trade Organization's Trade-Related Aspects of Intellectual Property Rights (TRIPS) agreement permitted the production and sale of cheaper, copycat alternatives to brand-name drugs—termed generics—by nations with inadequate patent protections. This provision removed the foundations of the original drug's monopoly, allowing free-market competition to drive down prices and expand patient access. The compromises outlined in the TRIPS agreement have far-reaching implications for public health in the developing world. Yet questions remain: By simply dismantling monopolies, are improved health outcomes assured? Can generics be completely trusted, as they are mere replicas of life-saving treatments? With rapid biopharmaceutical innovations, what is the future of access to affordable medicines? (Health Organization, 2022)

Similar to small-molecule chemical drugs, biologics (or biopharmaceuticals) are products prescribed for the treatment of medical conditions. Whereas chemical drugs are synthesized through elaborate chemical processes that yield predictable architectures, biologics are composed of complex macromolecules—most commonly proteins—that are biologically engineered in living cells. Biologics tend to be larger in size, costlier to develop and manufacture, and generally target high-unmet-need disease indications. Biologics accrue the same patent protections as chemical drugs, thus granting brand biologics monopoly rights. However, upon expiry of the brand drug's patent, a new class of drugs—biosimilars—enter the market. The anticipated arrival of biosimilars, analogous to generics in the chemical drug market, prompted nations to establish a regulatory framework to ensure the safety and efficacy of biosimilars in comparison to their brand biologics. Such regulations are often unique to the individual healthcare systems and political economies of nations, outlining differences in biosimilar development and market-entry scenarios across continents. Drug regulation is designed to protect patients from unsafe and ineffective treatments while encouraging pharmaceutical innovation. However, drug regulation is inherently paradoxical. Pharmaceuticals are not innocuous substances. But poor health outcomes impose direct economic losses, particularly on developing nations, fostering a gradual race toward increasingly stringent drug approvals and market-entry barriers. These drug approvals are wrought with complexity, ambiguity, and a shifting landscape, especially in the age of rapidly advancing technologies. This complexity can give rise to unintended consequences: unimaginable human catastrophes, as epitomized in the thalidomide tragedy; or calculated risks that benefit the wealthy few while neglecting the impoverished many (Singh, 2023). Biologics are a relatively new class of biopharmaceuticals, having been introduced to the market in the early 1980s. The first brand biologic—Recombinant DNA Human Insulin—was approved by the US Food and Drug Administration in 1982 and subsequently by the European Medicines Agency in 1986. Brand biologics triggered a paradigm shift in the pharmaceutical industry by targeting complex disease mechanisms that inspired blockbuster biologics—good-for-all drugs promising $1 billion annual sales. Ripple effects burgeoned biosimilars, or generic biologics. The first biosimilar to be approved by the European Medicines Agency was Omnitrope, a growth hormone, in 2006. The FDA approved its first biosimilar—Zarxio (filgrastim)—in 2015. Subsequently, 43 biosimilars have been approved in the US and 58 in the EU as of March 2023 (Eleryan et al., 2016). Commercial concerns do exist vis-à-vis competitive markets; however, empirical evidence suggests that biosimilars incentivize healthcare providers to switch patients from brand biologics to biosimilars, resulting in substantially lower treatment expenditures. Consider the oncology care therapy class comprising Avastin (bevacizumab), a brand biologic. With the market entry of biosimilar bevacizumab (Mvasi) in 2017, Medicare expenditures declined by $975 million. Nonetheless, patient-switching concerns abound despite seemingly identical chemistries. Biosimilars are biopharmaceuticals too, meaning they are similar but not identical to their brand biologics, developed through deliberate design, planning, and conduct. These differences are clinically noninferior when it comes to drugs' safety and efficacy.

7.2.2 Definition and key differences

In the current discourse regarding access to affordable medicines, the terms "generic drugs" and "biosimilars" are cited frequently, yet they remain poorly understood. Precise definitions of these terms are essential for framing the discussion of their importance. Generic drugs are pharmaceutical products that are bioequivalent to their branded counterparts and are marketed under their chemical names without any brand name. In contrast, biosimilars are pharmaceutical products that are highly similar to, but not identical to, their respective innovator biologics. There are key differences between the two classes of drugs, which stem from differences between small-molecule chemically synthesized drugs and large-molecule biologics (Eleryan et al., 2016). These differences are fundamental to understanding the differences in regulatory approvals of generic drugs and biosimilars.

The differences between generic drugs and biosimilars also have implications for healthcare professionals' prescribing practices. Since generic drugs are bioequivalent to the innovator drugs, switching between the two creates no difference in therapeutic effect. However, in the case of biosimilars, although they are highly similar to their respective innovator biologics, they are not bioequivalent. Therefore switching from a branded biologic to a biosimilar or between biosimilars creates uncertainty with regard to therapeutic effect due to the legally allowed differences in antibody structure based on the differences in manufacturing processes. In fact, manufacturers of biosimilars utilize their own proprietary and unique processes for biosimilar production that are often different from those of the innovator biologics. These differences in manufacturing processes result in very different cost structures for biosimilars compared to generic drugs. This is why biosimilars are usually priced only 20%–30% lower than their innovator counterparts, while generics are generally priced 70%–80% lower than the branded drugs. Because of differences in the biomedical design and development of biosimilars and biologics, there are concerns regarding quality and efficacy. However, the similarity testing requirements mandated by the US FDA and the European Medicines Agency have been implemented to ensure that biosimilars are safe alternatives to innovator biologics. With the advent of biosimilars, there is considerable confusion among healthcare professionals regarding safety, efficacy, design, and development. This confusion is partially due to unique terminologies and differences in the biopharmaceutical developmental process as compared to small-molecule nonbiologic agents. There are also political, financial, and economic reasons why healthcare professionals need to better understand biosimilars. (Calamia & Abraham, 2023)

To address these issues, the most common terms used to refer to the biopharmaceutical development process are defined first. Then, an overview of the fundamental differences in the design, development, and manufacturing processes of biologics/biosimilars and nonbiological agents/generic drugs is provided, along with relevant implications for the healthcare system. Finally, a brief history of biosimilars is presented, along with reasons why physicians and patients need to be educated and informed about them, to enhance discussion amongst healthcare providers, improve patient education and compliance, and ensure patient safety.

7.2.3 Regulatory framework and approval processes

The safety, efficacy, and quality of medicinal products are primarily determined by their active pharmaceutical ingredients (APIs). As a pharmaceutical product is developed, its API is manufactured and formulated in conjunction with other excipients into a drug product (DP). DP manufacture is generally an operation that combines APIs with excipients and processes them into a final dosage form, such as tablets, capsules, solutions, etc. A drug master file can be submitted to the FDA to protect the confidentiality of proprietary information at a facility used for drug product manufacture. A pharmaceutical company must hold the new drug application (NDA) or abbreviated new drug application (ANDA) for a DP. When a company's NDA/ANDA is approved, it is granted exclusive marketing rights for a specified period. After this period expires, other companies may submit their own NDAs/ANDAs for the same DP (Hasanah & Susanti, 2023).

A medicinal product can be a chemical entity (small molecule) or a biological (large molecule). Since the majority of drug losses occur at the patenting stage, it is imperative to understand a pharmaceutical patent and the tools to overcome it. To protect a pharmaceutical invention, a comprehensive patent strategy needs to be implemented alongside a development strategy. The groundwork for this strategy is laid long before any covalent modifications are made to the Invention. It is imperative to understand how intellectual property will be managed in the pharmaceutical alliance prior to research collaboration. Generics and biosimilars are regulated differently, as expounding on one will not clarify the other. Given the high burden of disease and healthcare expenditures, there remains a pressing need to understand how regulatory decisions shape the market for affordable medication (Rahman Kabir et al., 2019).

The robust regulatory framework for the approval of generic drugs and biosimilars is critical in ensuring patient safety and the efficacy of drugs. Health authorities perform stringent oversight of the approval of these pharmaceutical products. A generics company can copy a chemical drug once its patent and data exclusivity have expired. To enter the market, a generic company must demonstrate bioequivalence to the innovator drug under similar conditions. A biosimilars company can copy a biological drug once its patent has expired. However, the complexity of biological drugs means that biosimilars must go through a different regulatory path than generics. A biosimilars company must provide extensive comparability data to show that a proposed biosimilar is similar to the innovator biological drug regarding quality, efficacy, and safety (Kanter & Feldman, 2012).

Countries with recent biosimilars regulations generally model these after preexisting frameworks in other countries. However, key inconsistencies exist within the biosimilars regulatory framework, such as the choice of reference product and comparability study designs. The emergence of globally consistent biosimilars approval processes would allow countries to more easily adopt biosimilars, thereby meeting public health goals. In countries with high drug expenditures, the biosimilars market is a growing response to the expiry of original drug patents. The first generics entered the pharmaceutical market around ten years after the development of the innovator drug. Generics dramatically lowered the market price of the drug; for example, in the US, the market price fell by an average of 88% (i.e., from $1111 to $130 postgeneric entry). With the advent of the biosimilars, it remains to be seen how similarly the market will respond. The market prices of the initially launched biosimilars in the EU lowered the market price of the innovator drug by an average of 34% (i.e., from €11092 to €7295). (Car et al.2023)

The approval of generics and biosimilars is essential in maintaining the public health goal of access to affordable drugs, having historically been previously disadvantaged. A thorough understanding of these regulatory frameworks and the challenges converging on them is essential for equitable drug access. Currently, both biosimilars and generics face common challenges in bringing drugs to the market; despite these drugs being similar to preexisting drugs, the approval process has extended delays. Importantly, regulatory decisions heavily shape the market for affordable medication. In consideration of prior knowledge, it is hence essential to provide an overview detailing how regulatory practices directly affect the availability of affordable medication. A summary of the approval of generics and biosimilars is first presented, highlighting differing approaches and common ground. Considerable attention is then drawn to the most discussed issue across approval types and continents: delays in the approval process. Finally, an overview of how understandings of the regulatory framework can shape the market for affordable medication is presented.

7.3 Economic and market dynamics of generic drugs and biosimilars

This section examines the economic effects and market dynamics of generic drugs and biosimilars and their impacts on the healthcare system. Starting with an understanding of the cost savings that these pharmaceutical alternatives can bring to the healthcare system, the emphasis is on how those savings can help make treatments more affordable. Statistical evidence is provided to illustrate the effects of generics on the price reductions and expansion of the market share of the original drug. Similarly, how biosimilars impact affordability is evaluated, with trends showing the gradual uptake of biosimilars by the market after the first product was approved in 2013.

Competitive drug pricing is at the heart of affordability, and this section examines how market forces come into play to encourage competition, focusing on how accessibility relates to pricing strategies. Here, too, statistical trends are shown to demonstrate the gradual impact of generics and biosimilars on the competitive landscape. Discussing shifts in prescribing patterns from originator drugs to alternatives, the analysis shows that these trends indicate increased uptake of generics and biosimilars, though the process may remain slow in some therapeutic areas. Lastly, the impact of generics and biosimilars on innovation in the pharmaceutical industry is examined, outlining potential drawbacks to consider in the wake of these positive impacts on access. Identifying the key drivers behind the growth of the generics and biosimilars sector, patent expirations and a greater need for cost-effective medications are argued as the primary factors fostering this development (Lynch, 2017).

7.3.1 Cost savings and affordability impact

The financial aspect of generic drugs and biosimilars is examined in more depth here. How much might patients and healthcare systems save if generics and biosimilars were used instead of the original versions? There is strong evidence that employing these alternatives can lead to substantial cost reductions (Socal et al., 2022). During the 1990s, the discussion primarily centered on generics, though biosimilars were added in the 2000s. However, biopharmaceuticals remain a small fraction of the total drug market share, with biologics accounting for only 10% of all reimbursed pharmaceuticals. Nevertheless, the gradual uptake of biosimilars is contributing to a significant decrease in overall biopharmaceutical expenditure.

Biosimilars led to a dramatic reduction in spending on anti-TNF-biologics used to treat inflammatory bowel disease, even in small countries with few prescribers, where one might be concerned about the effect on quality. Detailed case studies and statistics make it abundantly clear how much out-of-pocket costs can fall if generics are used instead of originals (Lynch, 2017). Nonetheless, it is not only the patient's pocket but also a substantial reduction in overall healthcare spending that has come with generics. Public healthcare systems would pay €2.8 billion more each year if generics were not used, and in some countries, almost all of the increase in public healthcare costs would be eliminated if generics were taken into account. Concerns about prioritizing quality over affordability are addressed here. By showing how price developments have evolved over time, it is demonstrated that even after a decade of copying, the impact on affordability persists, and that policymakers' efforts to safeguard generics' use have been crucial.

The conclusion is that a functioning generics and biosimilars market is vital for ensuring affordable healthcare. This is an important basis in the analysis of AI's impact on the pharmaceutical industry regarding drug discovery, formulation development, and patient adherence, focusing on generics and biosimilars. Generics and biosimilars are expected to have the same chemical and biological properties as their reference medicinal product, which is a prerequisite for their market authorization.

7.3.2 Market trends and growth drivers

This section discusses current market trends affecting the growth of generic drugs and biosimilars, based on in-depth analysis of the global generic drugs and biosimilars market from 2020–30. The examination includes several industry and market components, such as acceptance and consumption rates of generic drugs and biosimilars, as well as forecasts, across the pharmaceutical industry. A thorough understanding of current trends and their eventual outcomes allows for informed resource investment or risk diversification decisions (Rahman Kabir et al., 2019). Key aspects of the industry are also explored, providing essential knowledge for stakeholders such as manufacturers, service providers, and financial institutions. In recent years, there has been a substantial increase in consumer acceptance and a growing shift towards generics and biosimilars in various therapeutic areas. This, along with patent expiries of leading blockbuster drugs, is driving market growth. Technological advances in manufacturing processes are also playing a crucial role in enhancing production efficiency. Emerging market competitors with readily accessible production plants are introducing new processes that reduce costs and increase system flexibility. Healthcare policies designed to encourage the uptake of these drugs are actively impacting consumer perception and promoting adoption. The overall generic drugs and biosimilars market is also significantly supported by expanding markets in developing nations, where, despite competitive pressures on pricing and availability, profound growth in consumption is expected through the widespread introduction of low-cost formulations.

7.4 Clinical and therapeutic equivalence

Clinical and therapeutic equivalence must be satisfied for generic drugs, biosimilars, and their branded counterparts, ensuring they will provide similar therapeutic outcomes. In the case where generics/biosimilars deliver similar efficacy and safety compared to their originators, these medications can be interchangeable (Rahman Kabir et al., 2019). This section will examine in detail the equivalence of efficacy and safety and discuss how clinicians can prescribe generics and biosimilars without compromising patient safety. As with any medication, adequate clinical studies must be conducted to provide pre-market evidence of equivalent efficacy and safety. In addition, post-market surveillance is required to continually assess the safety of drugs in the general population (Webster et al., 2021). The public often overestimates the risks of novel medications, primarily because of high-profile drug withdrawal cases, while underestimating the potential hazards associated with widely used medications.

A significant misconception about biosimilars is that their clinical efficacy is inferior to that of their originators. This misconception stems from biosimilars being new entities for the public and the widely held misconception that any new drug must be superior to existing alternatives. Legislative policies mandating the testing of new drugs against existing alternatives are often misconstrued as an assurance of superiority in efficacy and safety. Concerns regarding the comparability between the originator biologic drug and biosimilar regarding efficacy, immunogenicity, and safety profile have a significant influence on regulatory decisions. As such, it is critical to clearly describe how comparability issues unique to biologics (as opposed to small molecules) are resolved to assure stakeholders (prescribers, patients) of the reliability and quality of biosimilars and ensure confidence in the therapeutic equivalence of these drugs.

With the rapid adoption of generic drugs and biosimilars in national health systems, it has become critical to define the respective roles of key stakeholders (physicians, pharmacists, health authorities, and policymakers) in ensuring generics/biosimilars are utilized effectively in treatment while safeguarding patient health. As with any newly marketed drugs, concerns must be addressed regarding the safety of generics/biosimilars in the post-market setting and the continued physician involvement in patient monitoring following treatment switches from originators to generics/biosimilars. Three basic principles should govern how physicians integrate generics/biosimilars into their practice: patient rights; quality assurance; and the prioritization of care over economic considerations (Cheng et al.2022).

7.4.1 Efficacy and safety considerations

Efficacy and safety are critical considerations when discussing generic drugs and biosimilars. Generic drugs are copies of brand-name products that have lost their patent protection, while biosimilars are copies of biologic medications that have also lost their patent protection, but are produced through living organisms. Despite differences in production processes, both alternatives must demonstrate comparable effectiveness compared to their brand-name counterparts. Here, clinical trial data from different jurisdictions are presented to support the claim that generic drugs and biosimilars are as effective and safe as their brand-name versions (Vulto & Crow, 2012).

To mitigate the effects of an impending patent cliff for monoclonal antibodies in the United States, the Biologics Control and Safety Act was amended to allow biosimilars to enter the market. While there are concerns about switching to a generic or biosimilar medication, it is essential to analyze whether the risks outweigh the benefits. What happens when a patient is switched to a generic alternative? These questions are comprehensively analyzed with respect to patient experiences and pre- and post-marketing observational studies that inform the discussion of the safety profile and clinical outcomes (Lynch, 2017).

In light of these considerations, the ethical imperatives surrounding prescribing practices are reviewed. European Union regulators require that doctors maintain a record of the innovator product unless it is "clear that a biosimilar will be used," and that the name of the biosimilar product must be provided. This is to ensure monitoring of patient response postswitch and prevention of inadvertent substitution with another biosimilar. However, in the European Union, where many biosimilars were approved simultaneously, it is difficult to see how these safeguards would prevent switching between biosimilars. Regulatory requirements state that all biosimilars must undergo rigorous testing before being approved, which should instill confidence in their safety. Regarding generics, the panel is reminded that there is a role for healthcare providers, as is currently the case with the biosimilar pathway—to monitor patient responses postswitch and consider switching back to a different brand if there are safety issues. Nevertheless, the intent is to ensure that efficacy and safety considerations are at the forefront of discussions surrounding generics and biosimilars (Molnár-Gábor et al.2022).

7.5 Challenges and opportunities in adoption

Generic drugs and biosimilars have the potential to significantly enhance access and affordability in the pharmaceutical industry, but their widespread acceptance and adoption face challenges that must be addressed. This section reviews the challenges and opportunities surrounding the acceptance of these medications. It begins by exploring the factors influencing physician and patient acceptance of the alternatives, focusing on misconceptions and knowledge gaps that hinder wider adoption. Efforts made to improve understanding of these medications through educational initiatives are also analyzed (Rahman Kabir et al., 2019). The focus then shifts to the opportunities available for enhancing accessibility, particularly in regard to the competitive nature of the pharmaceutical market. While market competition is often seen as a means to improve availability, it can also complicate pricing decisions. Nonetheless, competitive environments may create openings to enhance accessibility through partnership models or subsidization. The role of patient advocacy groups in facilitating the adoption of generics and biosimilars is also discussed (Lynch, 2017). Ultimately, this section aims to provide a balanced overview of both the obstacles faced and the pathways to wider acceptance of these alternatives.

7.5.1 Physician and patient acceptance

Focusing on the impact on acceptance of generics and biosimilars by physicians and patients, several studies related to attitudes among both target groups are analyzed. Although pharmaceutical companies, health authorities, and society expect that physicians will prescribe alternatives to originators, patients will usually benefit only if prescribers accept these alternatives. Studies on factors influencing the prescribing habits of physicians reveal that personal experience and the quality of the drug, both perceived and scientific, are often the most important factors to influence prescribing behavior (Binder & Zeitlinger, 2023). The need for ongoing education is essential to address widely cited and prevalent concerns and misconceptions that involve the quality of these alternatives to originators. Nevertheless, studies show that once patients trust their physician, they will accept whatever drug the physician is prescribing. The majority of patients prefer generics to no treatment, even if they consider generics to be of lower quality (Sarnola et al., 2020). Nevertheless, concern remains about the ability of generics to perform as well as the innovator formulation.

There is also an indication that once patients trust their physician, they will accept whatever medication the physician prescribes. The majority of patients prefer generics to no treatment, even if they consider generics to be of lower quality. However, there is still concern that generics may not perform as well as the innovator formulation. It is therefore the responsibility of healthcare professionals to ensure that patient choices are based on informed consent, making patient education and the professional's own choice of treatment options paramount. Several examples of successful strategies to enhance acceptance of generics are provided. The strategies include, but are not limited to, explaining the economic impact of generics, providing written information, and using posters in waiting rooms. In addition to strategies, some barriers to acceptance, such as regulatory uncertainties, institutional policies, and anxiety about liability, are also presented. The purpose is to highlight and identify the most critical aspects and factors affecting acceptance to enable more dependence on these alternative medications.

7.5.2 Market competition and pricing strategies

The discussion primarily revolves around market competition concerning generic drugs and biosimilars. Competition is the very basis of a market; if a commodity is being produced on a large scale by many manufacturers, it leads to competition among them to sell their products. In such a scenario, the price of the commodity is bound to decrease while the choice increases for the consumer. In the pharmaceutical industry, competition among manufacturers of generic drugs and biosimilars creates an impact of lower prices and greater choice on the consumer (Dickson & Kent, 2021). This is how the market dictates pricing strategy for all companies. Those companies that fail to remain competitive in pricing may have to bear a loss in their market share, which may drastically affect their sales performance.

When market competition is forced to happen, companies adopt strategies like discounting, bundled offers, etc., to ensure that they remain competitive in pricing. Consider the example of the generic market in the US. Consequently, when a generic version of a drug enters the market, the brand version is so severely discounted that it makes the previous lowest-priced option seem exorbitant. Similarly, if a biosimilar is introduced, the originator's discount to remain competitive will automatically have to match that of the biosimilar (Danzon & Chao, 2000). Such competitive pricing can often happen where regulatory policies do not interfere with a drug's pricing. It is believed that drugs should be affordable to everyone; hence, the government must intervene in pricing decisions. However, drug affordability and the industry's drive to make profits are two ends of the same stick.

If the pricing of drugs is left entirely to market competition, it will be favorable for the consumer, but then it is possible that companies may not find it lucrative to invest in innovative research since the very basis of competition is that the drug would be guaranteed to be off-patent after a certain period. Competition happens to drive innovation in a sector. If there is no competition, it can be detrimental for the consumer; for example, the industry may research a drug that is ineffective but very costly simply because it can be sold at a premium price. So, the question then arises: how much competition is good for an industry? This is the aspect that needs to be studied with respect to competition in generic and biosimilar markets.

7.6 Technological innovations in manufacturing and quality assurance

Advancements in technology profoundly impact the manufacturing and quality assurance of generic drugs and biosimilars. Innovations in production techniques, including automation and more sophisticated quality control systems, enhance efficiency levels, as companies can scale up production and launch new products with lower resource demands (Rantanen & Khinast, 2015). Furthermore, enhanced analytical testing methods can create new forms to contribute to safety/performance metrics beyond what was previously possible. For example, molecular imaging or measurements of surface/free energies could address toxicity concerns associated with certain nanoscale delivery systems. Demonstrating the impacts of numerical modeling is paramount. As an illustration, computational fluid dynamics can model how the inner workings of a precision spray dryer affect microparticle formation, helping mitigate the risk of invalidating a key quality control measure. Although currently focused on small-molecule drugs, the technology can help streamline biosimilar production while meeting regulatory obligations to demonstrate bioequivalence. Changes in upstream/fermentation stages that affect the critical quality attributes of the final drug product can be tracked using sophisticated analytics. Drug integrity must remain paramount in the face of rapidly evolving digital technologies for managing supply chains and tracking drugs from factory to pharmacy. The 2009 H1N1 pandemic experience prompts vigilance regarding cyber-threats targeting drug production, distribution, or design; reliability and security measures adopted by the aerospace industry could serve as models for pharmaceuticals. Continual investments in emerging technologies deliver improved manufacturing sustainability, cost-effectiveness, and product accessibility (Nicholson II Price, 2014). As a good manufacturing practice (GMP) requirement, automated systems controlling drug production and QA must be validated to prevent data manipulation opportunities that compromise product quality and safety. Describing how emerging techs help address GMP worries can support calls for vigilance regarding their use in generics. Public trust is vital for the quality of all medications, although perhaps especially generics. Developing new processes/analyses requiring jurisdictions to recalibrate QA approaches highlights how techs/tech innovations can bolster public confidence in generics. Emphasizing how pharma innovations could help countries improve drug access showcases the public health benefits of competitively manufacturing exports. Ultimately, technologies/tech innovations will transform how drugs are produced, making production more efficient and products more reliable, safer, and effective.

7.7 Role of artificial intelligence in drug development and distribution

Efforts to make essential medicines available, affordable, and accessible for all have focused largely on strengthening the generic drug and biosimilar product markets. Pharmaceutical innovations, on the other hand, deal with the opposite side of the equation: cost explosion, overly monopolistic power, and pharmaceutical market cartelization. These issues become more pressing in the era of AI innovations, both for fairer and better access to the AI-enabled pharmaceutical innovations, and for considering the AI's potential role in rejuvenating and innovating the whole process from drug development to access. Nevertheless, there are still many unknowns and challenges regarding how access and affordability should be guaranteed for future pharmaceutical innovations, particularly for the emerging vital AI-enabled technologies involving deep learning and large language models. Addressing this knowledge gap would be the first step in analyzing the impact of the generic drug and biosimilar product markets on access and affordability under the AI-driven pharmaceutical industry (Mhazo & Maponga, 2021).

AI technologies have the potential to transform every step of drug development and distribution, from the initial discovery of the API to the final delivery of the pharmaceutical product. APIs are the "drugs" that make a pharmaceutical product effective and safe. Drug discoveries usually focus on finding small molecules that modulate the function of a disease-related protein target. The feasibility of a discovery based on a compound's pharmacological activity within a target can be theoretically evaluated by modeling the target's interaction with the compound. In the early stages of a compound's development, such in silico predictive modeling alone can save enormous resources for high-throughput biochemical screening, which is usually time-consuming and expensive. Using a druggable crystal structure of the target, AI technologies can build up homology 3D structures of temporally unresolved targets and then generate the ligand-binding pocket models for virtual screening. It has been demonstrated that deep generative models can also be used to de novo design drug-like compounds to fit a desired target. AI technologies can optimize lead compounds to iteratively improve their pharmacokinetic profiles and predict toxicity liabilities for selecting the most promising candidates for further development. AI technologies are transforming drug design by not only enhancing the chance of finding good binders but also generating novel molecular structures with desired target binding properties (Ioana Visan & Negut, 2024).

7.8 Global regulatory landscape and harmonization efforts

The market introduction of generic drugs and biosimilars is largely determined by national legislation and public policies, which frame the market for generics and biosimilars with very different country-specific settings at present. As a consequence, generics and biosimilars may offer no as opposed to many competitive price alternatives in some countries. The currently observed outcome of such country-specific frameworks is in part due to the complexity of regulation and the interplay of many factors determining how effective a market for generics and biosimilars can be in a certain country (Rahman Kabir et al., 2019). However, a globalized economy and worldwide trade put national frameworks under pressure. Regulatory processes need to be facilitated and harmonized to effectively ensure market access across countries. A prerequisite for market access is the unrestricted right to apply for a market authorization. The obligation to grant a market authorization generally requires a country to accept a marketing authorization made by another country, but usually under certain conditions that can vary substantially. These country-specific treaty obligations can greatly affect the duration of regulatory processes, resulting in time delays of market access that can range from one month to several years (Lynch, 2017).

Market access and market introduction of generics and biosimilars are globally regulated by the WTO TRIPS agreement. Art. 27 of the TRIPS agreement allows every Member State to set its own standards of patent protection and gives a leeway of five years (plus transition periods for developing countries) for such regulations to be in place. Several countries have opted for very limited or no patent protection for pharmaceuticals. Brazil, Cuba, India, and Thailand, for example, historically lacked patent systems for pharmaceuticals. Uruguay had a so-called industrial design law that covered some pharmaceutical compounds. A choice for strong patent protection is generally seen as restricting free competition and resulting in higher medicine prices (i.e., less access), especially in poor countries. Considering these trade-offs, countries find themselves in very different settings regarding access to medicines and affordability. These disparities could change the way countries balance between innovation incentives and access/affordability concerns. Similar to generics, differences in the trustworthiness of bioequivalence studies across countries dictate the need for regulatory effort on the part of the applicant, where, for generics, this may mean conducting clinical bioequivalence studies in each jurisdiction as opposed to one jurisdiction only (Patil et al.2024).

7.9 Case studies and success stories

A selection of case studies is presented to showcase success stories in the realm of generic drugs and biosimilars. Each case study illustrates unique challenges faced and how these challenges were effectively addressed, highlighting key learnings for stakeholders. The successes discussed here are those most directly linked to patient access and affordability. For each case, there is also an exploration of how these successes could potentially be scaled to other demographics and healthcare systems. Patient and healthcare provider testimonials have been included to reflect real-world experiences, the good, the bad, and the ugly; all account for learnings that can strengthen future efforts. Finally, the acceleration of these success stories through government policies is considered. By sharing these case studies, the intent is to inspire confidence that the adoption of generics and biosimilars can transform the pharmaceutical landscape. The hope is that stakeholders will find the impetus to act on these learnings, and these stories will compel wider interest in generics and biosimilars (Rahman Kabir et al., 2019). Throughout the world, biological therapies are being used to treat both chronic and life-threatening diseases, from cancer and autoimmune disorders to rare genetic disorders. Biologics fall into the category of high-cost pharmaceuticals, which have significantly increased drug expenditures for both public health systems and individual patients in need. Consequently, these high-cost therapeutics promote issues that require addressing with regard to controlling healthcare costs and accessibility of the drugs to patients. The introduction of biosimilars to the pharmaceutical market has signaled highly potential cost savings for patients who require treatment with biologics (Lynch, 2017).

7.10 Future directions and emerging trends

This narrative tackles some future directions and emerging trends pertinent to generics and biosimilars. The discussion is not intended to be exhaustive but focuses on areas deemed to be important growth opportunities, particularly influenced by advancing technology or novel market access strategies. There is a strong belief that patient-centric drug delivery systems could evolve as a key area to enhance patient outcomes, combined with generics, whereas biosimilars could benefit from the currently evolving healthcare policies driving the adoption of similar systems (Kabir et al., 2019). However, it is recognized that many described changes take years or decades to materialize and will require collaborative efforts from all industry stakeholders and regulators to shape the desired future landscape.

While this narrative highlights ongoing research endeavors focusing on particular generics and biosimilars aspects, it is also acknowledged that some areas remain largely unaddressed, particularly patient education and awareness initiatives. Still, such activities are regarded as the backbone for further ensuring a successful future for generics and biosimilars. Societal trends and consumer behavior are briefly considered when projecting various anticipated shifts affecting market growth. Ultimately, this narrative aims to project a positive vision regarding the future of access and affordability in pharmaceutical care (Lynch, 2017).

AI disclosure

During the preparation of this work, the author(s) used Paperpal for language editing. After using this tool/service, the author(s) reviewed and edited the content as needed and take(s) full responsibility for the content of the publication.

References

Binder, L. & Zeitlinger, M. (2023). Perception of pharmacological equivalence of generics or biosimilars in healthcare professionals in Vienna.

Calamia, M., & Abraham, I. (2023). The economics of biosimilars and challenges to biosimilar adoption in low- and middle-income countries. *Expert Opinion on Biological Therapy*.

Car, E., Vulto, A. G., Houdenhoven, M. V., Huys, I., & Simoens, S. (2023). Biosimilar competition in European markets of TNF-alpha inhibitors: A comparative analysis of pricing, market share and utilization trends. *Frontiers in Pharmacology, 14*, 1151764.

Cheng, M., Adekola, O., Albia, J., & Cai, S. (2022). Employability in higher education: A review of key stakeholders' perspectives. *Higher Education Evaluation and Development, 16*(1), 16–31.

Danzon, P.M. & Chao, L. (2000). Does regulation drive out competition in pharmaceutical markets?

Dickson, S.R. & Kent, T. (2021). Association of generic competition with price decreases in physician administered drugs and estimated price decreases for biosimilar competition.

Eleryan, M. G., Akhiyat, S., Rengifo-Pardo, M., & Ehrlich, A. (2016). *Biosimilars: Potential Implications for Clinicians*.

Hasanah, A. N., & Susanti, I. (2023). Molecularly imprinted polymers for pharmaceutical impurities: Design and synthesis methods. *Polymers*.

Health Organization, W. (2022). Accelerating access to genomics for global health: promotion, implementation, collaboration, and ethical, legal, and social issues. A report of the WHO.

Ioana Visan, A. & Negut, I. (2024). Integrating artificial intelligence for drug discovery in the context of revolutionizing drug delivery.

Kanter, J. & Feldman, R. (2012). Understanding and incentivizing biosimilars.

Lynch, C. (2017). The U.S. biosimilar market: Ongoing policy challenges among key health care stakeholders

Mhazo, A. T., & Maponga, C. C. (2021). Agenda setting for essential medicines policy in sub-Saharan Africa: A retrospective policy analysis using Kingdon's multiple streams model. *Health Research Policy and Systems*.

Molnár-Gábor, F., Sellner, J., Pagil, S., Slokenberga, S., Tzortzatou-Nanopoulou, O., & Nyström, K. (2022). Harmonization after the GDPR? Divergences in the rules for genetic and health data sharing in four member states and ways to overcome them by EU measures: Insights from Germany, Greece, Latvia and Sweden. In *seminars in Cancer Biology, Vol. 84*. Academic Press, 271–283.

Nicholson II Price, W. (2014). Generic entry jujitsu: Innovation and quality in drug manufacturing.

Patil, N., Ranjan, A., Gaurav, Mukherjee, D., Panda, B.K., Diksha, & Singh, A. (2024). Navigating biosimilar regulatory pathways in emerging markets: Insights from Brics Nations. Applied Drug Research, Clinical Trials and Regulatory Affairs.

Rahman Kabir, E., Sherwin Moreino, S., & Kawsar Sharif Siam, M. (2019). The breakthrough of biosimilars: A twist in the narrative of biological therapy.

Rantanen, J. & Khinast, J. (2015). The future of pharmaceutical manufacturing sciences.

Sarnola, K., Merikoski, M., Jyrkkä, J., & Hämeen-Anttila, K. (2020). Physicians' perceptions of the uptake of biosimilars: A systematic review.

Shaikh, R., Yadav, K., Thummar, K., Maheriya, B., & Chauhan, S. (2025). Development of complex generics: Insights into trends, challenges, and market opportunities. *Journal of Generic Medicines* 17411343251313962.

Singh, D. (2023). A short appraisal of biological macromolecules as tethering excipients for improved drug delivery: Current advances. *Journal of Macromolecular Science*.

Socal, M.P., Cordeiro, T., F. Anderson, G., & Bai, G. (2022). Estimating savings opportunities from therapeutic substitutions of high-cost generic medications.
Vulto, A.G. & Crow, S.A. (2012). Risk management of biosimilars in oncology: Each medicine is a work in progress.
Webster, C.J., George, K.L., & Woollett, G.R. (2021). Comparability of biologics: Global principles, evidentiary consistency and unrealized reliance.
Wouters Olivier, J., G. Kanavos Panos., & M., Martin. (2017). Comparing generic drug markets in Europe and the United States: Prices, volumes, and spending.

CHAPTER 8

Over-the-counter medications: meeting consumer needs in the digital age

Sarah Abdulrahman Alajlan

Clinical Pharmacy Department, AlMaarefa University, Riyadh, Saudi Arabia

8.1 Introduction

Digital technology has become a key component of transformation in almost every industry in the twenty-first century, and the healthcare sector is no exception (Meskó et al., 2017). The area of pharmacy services, specifically the availability, distribution, and utilization of over-the-counter (OTC) drugs, has experienced substantial changes driven by digital innovation (Clark et al., 2017).

Traditional pharmacy practice was largely based on paper prescriptions, in-person interactions, and limited access to pharmaceutical advice outside clinical settings (Champagne & Leclerc, 2015). However, digital transformation has redefined how consumers interact with pharmaceuticals by placing products, information, and professional support directly at their fingertips (Shambhavi, 2022).

Pharmacy processes are now being streamlined through the integration of automation, artificial intelligence (AI), telepharmacy, mobile health applications, and electronic health records (Laranjo et al., 2018; Raza et al., 2022). These technologies have significantly expanded access to OTC medications while improving efficiency and consumer engagement (Zhang, 2023).

By 2026, the global digital pharmacy market is projected to reach approximately $35.33 billion, growing at an annual rate of 14.42%, reflecting the increasing reliance on digital solutions in healthcare delivery (Shambhavi, 2022; Zhang, 2023). This growth illustrates the pharmaceutical industry's shift toward meeting evolving consumer expectations through digital platforms (Hole et al., 2021).

Self-care and consumer empowerment are among the most notable outcomes of this transformation (May et al., 2023). Patients are increasingly informed, connected, and proactive, using digital tools to research symptoms, compare treatment options, and access virtual consultations (Aboueid et al., 2021; Millenson et al., 2018). As a result, individuals have transitioned from passive recipients of care to active participants in managing their own health (Meskó et al., 2017).

The Future of Pharma Across All Sectors in the Artificial Intelligence Era. DOI: https://doi.org/10.1016/B978-0-443-40572-3.00007-1

Through e-commerce platforms and mHealth technologies, OTC medications have become more accessible than ever (Zhou et al., 2019). Consumers can now read reviews, compare costs, set medication reminders, and monitor treatment outcomes using mobile applications and wearable devices (Zhang, 2023; Zhou et al., 2019).

The COVID-19 pandemic further accelerated the adoption of digital pharmacy services, with online pharmacies, teleconsultations, and remote care becoming essential during periods of lockdown and healthcare system strain (Haydon et al., 2021; Pharmaceutical Technology, 2021). This shift was particularly beneficial for individuals in rural or underserved areas, where access to healthcare services is often limited (IMARC Group, 2023).

AI and data analytics have emerged as central drivers of this transformation, enabling personalized recommendations and predictive healthcare solutions (Raza et al., 2022). AI systems can analyze patient data, behavioral patterns, and purchasing history to suggest appropriate OTC products tailored to individual needs (Laranjo et al., 2018).

Despite these advancements, the increasing availability of OTC medications through digital channels raises concerns about safety and appropriate use (Algarni et al., 2021). The need for digital health literacy is becoming increasingly important, as consumers must be able to evaluate online health information critically (Çetin & Gümüş, 2023).

Additionally, the widespread use of social media as a source of health information has contributed to the spread of misinformation, which may influence consumer decision-making (Smailhodzic et al., 2016; Ventola, 2014). Regulatory bodies face the ongoing challenge of ensuring that digital platforms provide accurate, evidence-based information while protecting consumer safety (Lifshitz et al., 2020).

Furthermore, disparities in access to digital technologies continue to create a digital divide, particularly among elderly populations and individuals with limited socioeconomic resources (Akpan et al., 2024). Addressing these inequalities is essential to ensure that the benefits of digital health innovations are equitably distributed (IMARC Group, 2023).

8.2 Background

OTC medications, which can be obtained without a prescription, represent a fundamental component of modern healthcare systems by enabling individuals to manage minor health conditions independently (May et al., 2023). These products are widely used for common ailments such as colds, allergies, headaches, and gastrointestinal disturbances, contributing significantly to self-care practices and reducing pressure on healthcare services (Bradley et al., 1998; May et al., 2023).

The accessibility and affordability of OTC medications make them a cornerstone of patient autonomy and health literacy, allowing individuals to take a proactive role in managing their health (Meskó et al., 2017). However, despite these benefits, the widespread availability of OTC medications raises important concerns regarding misuse, inappropriate self-medication, drug interactions, and lack of professional guidance (Algarni et.al., 2021; Holden et al., 2019).

A cross-sectional study examining public attitudes and behaviors reported that approximately 24.6% of individuals frequently use OTC medications, highlighting the high prevalence of self-medication practices (Alharthi et al., 2025). While patients generally respond positively to physicians recommending OTC treatments, they may be less receptive to pharmacist interventions such as therapeutic substitution, indicating variability in trust and decision-making behavior (Alharthi et al., 2025; Bradley et al., 1998).

International studies further demonstrate diverse patterns of OTC use. For instance, research conducted in Poland revealed that a significant proportion of individuals purchase OTC medications infrequently, yet over half reported usage of OTC cold remedies, emphasizing the role of seasonal and situational factors (Cybulski et al., 2018). Additionally, many participants expressed a preference for purchasing OTC medications exclusively from pharmacies, underscoring the perceived importance of professional oversight (Cybulski et al., 2018).

A systematic review investigating OTC misuse, abuse, and dependency identified pooled rates of 16.2% for misuse, 2.0% for abuse, and 7.2% for dependency, indicating that nonprescription medications are not without risk (Algarni et al., 2021). Certain drug categories, including analgesics, sedative antihistamines, and dextromethorphan-containing cough products, were frequently associated with problematic use (Carney et al., 2018; Algarni et al., 2021). These findings highlight the potential for both psychological and physical harm, including severe outcomes such as hospitalization or death (Algarni et al., 2021).

Consumer behavior is also influenced by socioeconomic and cultural factors. Studies conducted in Japan found that consumers often prefer branded OTC products, with advertising playing a significant role in shaping purchasing decisions (Aoyama et al., 2012). Additionally, individuals from lower socioeconomic groups may prioritize cost and accessibility over clinical effectiveness when selecting medications, potentially increasing the risk of inappropriate use (Aoyama et al., 2012; Habash & Al-Dmour, 2020).

In the context of Saudi Arabia, research indicates widespread use of OTC medications, particularly analgesics such as diclofenac (Alshahrani et al., 2020). Misuse of OTC medications, including antihistamines, dextromethorphan, and codeine-containing products, has been reported, often driven by self-management practices and, in some cases, nonmedical use (Algarni et al., 2022). Community pharmacists have highlighted concerns regarding frequent misuse and have advocated for stricter regulatory control and reclassification of high-risk medications (Algarni et al., 2022).

Among parents, OTC medication use is also highly prevalent. A study conducted in Jeddah found that 58.8% of parents purchased OTC medications for their children, with family physicians serving as the primary source of information for 37.3% of respondents (Mirdad et al., 2023). This highlights the continued importance of healthcare professionals in guiding safe medication practices, even within the context of self-care.

The increasing digitization of healthcare has further transformed access to OTC medications. Online pharmacies, mobile applications, and telehealth services allow consumers to obtain medications without visiting physical pharmacies, enhancing convenience and accessibility (IMARC Group, 2023). However, this shift introduces new challenges, including reduced pharmacist supervision, increased exposure to misinformation, and risks associated with counterfeit or substandard products (Lifshitz et al., 2020).

8.3 Self-care in the digital age: the role of online information in over-the-counter decision-making

The digital transformation of healthcare has fundamentally reshaped how individuals access and utilize health information, particularly in the context of self-care and OTC medication use (Meskó et al., 2017). Increasingly, consumers rely on online platforms to research symptoms, evaluate treatment options, and make informed decisions before seeking professional medical advice (Aboueid et al., 2021; Millenson et al., 2018).

Trusted digital resources, such as WebMD and the Mayo Clinic, have become primary sources of health information, offering accessible and user-friendly guidance for managing common conditions

(Millenson et al., 2018). This shift reflects a broader movement toward patient autonomy, convenience, and proactive health management (May et al., 2023).

Search engines, mobile health applications, and online forums play a critical role in shaping consumer behavior across all age groups, not only among younger digital natives (Zhou et al., 2019). As a result, digital health literacy has emerged as a key determinant of safe and effective self-care, influencing individuals' ability to critically evaluate and apply health information (Çetin & Gümüş, 2023).

AI-powered symptom checkers and health platforms further illustrate this transformation, providing personalized recommendations based on user-reported symptoms (Laranjo et al., 2018). These tools enhance convenience and accessibility, enabling users to make quick decisions regarding OTC medication use without immediate clinical consultation (Aboueid et al., 2021).

However, the increasing reliance on digital information raises concerns regarding accuracy, reliability, and the potential for misdiagnosis (Millenson et al., 2018). Inaccurate or misleading information may lead to inappropriate medication use, delayed treatment, or worsening health outcomes (Ventola, 2014).

Therefore, ensuring the quality of digital health content is essential for supporting safe self-care practices. Public health initiatives and regulatory frameworks must focus on improving health literacy and promoting evidence-based information to mitigate these risks (Çetin & Gümüş, 2023; Lifshitz et al., 2020).

8.4 Social media influence on over-the-counter medication choices

Social media platforms have become highly influential in shaping consumer health behaviors, including decisions related to OTC medications (Smailhodzic et al., 2016; Ventola, 2014). Platforms such as TikTok, Instagram, and YouTube serve as major channels for sharing health information, product reviews, and personal experiences (Gaysynsky et al., 2024).

These platforms are particularly impactful among younger populations, who often rely on peer recommendations and influencer content when making decisions about health products (Alalwan, 2018). User-generated content, including short videos and product demonstrations, can significantly influence perceptions of effectiveness and safety (Whiting & Williams, 2013).

However, the credibility of such information is often questionable, as influencers may lack formal medical training and may promote products for commercial purposes (Ventola, 2014). This creates a risk of misinformation, exaggerated claims, and inappropriate self-medication practices (Smailhodzic et al., 2016).

Despite these challenges, social media also presents opportunities for health promotion and education. When leveraged appropriately, it can be used to disseminate accurate information, correct misconceptions, and encourage responsible use of OTC medications (Gaysynsky et al., 2024).

8.5 Mobile health apps and digital tools in over-the-counter decision-making

The evolution of digital healthcare has extended significantly into mobile health (mHealth) applications and digital tools, which now play a central role in shaping consumer decision-making regarding OTC medications (Meskó et al., 2017; Zhou et al., 2019). These applications offer a wide range of functionalities, including symptom assessment, medication tracking, adherence reminders, and personalized recommendations, thereby enhancing patient engagement and autonomy (Raza et al., 2022; Zhou et al., 2019).

Symptom checker platforms such as Ada, WebMD Symptom Checker, and Healthily provide immediate, data-driven assessments based on user-reported symptoms, often accompanied by recommendations for OTC treatments (Aboueid et al., 2021). These tools are particularly valuable for managing non-urgent health conditions, including colds, headaches, digestive issues, and minor skin conditions, enabling faster and more convenient decision-making (Millenson et al., 2018).

In addition, digital pharmacy platforms integrate these tools with e-commerce capabilities, allowing consumers to consult healthcare professionals virtually, receive personalized OTC product recommendations, and have medications delivered directly to their homes (IMARC Group, 2023). This integrated approach enhances accessibility, especially for individuals with mobility challenges or those residing in remote areas (Haydon et al., 2021).

However, despite their benefits, concerns remain regarding the reliability and accuracy of these digital tools. Variability in symptom interpretation, particularly when users provide incomplete or inaccurate information, can lead to misdiagnosis and inappropriate medication use (Millenson et al., 2018). Furthermore, issues related to data privacy and limited regulatory oversight continue to pose challenges for widespread adoption (Lifshitz et al., 2020).

8.6 Saudi Arabia, the Gulf Cooperation Council, and the Global Online Pharmacies Regulatory Environment

The rapid expansion of digital pharmacy services has necessitated the development of robust regulatory frameworks to ensure consumer safety and maintain the integrity of pharmaceutical systems (Lifshitz et al., 2020). Globally, regulatory bodies have implemented various strategies to monitor online pharmacies, protect consumers, and prevent the distribution of counterfeit or substandard medications (Lifshitz et al., 2020).

In developed regions such as North America and Europe, regulatory systems emphasize licensing, prescription validation, and data protection. In the United States, the Food and Drug Administration (FDA) collaborates with professional bodies to certify legitimate online pharmacies, ensuring adherence to quality and safety standards (Champagne & Leclerc, 2015).

Despite these efforts, the global online pharmacy landscape remains fragmented, with a significant number of unregulated platforms operating outside established legal frameworks (Lifshitz et al., 2020). The World Health Organization has reported that a substantial proportion of medicines sold online are substandard or falsified, posing serious risks to public health (Lifshitz et al., 2020).

In the Middle East, Saudi Arabia and the Gulf Cooperation Council (GCC) countries have made notable progress in developing regulatory systems for digital healthcare services (IMARC Group, 2023). These initiatives are aligned with broader national strategies, such as Saudi Arabia's Vision 2030, which promotes healthcare digitization and innovation (IMARC Group, 2023).

Saudi Arabia has implemented licensing requirements for online pharmacies, established guidelines for teleconsultations, and introduced electronic prescription systems to ensure safe medication practices (Aljadhey et al., 2015). These measures aim to enhance access while maintaining high standards of quality and patient safety.

8.7 Digital literacy and the consumer gap in accessing over-the-counter medications online

Digital literacy plays a critical role in determining the effectiveness and safety of OTC medication use in the digital age (Çetin & Gümüş, 2023). The ability to access, evaluate, and apply digital health information is essential for informed decision-making and responsible self-medication practices (Çetin & Gümüş, 2023).

Individuals with strong digital literacy skills are better equipped to navigate online pharmacy platforms, interpret health information accurately, and make informed purchasing decisions (Zhou et al., 2019). These populations often include younger, urban, and more educated individuals who are familiar with digital technologies and healthcare applications (Akpan et al., 2024).

Conversely, vulnerable populations, including older adults, individuals with limited education, and those living in rural areas, often face significant barriers to digital health access (Akpan et al., 2024). These barriers may include limited internet connectivity, lack of technical skills, and difficulty understanding complex health information (Çetin & Gümüş, 2023).

The digital divide not only affects access to healthcare services but also contributes to disparities in health outcomes, as individuals with lower digital literacy are more likely to rely on unreliable sources of information or engage in unsafe self-medication practices (Ventola, 2014).

To address these challenges, targeted public health interventions are required, including digital literacy training programs, simplified user interfaces, and increased collaboration between healthcare providers and digital platforms (Akpan et al., 2024).

8.8 Artificial intelligence-driven personalized over-the-counter recommendations

AI has emerged as a transformative force in healthcare, particularly in the personalization of OTC medication recommendations (Raza et al., 2022). AI-driven systems are capable of analyzing large volumes of health data, including symptom profiles, demographic characteristics, and behavioral patterns, to provide tailored healthcare solutions (Laranjo et al., 2018).

These technologies enable consumers to receive personalized product suggestions that align with their specific needs, improving both the efficiency and effectiveness of self-care practices (Raza et al., 2022). AI-powered chatbots and virtual assistants further enhance this experience by providing real-time guidance and answering health-related queries (Laranjo et al., 2018).

Future advancements are expected to incorporate data from electronic health records, genetic testing, and wearable devices, further enhancing the accuracy and relevance of recommendations (Zhang, 2023).

8.9 Integration with wearable technologies and smart devices

Wearable technologies are increasingly integrated into digital healthcare ecosystems, providing continuous monitoring of physiological parameters such as heart rate, temperature, and activity levels (Meskó et al., 2017). These devices offer real-time data that can be used to inform OTC medication decisions and improve health outcomes (Zhang, 2023).

For example, wearable devices detecting early symptoms of illness may prompt users to take appropriate OTC medications, enabling earlier intervention and improved symptom management (Zhou et al., 2019).

8.10 Predictive analytics for demand and supply optimization

Predictive analytics is transforming the management of OTC medication supply and demand by enabling data-driven decision-making (Zhang, 2023). By analyzing historical sales data, consumer behavior, and public health trends, digital platforms can accurately forecast demand for specific products (Raza et al., 2022).

This capability enhances inventory management, reduces shortages, and ensures the availability of essential medications during peak demand periods, such as seasonal illnesses or public health emergencies (Zhang, 2023).

8.11 Future trends and innovations in the digital over-the-counter medication market

The future of OTC medication access is closely linked to ongoing advancements in digital healthcare technologies (Meskó et al., 2017). Emerging innovations, including AI-driven platforms, wearable integration, and advanced analytics, are expected to further enhance personalization, accessibility, and efficiency (Raza et al., 2022).

However, the successful implementation of these technologies will depend on ethical considerations, regulatory oversight, and efforts to reduce disparities in digital health access (Akpan et al., 2024).

8.12 Conclusion

The digitization of healthcare has profoundly reshaped the landscape of OTC medication access, utilization, and consumer decision-making, transforming traditional healthcare delivery models into dynamic, technology-driven systems (Hole et al., 2021; Meskó et al., 2017). What once depended primarily on in-person consultations and pharmacist-led guidance has evolved into a decentralized ecosystem in which consumers are empowered to access health information, evaluate treatment options, and obtain medications through digital platforms (Aboueid et al., 2021; Millenson et al., 2018).

This transformation has significantly enhanced accessibility, convenience, and personalization, aligning with broader trends in healthcare that emphasize patient autonomy and proactive self-management (May et al., 2023). Through the integration of e-commerce, mobile health applications, AI, and wearable technologies, individuals can now make informed decisions about OTC medication use based on real-time data and personalized recommendations (Raza et al., 2022; Zhang, 2023). These advancements have not only improved healthcare efficiency but have also expanded access to underserved populations, particularly in regions where traditional healthcare services may be limited (IMARC Group, 2023).

However, the rapid expansion of digital health solutions also introduces significant challenges that must be carefully addressed to ensure safe and effective outcomes (Lifshitz et al., 2020). The widespread availability of health information online, combined with the influence of social media platforms, has contributed to the proliferation of misinformation, which may lead to inappropriate self-diagnosis and medication misuse (Smailhodzic et al., 2016; Ventola, 2014). The absence of direct pharmacist supervision in many digital transactions further increases the risk of unsafe medication practices, including incorrect dosing, drug interactions, and reliance on unverified products (Algarni et al., 2021).

Additionally, disparities in digital literacy present a critical barrier to equitable healthcare access, as certain population groups—particularly older adults, individuals with limited education, and those in rural areas—may struggle to navigate digital health platforms effectively (Akpan et al., 2024; Çetin & Gümüş, 2023). This digital divide not only limits access to healthcare services but also exacerbates existing health inequalities, highlighting the need for targeted interventions to improve digital inclusion and health literacy (Akpan et al., 2024).

From a regulatory perspective, the ongoing evolution of digital pharmacy services necessitates robust governance frameworks to ensure the safety, quality, and authenticity of OTC medications distributed through online platforms (Lifshitz et al., 2020). Countries such as Saudi Arabia and other GCC nations have made notable progress in implementing regulatory measures that support digital health innovation while safeguarding consumer protection, reflecting a commitment to balancing accessibility with patient safety (Aljadhey et al., 2015; IMARC Group, 2023).

Looking ahead, the integration of emerging technologies such as AI, predictive analytics, and wearable health devices is expected to further transform the OTC medication landscape by enabling more personalized, data-driven healthcare solutions (Meskó et al., 2017; Raza et al., 2022).

These innovations hold significant potential for improving health outcomes, optimizing resource utilization, and enhancing the overall patient experience.

In conclusion, the digital transformation of OTC medication access represents both a major opportunity and a critical responsibility. While technological advancements have empowered consumers and improved healthcare accessibility, their successful implementation depends on the development of evidence-based practices, effective regulatory oversight, and inclusive strategies that ensure equitable access for all populations. Ultimately, achieving a balance between innovation, safety, and accessibility will be essential for maximizing the benefits of digital health and ensuring that OTC medication use contributes positively to global public health outcomes.

References

Aboueid, S., Meyer, S., Wallace, J. R., Mahajan, S., & Chaurasia, A. (2021). Young adults' perspectives on the use of symptom checkers for self-triage and self-diagnosis: qualitative study. *JMIR Public Health and Surveillance, 7*(1), e22637. https://doi.org/10.2196/22637.

Akpan, I. J., Effiom, L., & Akpanobong, A. C. (2024). Towards developing a knowledge base for small business survival techniques during COVID-19 and sustainable growth strategies for the post-pandemic era. *Journal of Small Business & Entrepreneurship, 36*(6), 349–378.

Alalwan, A. A. (2018). Investigating the impact of social media advertising features on customer purchase intention. *International Journal of Information Management, 42*, 65–77.

Algarni, M., Jalal, Z., Hadi, M. A., & Alghamdi, S. (2022). Community pharmacists' views and experiences toward over-the-counter medicines misuse and abuse in Saudi Arabia: a qualitative study. *Frontiers in Pharmacology, 13*, 997342.

Alharthi, M. S., Alsulami, F. T., Fathelrahman, A. I., Alqarni, M. A., Alorfi, N. M., & Alzahrani, M. S. (2025). Attitudes and behaviors of the public toward over the counter (OTC) medications in the Western Region of Saudi Arabia: a cross-sectional study. *Healthcare, 13*(5), 472.

Aljadhey, H., Assiri, G. A., Mahmoud, M. A., Al-Aqeel, S., & Murray, M. (2015). Self-medication in Central Saudi Arabia: community pharmacy consumers' perspectives. *Saudi Medical Journal, 36*(3), 328–334.

Alshahrani, S. M., Alakhali, K. M., Al-Worafi, Y. M., & Alshahrani, N. Z. (2020). Awareness and use of over the counter analgesic medication: a survey in the Aseer region population, Saudi Arabia. *International Journal of Advanced and Applied Sciences, 7*(3), 130–134.

Aoyama, I., Koyama, S., & Hibino, H. (2012). Self-medication behaviors among Japanese consumers: sex, age, and SES differences and caregivers' attitudes toward their children's health management. *Asia Pacific Family Medicine, 11*, 1–9.

Bradley, C. P., Riaz, A., Tobias, R. S., Kenkre, J. E., & Dassu, D. Y. (1998). Patient attitudes to over-the-counter drugs and possible professional responses to self-medication. *Family Practice, 15*(1), 44–50.

Carney, T., Wells, J., Parry, C. D., McGuinness, P., Harris, R., & Van Hout, M. C. (2018). A comparative analysis of pharmacists' perspectives on codeine use and misuse–a three country survey. *Substance Abuse Treatment, Prevention, and Policy, 13*, 1–8.

Çetin, M., & Gümüş, R. (2023). Research into the relationship between digital health literacy and healthy lifestyle behaviors: an intergenerational comparison. *Frontiers in Public Health, 11*, 2149521.

Champagne, H.A., Leclerc, D.O., 2015. The road to digital success in pharma. McKinsey & Company. https://www.mckinsey.com/industries/lifesciences/our-insights/the-road-to-digital-success-in-pharma.

Clark, M., Clark, T., Bhatti, A., & Aungst, T. (2017). The rise of digital health and potential implications for pharmacy practice. *Journal of Contemporary Pharmacy Practice, 64*(1), 32–40.

Cybulski, M., Cybulski, L., Krajewska-Kulak, E., Orzechowska, M., & Cwalina, U. (2018). Preferences and attitudes of older adults of Bialystok, Poland toward the use of over-the-counter drugs. *Clinical Interventions in Aging, 13*, 623–632.

Gaysynsky, A., Heley, K., & Chou, W. Y. S. (2024). Social media and health in linguistically diverse communities: an examination of overlooked populations. *Journal of Health Communication* Advance online publication.

Habash, R., & Al-Dmour, H. (2020). Factors influencing the intention to buy over-the-counter medicines: empirical study. *International Journal of Pharmaceutical and Healthcare Marketing, 14*(2), 305–323.

Haydon, H. M., Smith, A. C., Snoswell, C. L., Thomas, E. E., & Caffery, L. J. (2021). Addressing concerns and adapting psychological techniques for videoconsultations: a practical guide. *Clinical Psychologist, 25*(2), 179–186.

Holden, R. J., Srinivas, P., Campbell, N. L., Clark, D. O., Bodke, K. S., Hong, Y., & Callahan, C. M. (2019). Understanding older adults' medication decision making and behavior: a study on over-the-counter (OTC) anticholinergic medications. *Research in Social and Administrative Pharmacy, 15*(1), 53–60.

Hole, G., Hole, A. S., & McFalone-Shaw, I. (2021). Digitalization in the pharmaceutical industry: what to focus on under the digital implementation process? *International Journal of Pharmaceutics: X, 3*, 100095. https://doi.org/10.1016/j.ijpx.2021.100095.

IMARC Group. 2023. GCC e-pharmacy market: industry trends, share, size, growth, opportunity and forecast 2024–2032. IMARC Services Private Limited. https://www.imarcgroup.com/gcc-e-pharmacy-market.

Laranjo, L., Dunn, A. G., Tong, H. L., Kocaballi, B. B., Chen, J., Bashir, R., Surian, D., Gallego, B., Magrabi, F., Lau, A. Y. S., & Coiera, E. (2018). Conversational agents in healthcare: a systematic review. *Journal of the American Medical Informatics Association, 25*(9), 1248–1258. https://doi.org/10.1093/jamia/ocy072.

Lifshitz, A., Arrieta, O., Burgos, R., Campillo, C., Celis, M.Á., Llata, M., Domínguez, J., Halabe, J., Islas, S., Jasso, L., Moreno, M., Plancarte, R., Reyes-Sánchez, A., Ruiz-Argüelles, G., Soda, A., Verástegui, E., & Sotelo, J. (2020). Self-medication and self-prescription. *Automedicación y Autoprescripción. Gaceta Médica de México, 156*(6), 600–602. https://doi.org/10.24875/GMM.M21000456.

May, U., Bauer, C., Schneider-Ziebe, A., & Giulini-Limbach, C. (2023). Self-care with non-prescription medicines to improve health care access and quality of life in low- and middle-income countries: systematic review and methodological approach. *Frontiers in Public Health, 11*, 1220984.

Meskó, B., Drobni, Z., Bényei, É., Gergely, B., & Győrffy, Z. (2017). Digital health is a cultural transformation of traditional healthcare. *mHealth, 3*, 38. https://doi.org/10.21037/mhealth.2017.08.07 Article.

Millenson, M. L., Baldwin, J. L., Zipperer, L., & Singh, H. (2018). Beyond Dr. Google: the evidence on consumer-facing digital tools for diagnosis. *Diagnosis, 5*(3), 95–105. https://doi.org/10.1515/dx-2018-0009.

Mirdad, O. A., Esheba, G. E., Mousa, A. H., Nukaly, H. Y., Alhindi, Y. Z., Hariri, N. H., & Alsanosi, S. M. (2023). Over-the-counter medication use among parents in Saudi Arabia. *International journal of Environmental Research and Public Health, 20*(2), 1193.

Pharmaceutical Technology. 2021. COVID-19 accelerated digital transformation of the pharma industry by five years: Poll. https://www.pharmaceutical-technology.com/news/covid-19-accelerated-digital-transformation-of-the-pharma-industry-by-five-years-poll/.

Raza, M. A., Aziz, S., Noreen, M., Saeed, A., Anjum, I., Ahmed, M., & Raza, S. M. (2022). Artificial intelligence (AI) in pharmacy: an overview of innovations. *Innovations in Pharmacy, 13*(1). https://doi.org/10.24926/iip.v13i1.4710.

Shambhavi. 2022. Digital pharmacy on the rise: transforming the pharma sector. Brillio. https://www.brillio.com/digital-pharmacy-on-the-rise-transforming-thepharma-sector/.

Smailhodzic, E., Hooijsma, W., Boonstra, A., & Langley, D. J. (2016). Social media use in healthcare: a systematic review of effects on patients and on their relationship with healthcare professionals. *BMC Health Services Research, 16*(1), 442. https://doi.org/10.1186/s12913-016-1691-0.

Ventola, C. L. (2014). Social media and health care professionals: benefits, risks, and best practices. *Pharmacy and Therapeutics, 39*(7), 491–520.

Whiting, A., & Williams, D. (2013). Why people use social media: a uses and gratifications approach. *Qualitative Market Research: An International Journal, 16*(4), 362–369. https://doi.org/10.1108/QMR-06-2013-0041.

Zhang, X. (2023). Investment analysis based on intrinsic value in the information technology and pharmaceutical sectors for advancements in digital healthcare. *Finance and Economics, 1*(1). https://doi.org/10.56397/FE.2023.01.02.

Zhou, L., Bao, J., Setiawan, I. M. A., Saptono, A., & Parmanto, B. (2019). The mHealth app usability questionnaire (MAUQ): development and validation study. *JMIR mHealth and uHealth, 7*(4), e11500. https://doi.org/10.2196/11500.

CHAPTER 9

Medical devices and diagnostics: enhancing patient care and outcomes

Babar Bashir Chaudhri

Department of Cardiac and Thoracic Surgery, King's College Hospital London, Dubai, United Arab Emirates

9.1 Introduction

9.1.1 The importance of medical devices and diagnostics in modern patient care

Noncommunicable cardiovascular conditions and cancer account for over 70% of global mortality, most of which are detectable and modifiable through timely diagnostics and device-based interventions (Luciani et al., 2023). Medical devices are a significant part of therapeutic and preventive strategies for these illnesses (Aung et al., 2021). They range from life-sustaining technologies such as pacemakers, mechanical circulatory support devices, and dialysis machines to noninvasive imaging modalities and rapid diagnostic tests. These have improved survival and quality of life for patients with advanced disease. Diagnostics serve as tools for confirmation and clinical event prediction, enabling proactive, bespoke, personalized care. Early detection of atrial fibrillation (AF) via wearable ECG monitors, for example, can allow for the timely initiation of anticoagulants, preventing strokes and reducing long-term healthcare costs (Reiffel et al., 2020). Medical devices have become integrated with healthcare delivery systems. Innovations in telemetry, implantable sensors, and miniaturized monitors coupled with clinical decision support tools enable remote patient management at scale, such as early warning systems for nursing care (Gallo et al., 2024). These are increasingly important in the post-pandemic world, where resource efficiency, decentralized care, and real-time analytics are important. The success of such further integration and convergence will rely on the synergistic use of artificial intelligence (AI). Diagnostics and devices are increasingly reactive, predictive, adaptive, and intelligent.

9.1.2 The artificial intelligence era: convergence of pharma, devices, and diagnostics

Deepening integration between pharmaceuticals, diagnostics, and devices represents an ongoing convergence of technologies in medicine. This is driven by artificial intelligence integrating disparate data streams, enabling real-time interpretation and decision-making (Manickam et al., 2022). Examples include algorithmic triage of radiology images and deep-learning models embedded in cardiac rhythm monitors that predict decompensation before symptom onset (Knop

The Future of Pharma Across All Sectors in the Artificial Intelligence Era. DOI: https://doi.org/10.1016/B978-0-443-40572-3.00003-4

et al., 2022). Medtronic's HeartLogic algorithm uses data from cardiac resynchronization therapy devices to predict heart failure events up to six weeks in advance, allowing clinicians to adjust therapy (De Juan Bagudá et al., 2022; Santini et al., 2020; Narang et al., 2021). Caption Health's AI-enabled imaging ultrasound guidance system allows non-specialists to acquire diagnostic-grade cardiac images, enabling broader access to advanced diagnostics (Narang et al., 2021; Liebo et al., 2011). Lucid Therapeutics is creating hybrid platforms that combine real-time monitoring with drug administration feedback loops, bridging the device–drug divide. Lucid's neuromodulation device for neuropsychiatric and cardiac disorders integrates biometric data and behavioral inputs to modulate therapy dynamically, thereby enabling closed-loop therapeutics (Sellers et al., 2024).

The convergence of pharma, devices, and diagnostics is enabling precision medicine. AI-curated diagnostic insights increasingly inform therapy selection, dosing, and timing, enhancing drug efficacy and reducing adverse events. Companion diagnostics are a new class of tests developed alongside specific therapies to stratify patients. This model is well-established in oncology (e.g., HER2 testing for trastuzumab use) (Bradley et al., 2021). It is gaining traction in cardiovascular, metabolic, and neurodegenerative conditions, where device-collected data may help guide real-time pharmaceutical interventions.

AI is transforming the business models that underpin the sector. The ability to generate and act upon real-world evidence (RWE) from medical devices is becoming a critical strategic asset. Regulatory agencies such as the FDA have recognized this. They have created novel pathways such as the Breakthrough Devices Program to expedite the development and approval of AI-enabled therapeutics and diagnostics. (U.S. Food and Drug Administration). Neuralink recently received breakthrough status for its speech restoration brain implant, which aids individuals impaired with ALS, stroke, and other neurological conditions (Cordero, 2025), (https://www.reuters.com/business/healthcare-pharmaceuticals/neuralinks-speech-restoration-device-gets-fdas-breakthrough-tag-2025-05-01/).

In summary, medical devices and diagnostics are no longer standalone entities. When fused with AI and aligned with pharmaceutical strategies, they enable a model of care that is predictive, precise, and personalized. This chapter explores this convergence with real-world applications in cardiovascular medicine, electrophysiology (EP), and digital diagnostics, and examines how AI is accelerating a shift to continuous real-time care.

9.2 Cardiovascular device landscape

9.2.1 Implantable devices

9.2.1.1 Bioprosthetic and mechanical heart valves

Implantable devices in cardiovascular medicine include a range of devices and implants. Heart valve prostheses are a good example and are used for patients with structural valve disease, valvular degeneration, or rheumatic heart disease. Two major categories dominate the heart valve field: bioprosthetic valves (typically made of porcine valves or bovine pericardial tissue) and mechanical valves (constructed from pyrolytic carbon and titanium alloys).

Bioprosthetic valves offer excellent hemodynamic performance, particularly in elderly patients, and eliminate the need for lifelong anticoagulation. They are increasingly used in surgical and transcatheter procedures (e.g., TAVR: transcatheter aortic valve replacement), and their use has expanded into younger cohorts due to patient preference for less burdensome therapy. Recent innovations include resilient polymer-based valves, such as Foldax's TRIA (George et al., 2025), which combine synthetic durability with tissue-like flexibility, aiming to overcome calcification and structural degeneration, limitations that have reduced bioprosthetic valve longevity to 10–15 years.

Mechanical valves offer long-term durability, often lasting several decades. They require strictly controlled anticoagulation with warfarin, due to the risk of thromboembolic events. This exposes patients to bleeding complications and necessitates frequent INR monitoring, which can impair quality of life. Mechanical valves remain the preferred option in younger patients (<60 years) and in those at high risk of reoperation. AI-enabled INR monitoring platforms and smart pill dispensers are beginning to reduce the burden of anticoagulation, offering more real-time tracking and safety.

Valve selection involves consideration of patient age and comorbidity, risk tolerance for anticoagulation, access to follow-up care, life expectancy, and risk of reintervention. The 2020 ACC/AHA guidelines, among others, have shifted toward shared decision-making models, recommending bioprosthetic valves in younger patients where lifestyle and bleeding risk outweigh concerns about durability (Vahanian et al., 2022; Otto et al., 2021).

A new class of heart valves is in development: polymeric heart valves. These are engineered using advanced polymers to create durable, cost-effective, and biocompatible alternatives to current mechanical and biological valves, aiming to address issues like calcification and lifelong replacement needs (Giaretta et al., 2024). AI is beginning to be applied to this field, with AI-powered chatbots providing patient education on heart valve conditions and treatments, and computational simulations and robotics being used to design, test, and manufacture these novel polymeric valves, optimizing their design and function (Becker et al., 2025).

AI is increasingly being used for postimplant surveillance. Acoustic and flow signal analysis from implantable heart valves, integrated with wearable monitoring systems, allows the early detection of valve degeneration, thrombosis, or endocarditis. These systems can alert clinicians and patients to subclinical complications before traditional symptoms or echocardiographic findings appear (Fritzsche et al., 2004; Lansac et al., 2025). AI-enhanced echocardiography platforms, such as those developed by Caption Health and Ultromics, can support nonexpert providers in community settings to assess valve function accurately, enabling timely referral and treatment (Upton & Strom, 2025; Akerman et al., 2025; Asch et al., 2022).

9.2.1.2 Left ventricular assist devices: evolution, impact, and patient outcomes

Left ventricular assist devices (LVADs) are pumps used to support the failing heart. They are transformative interventions in the management of end-stage heart failure. Heart failure is a common condition affecting over 64 million individuals globally and accounts for immense morbidity, mortality, and healthcare expenditure (Ødegaard et al., 2020). LVADs were initially developed as a technology to bridge patients with severe heart failure to heart transplantation. LVADs have evolved into durable, long-term therapies for patients who are ineligible for transplant, forming the foundation of destination therapy (Antonopoulos et al., 2024). In patients with severe heart failure, cardiac transplantation has been shown to provide considerable benefit. Since 1967, in excess of 140,000 total heart transplants have been performed, and 1-year survival is 81%; the annual mortality is 4% per year thereafter (Khush et al., 2018). The supply of donor hearts is limited, and demand exceeds the supply of donor hearts. Research has focused on mechanical circulatory support for patients with severe heart failure (Chaudhri, 2019).

The first-generation LVADs, such as Thoratec HeartMate I, were large, pulsatile-flow devices, externally located and prone to infection and mechanical failure. The development of electrically driven, miniaturized continuous-flow LVADs, namely, HeartMate II, marked a turning point in internal implantation, durability, miniaturization, and hemodynamic stability (McDonagh et al., 2021). Subsequent iterations, including the HeartMate 3 (Abbott), introduced fully magnetically levitated centrifugal pumps, significantly reducing shear stress, hemolysis, and thrombosis risks (Krabatsch et al., 2017).

HeartMate 3 is the dominant device in global clinical use, backed by robust data from the MOMENTUM 3 trial, which demonstrated superior survival free from disabling stroke or device reoperation compared to the earlier HeartMate 2 (Mehra, Goldstein, et al., 2022; Chatterjee et al., 2018). The CE Mark trial follow-up results of HeartMate 3 implantation showed high patient survival rates of 98%, 92%, 81%, and 74% at 1 month, 6 months, 1 year, and 2 years postimplantation. The trial period showed low postoperative complications such as thrombosis, bleeding, stroke, and infection. No pump thrombosis or malfunction was detected during the follow-up. Gastrointestinal bleeding was found to be 12% and 20% at 1 and 2 years postimplantation, respectively. Total overall stroke rates were 18% and 24% at 1 and 2 years' time points, respectively. VAD implantation-associated infection rates were 48% and 52% at 1 year and 2 years postimplantation (Schmitto et al., 2017).

LVADs have redefined survival expectations in advanced heart failure. One-year survival now exceeds 80%, with many patients achieving functional Class II status on the NYHA scale, returning to work, or engaging in physical activity. Furthermore, recent data support improved health-related quality of life with significant gains in mobility, symptom burden, and independence (Lesyuk et al., 2018; Mehra, Nayak, et al., 2022).

LVADs may allow reverse remodeling, which is partial recovery of left ventricular structure and function, in addition to providing support. A small subset of patients, particularly younger individuals with nonischemic cardiomyopathies, can achieve sufficient myocardial recovery to allow device explantation (Birks et al., 2020; Bonios et al., 2018). Cardiac transplantation, nonetheless, is still the best long-term therapy for patients with medically refractory end-stage heart failure (Lund et al., 2016). It is a durable treatment with 90 % one year survival and a median survival of 10–16 years. With further improvements in technology, in particular with the development of fully implantable systems, it is expected that survival with LVADs will exceed that of cardiac transplantation (Pya et al., 2019).

Driveline infections (DLI) are an important cause of device attrition. A metaanalysis of 21 studies (5393 patients) reported a 6-month DLI rate of 11.9% for HeartMate 3, compared to 9.1% and 7.2% for the Heartware HVAD and HeartMate II, respectively. Extrapolating to 1 year and considering additional registry data, DLIs in continuous-flow VADs typically occur at rates of 10%–20% per patient year (Mehra, Goldstein, et al., 2022). Supporting registry data (INTERMACS, EUROMACS, IMACS, etc.) report 9%–11.2% per year for DLIs overall. HM3 sees approximately 11.9% at 6 months, which corresponds to roughly 20% per year in most clinical settings (Kirklin et al., 2017; Kormos et al., 2019; Molina et al., 2021; Teuteberg et al., 2013).

There is ongoing development of fully implantable LVADs that eliminate percutaneous DLIs, which are the main weaknesses of current systems. The FIVAD (Fully Implantable Ventricular Assist Device) program at Texas Heart Institute and other private R&D initiatives are pursuing wireless energy transfer and transcutaneous charging technologies. Calon Cardio UK MINIVAD is an emerging device with enormous potential. This device has been iteratively tested and optimized with computational flow analysis using Formula 1 technology (Westaby, 2022).

9.2.1.3 Artificial intelligence integration in left ventricular assist device management

Recent advances have focused on AI-enhanced LVAD management, particularly in predicting decompensation, early pump thrombosis, or DLI. AI models embedded within LVAD platforms, such as Abbott's HeartMate 3, use telemetry data to guide therapy optimization and reduce adverse events (Rogers et al., 2017). The HeartMate 3 LVAD by Abbott is the market-leading ventricular assist device for end-stage heart failure, incorporating advanced telemetry and self-regulating rotor dynamics through full magnetic levitation. AI integration has elevated its capabilities from mechanical support to proactive clinical monitoring (Nair, 2022). Telemetric data (flow, speed, power, pulsatility index) is analyzed using machine learning (ML). AI alerts pump thrombosis risk, low flow events, and early signs of right heart failure. Abbott's remote platform (Merlin.net) allows AI-based monitoring and alerts to heart failure clinics (Manyam et al., 2023). This integrates with mobile patient apps to track symptoms and fluid intake (Moscato et al., 2021; Quartieri et al., 2023). Next-generation prototypes aim for fully implantable wireless LVADs with AI to self-regulate pump output based on physiologic demand, for example, Calon Cardio UK MINIVAD.

9.2.1.4 Total artificial hearts

A total artificial heart (TAH) is a mechanical device that completely replaces the heart's ventricles and valves, performing both right and left heart functions in patients with end-stage biventricular heart failure. It provides pulsatile flow by pneumatic or electromechanical power systems to drive the pumps and includes sensors that adjust flow based on the patient's activity level. Unlike LVADs, which assist only one side of the heart, usually the left ventricle, TAHs provide full cardiac replacement after surgical removal of the native ventricles (cardiectomy). They are used mainly as a bridge to heart transplantation or, in very select cases, as destination therapy (Cook et al., 2015).

In 1969, Denton Cooley implanted the first TAH, the Liotta–Cooley device, in a human patient at the Texas Heart Institute. The patient survived for 64 hours before receiving a donor heart (Cooley et al., 1969). Subsequently, the Jarvik-7 became the first TAH approved for clinical use. In 1982, Dr. William DeVries implanted the Jarvik-7 in a patient with severe heart failure, who survived for 112 days (Devries et al., 1984). The device's durability and complications, including thromboembolism and infection, limited widespread use. There are two major TAH devices in use currently:

1. SynCardia TAH: FDA-approved and CE-marked TAH, originally based on the Jarvik-7 design. It replaces the native ventricles and is pneumatically driven, available in 50cc and 70cc versions to accommodate patient size. It has been used in over 2000 patients worldwide (Devries et al., 1984; Copeland et al., 2004; Molina et al., 2021).
2. CARMAT TAH (Aeson): A next-generation, bioprosthetic TAH with a self-regulating mechanism that mimics the native heart's physiology. It includes biological valves and sensors to adapt flow to the patient's activity level. The CARMAT TAH received CE marking in 2020 and early clinical use suggests improved biocompatibility and physiological control (Mohacsi & Leprince, 2014; Potapov et al., 2019).

TAHs are primarily indicated for patients with biventricular heart failure who are not candidates for durable LVAD therapy. These patients typically have severe right ventricular failure, postmyocardial infarct mechanical complications such as ventricular septal defect, restrictive or infiltrative cardiomyopathies, or complex congenital heart disease. Most cases involve use as a bridge to transplant, though destination therapy is being explored in limited settings where transplantation is contraindicated (Diyar et al., 2023). The INTERMACS (Interagency Registry for Mechanically Assisted Circulatory Support) classification system is used to assess severity and timing of intervention. TAHs are generally indicated in most severe INTERMACS categories and critically ill patients (Kormos et al., 2019; Teuteberg et al., 2013; Molina et al., 2021). Survival outcomes with TAH support vary by device and center experience. For the SynCardia TAH, bridge-to-transplant survival rates are approximately 79% at one year and 60%–70% at two years. The CARMAT TAH, though in early-phase clinical trials, has demonstrated promising survival and lower thrombogenicity and hemolysis compared to earlier devices. Common complications include bleeding, infection, stroke, and device malfunction, although CARMAT shows reductions in adverse events (Mohacsi & Leprince, 2014). TAHs remain a niche therapy for patients with biventricular heart failure who lack other options. As technology advances and biocompatibility improves, TAHs may play an increasing role in end-stage heart failure management in destination therapy.

9.2.1.5 CARMAT Aeson total artificial heart

The CARMAT Aeson TAH is a TAH system, which provides a long-term, biocompatible, fully implantable alternative to donor heart transplantation. It is hydraulically driven, with dual silicone-oil diaphragms mimicking native heart chambers, driven by miniature motors and hydraulic fluid. The inner membranes and valves are lined with bovine pericardium, which promotes haemocompatibility and reduces thrombosis risk. Embedded pressure sensors balance output between left and right chambers, dynamically modulating stroke volume and rate, mimicking the physiological Frank–Starling mechanism (Yokota et al., 2024). It has an external controller and battery pack to provide power and patient mobility. This device was designed and refined from 1993 onwards by Professor Alain Carpentier and Matra Defense. Initial trials in man in 2013 demonstrated around 70% six month survival in 10-patient cohorts, with zero disabling strokes, GI bleeding, or DLIs (SynCardia ~54%–62%). The EFICAS Study (Europe), reported in early 2024, showed 49 of 52 planned implants completed, with interim success at 75% survival at six months (Han, 2021). The CE-mark is anticipated in 2025. The first U.S. FDA Early Feasibility Study (EFS) implant was performed at Duke in 2021 (Han, 2021). The FDA has approved the second cohort of 7 more patients, with expected recruitment in late 2025, and is aiming for pre-market approval (PMA) submission in 2027. As of Q1 2025, 108 implants have been done in Europe. Aeson offers near-physiologic perfusion (4.3–7.3 L/min) with physiological pulsation and autoregulation (Schroder et al., 2023). Research shows minimal hemolysis and thrombosis with excellent biocompatibility. R&D is ongoing with enhanced controller algorithms, wireless power, and AI-driven pump adjustments based on sensor networks and patient activity. CARMAT has faced financial pressure, with recent Reuters reports indicating insolvency risk due to the need for €3.5 M in funding by June 2025. Its commercial rollout in Europe is contingent on EFICAS results (Lille, n.d.) and reimbursement, while U.S. expansion hinges on FDA PMA approval. If successful, it may offer a durable mechanical alternative to donor hearts for high-risk heart failure patients.

9.2.2 Electrophysiology devices

9.2.2.1 Pacemakers, defibrillators, and catheter ablation systems

Pacemakers are the oldest forms of implantable cardiac technology, first deployed in the 1950s (Weirich et al., 1957). They were designed to correct bradyarrhythmias via fixed-rate pacing. They have evolved into highly programmable, bi-directional communication systems that adapt to patient physiology (Koulouris & Cascella, 2025). EP is an important field of modern cardiology, providing diagnostic modalities and therapeutic interventions for heart rhythm disorders and heart failure. There are new miniaturized, intelligent, and remote-enabled EP devices, pacemakers, automatic implantable cardioverter-defibrillators, and catheter ablation systems. These technologies prolong survival and significantly improve the quality of life for patients with AF, ventricular arrhythmias, or advanced conduction disease.

Leadless pacemakers, such as the Micra system by Medtronic and Aveir by Abbott (Nakano et al., 2025), are implanted directly into the right ventricle via transcatheter delivery. This eliminates surgical pockets in the chest wall and leads, which are associated with infection, lead failure, and venous occlusion (El-Chami et al., 2016). Clinical trials show comparable safety and pacing efficacy with fewer complications compared to a traditional dual-chamber system (Andreae et al., 2025). Dual-chamber leadless pacing is being developed, where multiple units communicate wirelessly within the heart. Abbott's Aveir DR system, approved in 2023, was the first and is expected to result in completely leadless, synchronized pacing (Nakano et al., 2025).

Modern pacemakers incorporate adaptive algorithms that adjust pacing based on sensed physical activity, respiration, and heart rate variability (HRV). Advanced systems also predict the onset of AF or heart failure decompensation using AI-derived signal analytics. Boston Scientific's SmartCRT optimizes lead configuration dynamically, improving synchrony in cardiac resynchronization therapy (García-Bolao et al., 2025). AI plays a central role in continuous rhythm monitoring, early decompensation detection, and predictive analytics. Devices upload data to cloud-based platforms that apply ML to detect impending heart failure exacerbation, new-onset AF, lead malfunction, or battery depletion. Patients may benefit from proactive management, reducing admissions to the hospital, emergency visits, and monitoring costs (Svennberg et al., 2025). Consumer wearables such as Apple Watch are expanding screening and data collection to millions of people.

9.2.2.2 Implantable defibrillators: preventing sudden cardiac death

Implantable defibrillators (ICDs) are implanted in patients at risk for life-threatening ventricular arrhythmias. These devices sense life-threatening rhythms such as ventricular tachycardia (VT) or ventricular fibrillation. They deliver electrical shocks or anti-tachycardia pacing (ATP) to restore normal rhythm (Demir et al., 2025; Kołodziejczak et al., 2017; Svennberg et al., 2025).

ICDs normally require transvenous leads, which result in lifetime risks of thrombosis and infections. The subcutaneous ICD (S-ICD), such as the EMBLEM S-ICD System by Boston Scientific, avoids venous implantation (Hrymniak et al., 2025). The defibrillation coil is placed in a subcutaneous pocket, reducing infection risk and making it suitable for younger or high-risk patients. New systems are incorporating ATP as well (Svennberg et al., 2025).

AI-driven detection algorithms are used by ICDs to distinguish between benign and malignant rhythms, reducing inappropriate shocks. SmartShock Medtronic uses a composite of rhythm discrimination tools, which include rate, onset, stability, and morphology analyses, to reduce false positives by 70% (Svennberg et al., 2025; Tjong & Koop, 2018). Integration with cloud-based platforms such as CareLink and Latitude allows remote interrogation, threshold adjustments, and alerts clinicians in near real-time of arrhythmias.

9.2.2.3 Catheter ablation systems

Ablation systems are used for AF, supraventricular tachycardias, and certain VT. These treat arrhythmogenic foci or disrupt aberrant conduction pathways via radiofrequency (RF) or cryoablation energy.

Advanced EP labs deploy AI-enhanced 3D electroanatomical mapping systems, such as CARTO 3 (Biosense Webster), EnSite Precision (Abbott), and Rhythmia (Boston Scientific) (Rattka et al., 2025; Yokota et al., 2025; Ballı et al., 2024; Costea et al., 2025). These platforms integrate electrical signals, anatomical data, and real-time navigation to create high-resolution maps of the heart to guide ablation catheter placement. AI-based algorithms identify low-voltage areas, complex fractionated electrograms, and rotors critical to sustaining arrhythmias, which are targets for ablation. The LATITUDE system combines ML to track lesion completeness and transmurality to guide durable pulmonary vein isolation.

9.2.3 Hemodynamic implants and shunting technologies

Hemodynamic regulation plays a critical role in the management of chronic heart failure, pulmonary hypertension, and neurocardiogenic syndromes. Current drug therapies may often reach a ceiling in efficacy in advanced-stage patients. A new class of implantable hemodynamic devices (Svennberg et al., 2025) and interatrial shunting technologies has emerged. These improve outcomes by physically modulating the circulatory system and altering autonomic balance. Examples include interatrial shunts, venous modulators, and neurostimulators, which are AI-integrated or feedback-responsive.

The V-Wave Ventura Interatrial Shunt is a catheter-delivered, self-expanding nitinol device that creates a controlled opening between the left and right atria. It offloads elevated left atrial pressure (LAP) in patients with heart failure with preserved or reduced ejection fraction (HFpEF/HFrEF) (Stone et al., 2024). The V-wave device allows a small volume of blood to flow from the left to the right atrium during periods of high LAP, effectively decompressing the left atrium, reducing pulmonary congestion, and improving symptoms. The pivotal RELIEVE-HF trial (2020–24) showed promising results in a subgroup of HFrEF patients, with significant improvements in NYHA functional class, 6-minute walk distance, quality of life metrics (KCCQ score), and reduced hospitalization rates for decompensated HF. This benefit was more limited in HFpEF populations, safety endpoints were met, and no device thrombosis or systemic embolization was observed (Rodés-Cabau et al., 2024; Reed et al., 2024). V-Wave has been integrated with remote LAP monitoring platforms. AI-enabled algorithms allow dynamic flow modulation in next-generation implants, creating closed-loop systems that respond to real-time hemodynamic changes.

9.2.3.1 Neuroresponsive implants for cardiovascular and psychiatric modulation

Vagal stimulation reduces AF burden by improving autonomic tone. Early clinical trials show reductions in paroxysmal AF episodes, particularly in patients with high sympathetic drive (Krishna & Fasano, 2024; Karatela et al., 2023). It treats resistant hypertension via baroreceptor activation, reducing systemic vascular resistance. Its system tracks anxiety and emotional stress markers and tunes neurostimulation to reduce sympathetic arousal. Early pilots indicate improvements in generalized anxiety disorder and panic symptoms in patients with arrhythmia or palpitations. Parasym is an investigational device in the United States. It uses multi-sensor fusion to create a personalized autonomic profile for each user. The system can detect autonomic imbalance (e.g., excessive sympathetic tone), predict arrhythmic or hypertensive events, and deliver tailored neuromodulation in response. Parasym is developing a closed-loop implantable system for treating disorders linked to autonomic dysregulation, resistant hypertension, AF, anxiety, and depression (Fang et al., 2016). The core system comprises an implantable neurostimulation lead targeting vagal or baroreceptor pathways, a biometric sensor array measuring HRV, blood pressure, respiratory rate, and galvanic skin response. It is partnered with a cloud-based AI engine that analyses physiologic and behavioral patterns to dynamically adjust stimulation parameters. The device is autonomous, adjusting stimulation amplitude, pulse width, and frequency based on patient state, with clinician oversight through a secure portal. Neuromodulation systems integrate with digital therapeutics (CBT apps) and wearables. AI engines enable subscription-based neuromodulation-as-a-service models, enhancing scalability while collecting real-world data for regulatory validation and pharma partnerships. These systems can be paired with digital CBT tools and wearables (e.g., Oura Ring, Apple Watch) for behavioral reinforcement. Sooma Medical has received FDA breakthrough device designation for its innovative at-home depression treatment device. Wave Neuroscience, a non-invasive neuromodulation Magnetic EEG Resonance Therapy (MeRT) system, also received Breakthrough Device Designation from the U.S. Food and Drug Administration (FDA) for adjunctive treatment of Post-Traumatic Stress Disorder (Park, 2023).

Adaptive implants that monitor and respond to real-time physiology to modulate therapy dynamically are being developed. These include adjustable shunt valves (e.g., for pulmonary hypertension), smart nerve stimulators for arrhythmia and anxiety cotreatment and implantable baroreflex stimulators integrated with cloud-based AI dashboards (Mas-Peiro et al., 2025; Perez et al., 2019; Strik et al., 2023; Mas-Peiro et al., 2025).

9.2.3.2 Artificial intelligence in pediatric cardiology

9.2.3.2.1 Artificial intelligence and the Fontan circulation

The Fontan operation, first described in 1971, is a palliative strategy for single-ventricle congenital heart disease, redirecting systemic venous return directly to the pulmonary arteries without a subpulmonary ventricle (Luo et al., 2025; Fontan & Baudet, 1971). Survival has improved substantially; however, morbidity remains high, with long-term outcomes limited by arrhythmias, Fontan failure, and Fontan-associated liver disease (FALD) (Pundi et al., 2015; D'Udekem et al., 2014; Rychik et al., 2019).

The Fontan Outcomes Registry for Collaborative Evidence (FORCE) incorporates more than 4700 patients across 45 centers, linking clinical, imaging, and outcomes data (Reddy et al., 2020). FORCE integrates nearly 7000 cardiac MRI and CT scans processed through deep-learning, automating ventricular segmentation, volumetric analysis, and 4D flow quantification (Yao et al., 2024; Frieberg et al., 2021; Liu et al., 2022). These AI pipelines provide reproducible measures and feed predictive models stratifying risk of Fontan failure, arrhythmia, and FALD (Liu et al., 2022). Radiomics and deep-learning approaches applied to MRI and CT can stage fibrosis, quantify congestion, and detect early hepatocellular carcinoma in FALD more accurately than visual inspection. Single-cell multiomics integrated with imaging phenotypes have begun to reveal pathways driving fibrosis and inflammation, highlighting therapeutic targets (Hu et al., 2024).

9.2.3.2.2 AI-enhanced electrocardiography

Parallel advances in AI applied to ECG analysis are reshaping pediatric diagnostics. A convolutional neural network trained on more than 92,000 ECG–echocardiogram pairs demonstrated robust performance in detecting left ventricular (LV) dysfunction, hypertrophy, and dilation, with AUROCs up to 0.94 and negative predictive values of 99% (Mayourian, Asztalos, et al., 2025; Mayourian, Geggel, et al., 2025; Mayourian, van Boxtel, et al., 2024).

Explainability methods identified physiologically plausible features: lateral T-wave inversion predicting LV dysfunction, deep S waves in V1–V2 with tall R waves in V6 indicating hypertrophy, and tall R waves across V4–V6 predicting dilation (Mayourian et al., 2025).

Further studies confirmed consistency across congenital cohorts, detecting biventricular dysfunction and mortality risk in repaired tetralogy of Fallot, and identifying secundum atrial septal defects (Mayourian et al., 2025; Mayourian, Gearhart, et al., 2024; Mayourian et al., 2025). AI applied to ECG images, rather than raw waveforms, achieved strong external performance, broadening deployment in resource-limited contexts (Sangha et al., 2023).

AI-enhanced ECG offers an inexpensive, non-invasive, and scalable screening modality capable of triaging echocardiography, accelerating diagnosis, and extending access to pediatric cardiology expertise in community and emergency settings (Sen & Ramakrishnan, 2024; Ren et al., 2025).

9.3 Diagnostics and monitoring innovations

9.3.1 Wearables, AI-enhanced imaging, and remote patient monitoring

Advances in diagnostics and monitoring technologies are enabling continuous predictive diagnostics outside clinical settings. AI is enabling the integration of data from sensors, imaging platforms, and patient-reported outcomes (PROs) into clinically valid insights. Wearables are becoming validated diagnostic tools capable of detecting arrhythmias, respiratory disorders, and metabolic decompensation (Perez et al., 2019). They serve as early warning systems, generating continuous physiological data by AI algorithms. Apple Watch Series 6–9 uses single-lead ECG and photoplethysmography for AF detection, validated in the Apple Heart Study (Perez et al., 2019). These wearables may integrate with EHR systems and physician dashboards through secure application programming interfaces, enabling physician-directed remote patient monitoring.

9.3.1.1 Cardiac telemetry and implantable monitors

Cardiac rhythm monitoring is especially advanced; Boston Scientific's LUX-Dx (Kahwash et al., 2025) and Biotronik's BioMonitor III provide long-term, subcutaneous ECG monitoring with wireless transmission to cloud-based dashboards (Lau et al., 2023). These insertable cardiac monitors (ICMs) are used for AF detection, especially after stroke, cryptogenic syncope investigation, and long QT and Brugada syndrome risk monitoring. They enable earlier detection of arrhythmias than conventional Holter monitors, reducing stroke risk and hospitalization rates (Lau et al., 2023).

Philips' BioTel Heart, Current Health (Best Buy Health), iRhythm's ZioXT (Schwennesen et al., 2024) combine wearable devices with AI algorithms to track pulmonary congestion, weight trends, respiratory rate, blood pressure, and HRV. This allows for decompensation alerts up to 7–10 days before overt symptoms, enabling preemptive diuretic therapy or clinic review and dramatically reducing readmission.

9.3.2 Imaging and procedural guidance

9.3.2.1 Artificial intelligence as the second observer in medical imaging

The integration of AI into imaging workflows has improved accuracy, speed, reproducibility, and access. AI is increasingly used to act as the second observer in medical imaging. Cardiac ultrasound, such as Caption Health (acquired by GE HealthCare) and Ultromics (Upton & Strom, 2025), uses deep learning to interpret echocardiograms for ejection fraction, strain patterns, and valvular disease, with diagnostic accuracy comparable to expert cardiologists. This enables access to echo-based diagnostics in primary care, remote clinics, and low-resource settings. AI is increasingly used in coronary CT angiography for plaque characterization (e.g., Cleerly Health), cardiac MRI interpretation for fibrosis and perfusion mapping (e.g., Arterys, Aidoc), nuclear cardiology image reconstruction and automated quantification (e.g., Syntermed) (Okwuosa et al., 2011; Williams et al., 2013). AI allows imaging to become more predictive and integrated by reducing inter-observer variability and enhancing diagnostic confidence.

Ultromics' EchoGo platform uses deep learning to analyze uploaded echocardiograms for assessment of global longitudinal strain, left ventricular ejection fraction, diastolic function, and valvular abnormalities. It can predict heart failure with preserved ejection fraction (HFpEF), assess myocardial toxicity in oncology patients, and identify early systolic dysfunction in asymptomatic individuals. It is FDA-cleared for heart failure risk prediction (Upton & Strom, 2025; Akerman et al., 2023). It improves diagnostic consistency across institutions and supports AI-powered clinical decision-making, notably in heart failure clinics (Malins et al., 2025; Akerman et al., 2025).

9.3.3 Predictive analytics and decision support

Data from wearables and imaging platforms is increasingly integrated with electronic health records (EHRs), PROs, and environmental and behavioral data. This supports AI-driven risk stratification, enabling early interventions in high-risk patients. QardioMD and validic impact integrate remote BP and ECG monitoring with predictive alerts. Eko AI analyses heart sounds from digital stethoscopes to detect murmurs, valvular disease, and heart failure with >90% sensitivity. Aidoc flags acute findings on radiology studies, such as pulmonary embolism or aortic dissection, directly in the PACS system for expedited triage (Brin et al., 2025).

Wearables and diagnostics also serve as generators of real-world data, supporting drug efficacy and adherence monitoring, value-based contracting, and population health analytics. Health systems are increasingly adopting these tools to monitor chronic disease populations at scale. Kaiser Permanente's AI-enabled RPM program for hypertension and diabetes has reduced emergency visits by 25% over 18 months (Gunn et al., 2024).

Practice Focus: What AI-Driven Devices Mean for Clinicians and Health Systems

For clinicians, AI-integrated devices offer earlier detection of deterioration, improved diagnostic confidence, and reduced cognitive burden through automated triage and decision support. However, effective adoption requires trust, transparency, and clear delineation of clinical responsibility. Human-in-the-loop design—where clinicians can interpret, validate, and override AI outputs—remains essential to safe practice.

For healthcare organizations, AI-enabled devices demand new operational capabilities, including data governance, cybersecurity, workflow redesign, and continuous performance monitoring. Health systems must invest in digital literacy, multidisciplinary governance structures, and post-market surveillance processes to ensure these technologies improve outcomes without exacerbating inequities or operational complexity.

9.4 Commercialization and regulatory strategies

FDA regulatory pathway for medical devices includes EFS and pivotal studies, which are key stages in the pre-market approval (PMA) or 510(k) process for moderate- to high-risk devices (Class II/III). These studies serve as stepping stones on the route to market in the United States (Table 9.1).

An EFS is a limited clinical investigation of a device early in development, typically before the device design has been finalized, for a specific indication (e.g., innovative device for a new or established intended use, repurposing of a currently available device for a novel clinical application). It may be used to evaluate the device design concept with respect to initial clinical safety and device functionality in a small number of subjects (fewer than 10 initial subjects) when this information cannot practically be provided through additional nonclinical assessments or when appropriate nonclinical tests are unavailable. FDA approval of an IDE application for an EFS, including certain first-in-human (FIH) studies, may be based on less nonclinical data than would be expected for a traditional feasibility or a pivotal study. This is because EFS are only appropriate when additional nonclinical testing would not provide the information needed to advance the developmental process. Information obtained from an EFS may guide device modifications. An EFS does not necessarily involve the first clinical use of a device.

Table 9.1 Food and Drug Administration (FDA) device pathway trials.

Stage	Description	Purpose
Presubmission (Q-Sub)	Informal feedback from FDA before formal submissions	Derisk study and align with FDA expectations
Early feasibility study	First-in-human study in the U.S.	To collect initial safety, performance, and design data
Pivotal study	Statistically powered trial	To generate definitive evidence of safety and effectiveness
Regulatory submission	510(k), de novo, or PMA	To obtain market authorization
Post-market surveillance	Registries, 522 studies, etc.	Ongoing safety/performance monitoring

A FIH study is a type of study in which a device for a specific indication is evaluated for the first time in human subjects. A traditional feasibility study is a clinical investigation that is commonly used to capture preliminary safety and effectiveness information on a near-final or final device design to adequately plan an appropriate pivotal study.

A pivotal study is then done. This is a clinical investigation designed to collect definitive evidence of the safety and effectiveness of a device for a specified intended use, typically in a statistically justified number of subjects. It may or may not be preceded by an early and/or a traditional feasibility study.

9.4.1 US FDA pathway overview: medical device development route to market

9.4.1.1 Early feasibility study

This is a clinical investigation of a device early in development, often prior to final design freeze, to evaluate the device concept in a small number of subjects (typically ≤15–30 patients). This requires Investigational Device Exemption (IDE) submission under 21 CFR Part 812. The FDA's EFS Program facilitates early access to FIH studies in the US (Table 9.2).

9.4.1.1.1 Key features

Submission requirements:

IDE application includes service description and development status, clinical protocol and justification, risk analysis, preclinical data, IRB approval, informed consent documentation: FDA EFS Guidance (2013).

Table 9.2 Early feasibility study- key features.

Element	Description
Objective	Explore design iterations, proof-of-concept, safety profile
Sample size	Small (≤15–30 subjects), may expand
Design flexibility	Allows protocol/design iteration under FDA oversight
Sites	Often 1–3 centers with strong clinical/research governance
Data use	To inform pivotal trial design, device modifications

Table 9.3 Pivotal studies—key features.

Attribute	Description
Study design	Prospective, multicentre, randomized or single-arm
Sample size	Statistically powered (hundreds of subjects)
Endpoints	Safety and effectiveness based on clinically meaningful outcomes
Duration	Often ≥12 months follow-up
Regulatory role	Forms primary evidence in PMA, de novo, or 510(k)
IDE requirement	Yes (same IDE process as EFS, but more extensive)

9.4.1.2 Pivotal studies

Pivotal studies provide primary clinical evidence needed for FDA clearance/approval. Typically, this is for pre-market approval PMA: Required for Class III devices. An FDA Class III medical device is a high-risk device that is regulated by the US Food and Drug Administration (FDA). These devices are typically life-supporting, life-sustaining, or pose a potential unreasonable risk of illness or injury. Due to the high risk associated with these devices, they require pre-marketPMA from the FDA before they can be marketed in the United States (Table 9.3).

Submission to FDA Pivotal IDE includes a detailed statistical analysis plan, inclusion/exclusion criteria, monitoring, adverse event reporting, and data safety plans, manufacturing data (often more complete than EFS). Real-World Examples include transcatheter mitral valve repair: EFS. Abbott MitraClip FIH trials were done in limited centers under IDE (Lindman et al., 2023). This was followed by iterative device optimization and procedural technique refinement. The pivotal trial (e.g., COAPT trial) was a randomized, multicentre trial with >600 patients (Stone et al., 2023). The FDA PMA was based on this pivotal data.

9.4.1.3 Navigating market access for AI-driven devices and diagnostics

The integration of AI into medical devices and diagnostics has introduced a host of opportunities and complexity in how these technologies are developed, regulated, reimbursed, and brought to market. AI-driven technologies are inherently iterative, data-dependent, and software-enhanced, functioning at the intersection of hardware, software, and services. Successful commercialization requires navigating a landscape that includes regulatory innovation, value-based pricing, and strategic partnerships (Tettey-Engmann et al., 2025).

9.4.1.4 The digital and device regulatory framework

To accommodate software-based and AI-augmented devices, the U.S. Food and Drug Administration (FDA) has introduced several key programs (FDA, 2021, 2019):

FDA Breakthrough Devices Program (BDP) expedites the review of devices that provide more effective treatment or diagnosis of life-threatening or irreversibly debilitating conditions. It is particularly suited for novel technologies such as V-Wave's interatrial shunt. The breakthrough designation provides early interaction with FDA teams, rolling data submission, and priority review. For standalone AI algorithms or cloud-based analytics (e.g., Caption Health, Aidoc), the FDA classifies them as Software as a Medical Device (SaMD). The agency is developing a Pre-Certification Pilot regulatory pathway that assesses the developer's software lifecycle quality rather than treating each software version as a separate product. In the European Union, the new Medical Device Regulation (MDR) enforces stricter rules for clinical evidence, post-market surveillance, and cybersecurity. AI-driven devices must now undergo robust clinical performance evaluations, even if they are software-only solutions (Proposal for a Regulation of the European Parliament and of the Council Laying Down Harmonised Rules on Artificial Intelligence Act and Amending Certain Union Legislative Acts 2021, n.d.).

9.4.1.5 Reimbursement pathways and value demonstration

Many medical devices lack established billing codes or DRG alignment, requiring novel reimbursement strategies. This is particularly true for AI software tools (e.g., image interpretation, arrhythmia prediction), integrated device + software packages (e.g., RPM platforms), and digital therapeutics (e.g., neuromodulation with behavioral feedback). CPT and HCPCS Codes have been created for remote patient monitoring (e.g., CPT 99453–99458) and AI-assisted imaging analysis (Category III CPT codes). Their uptake depends on payer education and clinical utility data. NTAP (New Technology Add-On Payment). In the U.S., CMS offers temporary add-on payments for innovative technologies under Medicare. The HeartMate 3 LVAD, for example, received NTAP status based on the MOMENTUM 3 data. Bundled Payments and Value-Based Models. Devices like V-Wave's shunt or HeartLogic monitoring must demonstrate reductions in readmissions, emergency visits, or downstream costs. RWE from RPM programs and health economics studies is increasingly used to negotiate outcomes-based contracts.

9.4.1.6 Strategic partnerships and pharma-diagnostics convergence

Many device companies are establishing partnerships with pharmaceutical firms or digital health providers to expand access and integrate into broader treatment paradigms. Parasym positions its neuroadaptive system as a digital companion to psychiatric and cardiovascular drug regimens, potentially improving drug adherence and measuring biomarker response (https://www.parasym.co/about-parasym.html). Ultromics partners with pharma companies to identify heart failure subtypes likely to respond to novel therapies (Akerman et al., 2023, 2025). Medtronic + Fitbit pilot programs aim to integrate wearable data into chronic disease management pathways. This convergence reflects a shift toward diagnostic-therapeutic ecosystems rather than single-point solutions. The capital environment for AI-enabled diagnostics and devices has been robust. V-Wave raised ~$130 M before its $1.7B acquisition by Johnson & Johnson. Lucid Therapeutics closed a $65 M Series B in 2023, backed by digital health and device investors. Aidoc, HeartFlow, and Eko each secured $50M–$150 M in funding rounds as they scale regulatory approval and commercial infrastructure. Investors are increasingly drawn to companies with regulatory momentum (e.g., FDA BDP or CE mark under MDR), proprietary AI pipelines, integrated device + cloud platforms, and real-world data capabilities.

9.5 Ethical and regulatory challenges: bias, transparency, and accountability in AI-driven medical devices

There are significant ethical and regulatory challenges with the integration of adaptive AI into medical devices. AI-enabled devices, especially those using ML, are designed to evolve through real-time data, diverging from static software and hardware medical devices. This dynamic behavior complicates traditional regulatory frameworks, which were not originally developed for self-learning systems (Kolfschooten and EU, 2021; Kolfschooten, 2023). AI systems often operate as “black boxes,” providing accurate outputs without interpretable reasoning. Explainable AI techniques aim to generate human-understandable justifications for algorithmic predictions. Technical evaluations of explainability (e.g., faithfulness to the model’s actual reasoning) and clinical relevance remain difficult to standardize (Sadeghi et al., 2024). This lack of interpretability can erode clinician trust, inhibit adoption, and compromise informed consent. Ethical concerns are further amplified by algorithmic bias, which propagates disparities in healthcare delivery. Bias arises from imbalanced training data or systemic oversights, resulting in poorer performance for underrepresented populations. AI diagnostic tools trained predominantly on high-quality academic center data, for example, may underperform in community hospitals with lower imaging resolution (Koçak et al., 2025).

The U.S. Food and Drug Administration (FDA) has introduced the Predetermined Change Control Plan (PCCP), enabling preapproval of algorithmic modifications within defined boundaries. This supports the safe adaptation of AI-based devices while maintaining regulatory oversight. The European Union's Artificial Intelligence Act introduces a layered risk-based approach, placing high-risk medical AI under enhanced scrutiny.

Post-market surveillance is critical to identifying and mitigating failures. Continuous learning AI models require innovation to ensure that evolving AI performance does not degrade or diverge from intended clinical outcomes. Regulatory authorities increasingly advocate for RWE frameworks, incorporating patient registries, clinician feedback, and longitudinal performance monitoring. The FDA and WHO emphasize lifecycle oversight as essential to safeguard safety, efficacy, and public trust. A comprehensive risk management framework is necessary to anticipate hazards specific to AI, such as dataset shift, algorithmic drift, and adversarial attacks. Traditional risk assessment tools designed for mechanical or deterministic software do not adequately address these AI-specific threats (Lekadir et al., 2025).

In the event of an adverse outcome from an AI-based device, accountability and liability may be unclear. It may not be entirely clear whether liability lies with the developer, the device manufacturer, or the clinician who trusted the output. This affects legal responsibility and the ethical doctrine of professional judgment and patient autonomy. Shared accountability frameworks and transparent clinical decision-support interfaces may help distribute responsibility without diffusing it (WHO, 2021; Zhou & Gattinger, 2024; Overgaard et al., 2023).

Informed consent is also affected. AI-enabled diagnostics or therapeutics may rely on data-driven associations that are unintelligible to both patient and provider. Without meaningful explanation, informed consent may be challenging to obtain. New models of layered or dynamic consent, where patients are informed about algorithmic updates, may provide a more ethical alternative. AI-based medical devices are frequently deployed in well-funded, urban hospitals but are absent from rural or under-resourced settings. This creates the risk of exacerbating existing health inequities. Global equity in AI deployment requires transparent performance benchmarking across diverse clinical contexts and patient populations. Ethical implementation also hinges on professional acceptance. Clinicians must understand, trust, and be able to override AI outputs when necessary. Seamless integration of AI into clinical workflows and decision trees is essential. Tools that explain recommendations, provide confidence metrics, and allow for clinician override are more likely to be used appropriately and ethically. Regulatory agencies, technical experts, ethicists, clinicians, and patient representatives must codevelop governance frameworks that protect patient rights without stifling innovation. The European Commission's High-Level Expert Group on AI represents important steps in this direction (EU Liability Rules for the Age of Artificial Intelligence March 2021 by the Authors for the Centre on, n.d.). The ethical and regulatory challenges of AI in medical devices require a system-wide approach that includes clear messaging and clarity of technical mechanisms, regulatory reform, robust surveillance, and fairness in deployment. These have to be systematically engaged with for AI to fully realize its transformative potential while remaining fully compliant with medical ethics.

9.6 Challenges and future outlook

AI holds enormous transformative potential for healthcare delivery. Its integration is impeded by critical clinical, regulatory, technical, and ethical challenges. One of the concerns is the limited wider utility of AI models, which are usually trained on relatively homogenous datasets. This results in diagnostic bias and reduced performance in diverse populations and real-world settings (Dankwa-Mullan, 2024). This raises concerns regarding the reproducibility and fairness of AI tools, especially in underrepresented patient groups. To address this, new multicentre clinical trials (e.g., via Caption Health and Ultromics) and federated learning approaches are emerging. These enable models to be trained across decentralized, diverse datasets and help preserve patient privacy. Regulatory agencies such as the FDA and EMA are moving toward harmonized performance metrics to standardize AI validation and enable trust.

Regulatory oversight remains another mission-critical process for adaptive algorithms that are continuously and periodically updated post-deployment. Current regulatory pathways for static algorithms are slow-moving and ill-suited to these dynamic systems. This raises concerns about version control, model drift, and interpretability. The FDA's Total Product Lifecycle framework incorporates prespecified algorithm change protocols, real-world performance monitoring, and developer accountability (FDA, 2021). In parallel, the EU's MDR mandates re-evaluation following significant change, potentially imposing additional compliance burdens on rapidly evolving AI tools.

AI systems introduce new vulnerabilities around data privacy, ownership, and ethical accountability. The EU's General Data Protection Regulation and the US Health Insurance Portability and Accountability Act provide foundational safeguards, and the WHO's Ethics Guidance on AI in Health addresses explainability, inclusivity, and equitable benefit-sharing (WHO, 2021). The future of ethical AI depends on human-in-the-loop systems that ensure clinical judgment remains paramount. The long-term trajectory for AI-enabled devices remains promising as stakeholders coalesce around shared standards for integration, reimbursement, and clinical adoption. Seamless incorporation into existing workflows is vitally important and mission critical (Palaniappan et al., 2024; Gurevich et al., 2023; Smith et al., 2024).

Many healthcare systems face barriers such as EHR fragmentation, alert fatigue, and clinician resistance. Solutions include HL7 FHIR-based APIs, human factors-informed design, and reimbursement models that reward AI-supported care (e.g., RPM CPT codes, NTAP) (Barbaria et al., 2023). Payers demand robust cost-effectiveness data, yet economic and policy uncertainties continue to limit uptake. This is especially the case in low- and middle-income countries. Emerging trends, which include autonomous implants, multimodal AI diagnostics, synthetic trial arms, and companion therapeutics, are creating a direction of travel toward predictive, preventive, and personalized medicine. AI-integrated devices are poised to become critical components of modern precision healthcare.

9.7 Conclusion

The integration of AI into medical devices and diagnostics is rapidly ongoing and an inflection point has been reached. AI is elevating these technologies from passive instruments to active agents of personalized care. They detect pathology, anticipate deterioration, guide interventions, and learn from patient outcomes in real time. Robust clinical validation, equitable access, ethical integrity, transparent regulation, and sustainable commercial models are essential to embed AI-enabled tools within standard clinical workflows. Addressing these challenges collaboratively is pivotal to transforming episodic, reactive care into a continuous, proactive ecosystem that allows for personalized, bespoke, precisely tailored care, which is also predictive and preventive.

Strategic Insight: From Discrete Devices to Continuous Care Ecosystems

AI-enabled medical devices are no longer isolated therapeutic tools; they are evolving into continuous care platforms that combine sensing, analytics, and intervention across the patient journey. Implantable devices, wearables, and diagnostic systems increasingly generate longitudinal data streams that inform predictive models, enabling earlier intervention, dynamic therapy adjustment, and proactive risk mitigation. This shift supports a transition from episodic, hospital-centered care toward decentralized, home-based, and outcome-driven models of healthcare delivery.

Strategically, this evolution reshapes value creation in the medical device sector. Competitive advantage now depends not only on hardware performance but also on data integration, algorithmic learning, regulatory adaptability, and interoperability with digital health ecosystems. Companies that successfully align device innovation with AI-driven analytics, real-world evidence generation, and reimbursement frameworks are positioned to become long-term partners in chronic disease management rather than single-product suppliers.

Key takeaways

- Medical devices and diagnostics are evolving from passive tools into intelligent, adaptive systems that support continuous, predictive, and personalized care.
- Artificial intelligence enables earlier detection of disease, improved monitoring, and real-time therapeutic adjustment across cardiovascular, neurological, and chronic conditions.
- Successful adoption of AI-driven devices depends on robust clinical validation, regulatory alignment, and human-centered design.
- Ethical governance, transparency, and equity are critical to sustaining trust and avoiding unintended disparities in AI-enabled healthcare.
- The future of medical devices lies in integrated diagnostic–therapeutic ecosystems, where devices, data, and decision support operate as a unified clinical infrastructure.

Editor's note

This chapter provides a technically rich and clinically grounded examination of how medical devices and diagnostics are being transformed through AI. Rather than treating AI as an abstract enabler, the author anchors innovation in real-world cardiovascular, EP, and diagnostic systems, illustrating how intelligence is embedded into devices that already shape everyday clinical practice.

From implantable circulatory support systems and EP platforms to AI-enhanced imaging, wearables, and remote monitoring infrastructures, the chapter demonstrates a decisive shift: devices are no longer passive instruments but adaptive participants in continuous care ecosystems. The discussion is strengthened by detailed attention to regulatory pathways, clinical validation, and post-market surveillance—areas often overlooked in future-oriented technology narratives.

Importantly, the chapter does not portray innovation as frictionless. Ethical accountability, algorithmic bias, explainability, and governance are treated as core design constraints rather than afterthoughts. This balanced perspective reinforces the book's broader message: sustainable healthcare innovation emerges at the intersection of clinical value, technological rigor, regulatory trust, and human judgment.

For readers, this chapter serves both as a state-of-the-art reference and as a strategic lens for understanding how AI-enabled devices will redefine patient care pathways, professional roles, and healthcare systems in the decade ahead.

Key takeaways

AI is transforming medical devices from reactive tools into predictive clinical partners. Implantable devices, wearables, and diagnostic platforms increasingly operate as intelligent systems capable of anticipating deterioration, supporting early intervention, and enabling continuous care beyond traditional clinical settings.

Clinical value emerges when intelligence is embedded into workflows, not layered on top of them. AI-enabled monitoring systems deliver impact only when integrated with clinician decision-making, multidisciplinary review processes, and human oversight—minimizing alert fatigue while maximizing actionable insight.

Device–diagnostic–pharma convergence is redefining precision medicine. The fusion of real-time device data, advanced diagnostics, and AI analytics enables individualized therapy selection, adaptive treatment adjustment, and outcome-driven care models across cardiovascular and chronic disease management.

Regulatory readiness and post-market surveillance are strategic enablers, not constraints. Successful AI-driven devices align innovation with lifecycle governance frameworks, RWE generation, and adaptive regulatory pathways to maintain safety, trust, and scalability.

Ethics, transparency, and equity determine long-term adoption. Addressing algorithmic bias, explainability, accountability, and access is essential for sustaining clinician trust and ensuring that AI-enabled devices improve outcomes across diverse populations.

The future of medical devices is human–AI collaboration. Intelligent systems augment clinical expertise rather than replace it—supporting clinicians in managing complexity while preserving professional judgment, patient autonomy, and compassionate care.

Mini case study vignette

From reactive monitoring to predictive care in advanced heart failure

Context: A large tertiary cardiac center in a high-income country manages a growing population of patients with advanced heart failure supported by implantable mechanical circulatory devices. Despite excellent surgical outcomes, the center faces persistent challenges related to unplanned readmissions, late detection of complications, and the burden of continuous outpatient monitoring.

The challenge: Clinical teams relied on scheduled follow-ups, patient-reported symptoms, and periodic device interrogations. Complications such as pump thrombosis, right heart failure, and infection were often detected after clinical deterioration, leading to emergency admissions and prolonged hospital stays. Clinicians expressed concern about alert fatigue from existing monitoring systems and limited confidence in interpreting complex telemetry streams.

The intervention: The center introduced an AI-enabled remote monitoring framework layered on top of existing implantable device telemetry. Continuous physiological signals (flow dynamics, power consumption, pulsatility indices, and patient-reported data via a mobile interface) were analyzed using machine-learning models trained on historical adverse-event patterns.

Rather than generating constant alerts, the system focused on risk trajectory prediction, flagging only clinically meaningful deviations from individualized baselines. Outputs were integrated into the heart failure clinic's workflow through a shared dashboard reviewed during weekly multidisciplinary meetings.

Outcomes: Within the first year of deployment:

Unplanned heart failure readmissions decreased significantly.

Clinicians reported earlier detection of device-related complications, often days before symptom onset.

Patient confidence improved, with many reporting a greater sense of safety and continuity of care.

Importantly, clinicians retained full decision authority; the AI system functioned strictly as a decision-support layer, not an autonomous controller.

Key insight: The case illustrates a central theme of this chapter: the clinical value of AI in medical devices lies not in replacing expertise, but in extending it across time, data, and uncertainty. When aligned with workflow, governance, and human oversight, intelligent devices can shift care from reactive rescue to proactive stability.

Learning activities

AI-enabled devices as continuous care platforms

Activity type: Individual (or pair work). **Estimated time:** 35–45 minutes. **Difficulty level:** Advanced (applied conceptualization). **Recommended placement:** After Section 3 (diagnostics and monitoring innovations)

Purpose

To help learners translate the chapter's content into a coherent "continuous care platform" logic, showing how devices + AI shift healthcare from episodic intervention to continuous prediction and proactive management.

Learning objectives

By completing this activity, learners will be able to:

Explain how AI transforms medical devices from standalone tools into continuous monitoring and decision-support platforms.

Identify the data pipeline (signals → analytics → clinical action) in a real device/diagnostic example from the chapter.

Evaluate clinical value and implementation requirements (workflow, governance, accountability).

Activity instructions

Select one system described in the chapter (choose one):

LVAD ecosystem (e.g., HeartMate 3 + telemetry + remote monitoring)

Implantable rhythm monitoring / ICM platforms

AI-enabled echo/imaging support (e.g., Caption Health / Ultromics)

Wearables + RPM (e.g., AF detection, remote HF monitoring)

Create a 1-page "Continuous Care Platform Map" with the following headings:

Clinical problem: What condition/event is targeted (e.g., HF decompensation, arrhythmia, valve degeneration)?

Inputs (data): What is measured? (signals, imaging, patient-reported data, etc.)

AI/analytics layer: What is predicted/detected/classified?

Decision pathway: Who acts on the output (patient/clinician/system) and how?

Outcome value: What improves (admissions, early detection, survival, QoL, cost)?

Implementation needs: Integration points (EHR/RPM dashboards), training, governance, and cybersecurity.

Add a short "risk & ethics" paragraph (120–180 words): Address **one bias risk**, **one explainability/trust issue**, and **one accountability question** relevant to your chosen system.

Deliverables

Deliverable A (Core): 1-page Continuous Care Platform Map (structured headings, bullet points allowed).

Deliverable B (short reflection): 120–180-word risk and ethics paragraph.

Suggested evaluation criteria (quick rubric)

Accuracy and relevance to chapter concepts (40%)

Clarity of the end-to-end pipeline (30%)

Realistic implementation/governance considerations (20%)

Quality of ethics reflection (10%)

Learning activity

Regulatory + market access simulation for an AI-driven device

Activity type: Team (3–5 learners). **Estimated time:** 45–60 minutes. **Difficulty level:** Expert (applied strategy and decision-making). **Recommended placement:** After Section 4 (commercialization and regulatory strategies)

Purpose

To train learners to think like device innovators and healthcare decision-makers by developing a structured route-to-market plan that integrates regulatory pathways, evidence strategy, and reimbursement logic for an AI-enabled device/diagnostic.

Learning objectives

By completing this activity, learners will be able to:

Distinguish between **EFS**, **pivotal studies**, and **post-market surveillance** requirements for high-risk and AI-enabled devices.

Propose an evidence strategy aligned with **FDA pathways** and the realities of AI iteration.

Identify reimbursement constraints and value demonstration logic (RPM codes, NTAP, outcomes-based contracts).

Activity instructions

Choose one use-case scenario (pick one):

Scenario A: AI-enabled implantable monitoring to predict HF decompensation

Scenario B: AI-guided ultrasound for nonspecialists in low-resource settings

Scenario C: Closed-loop neuromodulation for autonomic dysregulation (cardio + mental health overlap)

As a team, build a **2-page "Commercialization & Regulatory Brief"** containing: **(i) Product definition (short):** Intended use, target population, setting (hospital/home/community). **(ii) Regulatory strategy:**

Likely device classification (justify briefly)

Proposed trial sequence: **EFS → pivotal → post-market**

Key endpoints: safety + effectiveness (make them measurable)

One paragraph on AI-specific oversight (e.g., change control/lifecycle monitoring) **(iii) Market Access and Reimbursement:**

Who pays and why (payer logic)

What outcomes must be proven (reduced admissions, earlier detection, fewer strokes, etc.)

A short value proposition statement (max 80 words) **(iv) Risk and Ethics Snapshot:**

One bias risk and mitigation approach

One cybersecurity/privacy risk and mitigation approach

One accountability statement (who owns clinical decision responsibility)

Prepare a 3-minute pitch (spoken in class or recorded) summarizing your brief.

Deliverables

Deliverable A: 2-page commercialization and regulatory brief (structured with headings above).

Deliverable B: 3-minute pitch (slides optional; if slides used: max 3 slides).

References

Akerman, A. P., Porumb, M., Scott, C. G., Beqiri, A., Chartsias, A., Ryu, A. J., Hawkes, W., Huntley, G. D., Arystan, A. Z., Kane, G. C., Pislaru, S. V., Lopez-Jimenez, F., Gomez, A., Sarwar, R., O'Driscoll, J., Leeson, P., Upton, R., Woodward, G., & Pellikka, P. A. (2023). Automated echocardiographic detection of heart failure with preserved ejection fraction using artificial intelligence. *JACC: Advances, 2*(6), Available from https://doi.org/10.1016/j.jacadv.2023.100452, https://www.sciencedirect.com/journal/jacc-advances.

Akerman, A. P., Al-Roub, N., Angell-James, C., Cassidy, M. A., Thompson, R., Bosque, L., Rainer, K., Hawkes, W., Piotrowska, H., Leeson, P., Woodward, G., Pellikka, P. A., Upton, R., & Strom, J. B. (2025). External validation of artificial intelligence for detection of heart failure with preserved ejection fraction. *Nature Communications, 16*(1), Available from https://doi.org/10.1038/s41467-025-58283-7, https://www.nature.com/ncomms/.

Andreae, A., Breitenstein, A., & Piccini, J. P. (2025). Long-term management of leadless pacemakers. *European Heart Journal, Supplement, 27*, ii26. Available from https://doi.org/10.1093/eurheartjsupp/suae119, http://eurheartjsupp.oxfordjournals.org/.

Antonopoulos, M., Bonios, M. J., Dimopoulos, S., Leontiadis, E., Gouziouta, A., Kogerakis, N., Koliopoulou, A., Elaiopoulos, D., Vlahodimitris, I., Chronaki, M., Chamogeorgakis, T., Drakos, S. G., & Adamopoulos, S. (2024). Advanced heart failure: therapeutic options and challenges in the evolving field of left ventricular assist devices. *Journal of Cardiovascular Development and Disease, 11*(2). https://doi.org/10.3390/jcdd11020061, http://www.mdpi.com/journal/jcdd.

Asch, F. M., Munoz, V., & Ryan, V. Behalf of the WASE-COVID Investigators. (2022). Human versus artificial intelligence–based echocardiographic analysis as a predictor of outcomes: An analysis from the world alliance societies of echocardiography COVID study. *Journal of the American Society of Echocardiography, 35*.

Aung, Y. Y. M., Wong, D. C. S., & Ting, D. S. W. (2021). The promise of artificial intelligence: A review of the opportunities and challenges of artificial intelligence in healthcare. *British Medical Bulletin, 139*(1), 4–15. Available from https://doi.org/10.1093/bmb/ldab016, http://bmb.oxfordjournals.org/.

Ballı, Ş., Kanlıoğlu, P., & Akgun, G. (2024). Experience of left ventricular outflow tract arrhythmia ablation in paediatric patients using limited fluoroscopy and three-dimensional mapping technique. *Cardiology in the Young, 34*(5), 1026–1031. https://doi.org/10.1017/s1047951123003955.

Barbaria, S., Mahjoubi, H., & Rahmouni, H. B. (2023). A novel blockchain-based architectural modal for healthcare data integrity: Covid19 screening laboratory use-case. *Procedia Computer Science, 219*, 1436–1443. https://doi.org/10.1016/j.procs.2023.01.433.

Becker, T., Clark, A., Brinkman, W. T., Malaisrie, S. C., & Dasi, L. P. (2025). Computational modeling for aortic root replacement. *Journal of the Heart Valve Society, 2*(1), 68–80. https://doi.org/10.1177/30494826241312422.

Birks, E. J., Drakos, S. G., Patel, S. R., Lowes, B. D., Selzman, C. H., Starling, R. C., Trivedi, J., Slaughter, M. S., Alturi, P., Goldstein, D., Maybaum, S., Um, J. Y., Margulies, K. B., Stehlik, J., Cunningham, C., Farrar, D. J.,

& Rame, J. E. (2020). Prospective multicenter study of myocardial recovery using left ventricular assist devices (RESTAGE-HF [remission from stage D heart failure]) medium-term and primary end point results. *Circulation, 142*(21), 2016–2028. Available from https://doi.org/10.1161/CIRCULATIONAHA.120.046415, http://circ.ahajournals.org.

Bonios, M. J., Koliopoulou, A., Wever-Pinzon, O., Taleb, I., Stehlik, J., Xu, W., Wever-Pinzon, J., Catino, A., Kfoury, A. G., Horne, B. D., Nativi-Nicolau, J., Adamopoulos, S. N., Fang, J. C., Selzman, C. H., Bax, J. J., & Drakos, S. G. (2018). Cardiac Rotational mechanics as a predictor of myocardial recovery in heart failure patients undergoing chronic mechanical circulatory support a pilot study. *Circulation: Cardiovascular Imaging, 11*(4), Available from https://doi.org/10.1161/CIRCIMAGING.117.007117, http://circimaging.ahajournals.org/.

Bradley, R., Braybrooke, J., Gray, R., Hills, R., Liu, Z., Peto, R., Davies, L., Dodwell, D., McGale, P., Pan, H., Taylor, C., Anderson, S., Gelber, R., Gianni, L., Jacot, W., Joensuu, H., Moreno-Aspitia, A., Piccart, M., Press, M., ... Swain, S. M. (2021). Trastuzumab for early-stage, HER2-positive breast cancer: A meta-analysis of 13 864 women in seven randomised trials. *The Lancet Oncology, 22*(8), 1139–1150. Available from https://doi.org/10.1016/S1470–2045(21)00288-6, http://www.journals.elsevier.com/the-lancet-oncology/.

Brin, D., Gilat, E. K., Raskin, D., & Goitein, O. (2025). Evaluation of AI-based detection of incidental pulmonary emboli in cardiac CT angiography scans. *International Journal of Cardiovascular Imaging*. Available from https://doi.org/10.1007/s10554-025-03456-0, https://www.springer.com/journal/10554.

Chatterjee, A., Feldmann, C., Hanke, J. S., Ricklefs, M., Shrestha, M., Dogan, G., Haverich, A., & Schmitto, J. D. (2018). The momentum of HeartMate 3: A novel active magnetically levitated centrifugal left ventricular assist device (LVAD). *Journal of Thoracic Disease, 10*, S1790. Available from https://doi.org/10.21037/jtd.2017.10.124, http://jtd.amegroups.com/article/download/17467/13915.

Chaudhri, B. B. (2019). The current status of continuous flow left ventricular assist devices. *Advancements in Cardiovascular Research, 1*(5). https://doi.org/10.32474/acr.2019.01.000125.

Cook, J. A., Shah, K. B., Quader, M. A., Cooke, R. H., Kasirajan, V., Rao, K. K., Smallfield, M. C., Tchoukina, I., & Tang, D. G. (2015). The total artificial heart. *Journal of Thoracic Disease, 7*(12), 2172–2180. Available from https://doi.org/10.3978/j.issn.2072-1439.2015.10.70, http://www.jthoracdis.com/article/download/5756/5624.

Cooley, D. A., Liotta, D., Hallman, G. L., Bloodwell, R. D., Leachman, R. D., & Milam, J. D. (1969). Orthotopic cardiac prosthesis for two-staged cardiac replacement. *The American Journal of Cardiology, 24*(5), 723–730. https://doi.org/10.1016/0002-9149(69)90460-3.

Copeland, J. G., Smith, R. G., Arabia, F. A., Nolan, P. E., Sethi, G. K., Tsau, P. H., McClellan, D., & Slepian, M. J. (2004). Cardiac replacement with a total artificial heart as a bridge to transplantation. *New England Journal of Medicine, 351*(9), 859–867. https://doi.org/10.1056/NEJMoa040186.

Cordero (2025). Letter to the editor on 'the potential power of neuralink - how brain-machine interfaces can revolutionize medicine. *Expert Review of Medical Devices,* 1–2.

Costea, A. I., Khanna, R., Iglesias, M., & Rong, Y. (2025). Hospital readmissions following catheter ablation for atrial fibrillation with THERMOCOOL™ STSF/ THERMOCOOL™ ST catheter with CARTO™ 3 system versus TactiCath™ catheter with EnSite™ system. *Journal of Comparative Effectiveness Research, 14*(1), Available from https://doi.org/10.57264/cer-2024-0075, https://becarispublishing.com/loi/cer.

Dankwa-Mullan, I. (2024). Health equity and ethical considerations in using artificial intelligence in public health and medicine. *Preventing Chronic Disease, 21*. https://doi.org/10.5888/pcd21.240245.

de Juan Bagudá, J., Gavira Gómez, J. J., Iglesias, M. P., León, R. C., Pérez, V. E., Fernández, Ó. G., Gándara, N. R., Artaza, J. G., Molina, B. D., Gallego, A. M., Mateo, V. M., Martínez, J. G. M., Negrín, N. M., Salinas, G. L. A., Torres, L. G., Jiménez, J. F. D., Sánchez-Aguilera, P., Infante, E. D., Torres, M. F. A., ... Bodes, R. S. (2022). Remote heart failure management using the HeartLogic algorithm. RE-HEART registry. *Revista Española de Cardiología (English Edition), 75*(9), 709–716. https://doi.org/10.1016/j.rec.2021.09.015.

Demir, E., Köse, M. R., Şimşek, E., Orman, M. N., Zoghi, M., Gürgün, C., & Nalbantgil, S. (2025). Comparative analysis of implantable cardioverter-defibrillator efficacy in ischemic and non-ischemic cardiomyopathy in patients with heart failure. *Scientific Reports, 15*(1), Available from https://doi.org/10.1038/s41598-025-09074-z, https://www.nature.com/srep/.

Devries, W. C., Anderson, J. L., Joyce, L. D., Anderson, F. L., Hammond, E. H., Jarvik, R. K., & Kolff, W. J. (1984). Clinical use of the total artificial heart. *New England Journal of Medicine, 310*(5), 273–278. https://doi.org/10.1056/NEJM198402023100501.

Diyar, D. F., El Banayosy, A. B., Blume, Cowger, J. M. D., Hayward, C., Jorde, J. K., et al. (2023). The 2023 International Society for Heart and Lung Transplantation guidelines for mechanical circulatory support: A 10-year update. *The Journal of Heart and Lung Transplantation, 42*.

D'Udekem, Y., Iyengar, A. J., Galati, J. C., Forsdick, V., Weintraub, R. G., Wheaton, G. R., Bullock, A., Justo, R. N., Grigg, L. E., Sholler, G. F., Hope, S., Radford, D. J., Gentles, T. L., Celermajer, D. S., & Winlaw, D. S. (2014). Redefining expectations of long-term survival after the fontan procedure. *Circulation, 130*(11_suppl_1). https://doi.org/10.1161/circulationaha.113.007764.

El-Chami, M. F., Roberts, P. R., Kypta, A., Omdahl, P., Bonner, M. D., Kowal, R. C., & Duray, G. Z. (2016). How to implant a leadless pacemaker with a tine-based fixation. *Journal of Cardiovascular Electrophysiology, 27*(12), 1495–1501. Available from https://doi.org/10.1111/jce.13092, www.blackwellpublishing.com/journal.asp?ref=1045-3873.

EU liability rules for the age of Artificial Intelligence March 2021 by the authors for the Centre on. Regulation. (n.d.).

Fang, J., Rong, P., Hong, Y., Fan, Y., Liu, J., Wang, H., Zhang, G., Chen, X., Shi, S., Wang, L., Liu, R., Hwang, J., Li, Z., Tao, J., Wang, Y., Zhu, B., & Kong, J. (2016). Transcutaneous vagus nerve stimulation modulates default mode network in major depressive disorder. *Biological Psychiatry, 79*(4), 266–273. https://doi.org/10.1016/j.biopsych.2015.03.025.

FDA (2021). Artificial Intelligence/Machine Learning (AI/ML)-based software as a medical device action plan.

Fontan, F., & Baudet, E. (1971). Surgical repair of tricuspid atresia. *Thorax, 26*(3), 240–248. https://doi.org/10.1136/thx.26.3.240.

Frieberg, P., Plug, S., Poot, D., van der Laan, M., & Hazekamp, M. (2021). Computational fluid dynamics support for Fontan surgical planning. *Frontiers in Physiology, 12*, 747960. https://doi.org/10.3389/fphys.2021.747960.

Fritzsche, D., Eitz, T., Grimmig, O., Brensing, A., Minami, K., & Körfer, R. (2004). Home monitoring of patients after prosthetic valve surgery - experimental background and first clinical attempts. *Thoracic and Cardiovascular Surgeon, 52*(4), 211–217. https://doi.org/10.1055/s-2004-820900.

Gallo, R. J., Shieh, L., Smith, M., Marafino, B. J., Geldsetzer, P., Asch, S. M., Shum, K., Lin, S., Westphal, J., Hong, G., & Li, R. C. (2024). Effectiveness of an artificial intelligence-enabled intervention for detecting clinical deterioration. *JAMA Internal Medicine, 184*(5), 557–562. Available from https://doi.org/10.1001/jamainternmed.2024.0084, http://archinte.jamanetwork.com/issues.aspx.

García-Bolao, I., Gardner, R. S., Gras, D., D'Onofrio, A., Mark, G., Nair, D., Lellouche, N., Novak, M., Lo, R., Chew, E., Wright, D., Kaplan, A., Bertini, M., Veraghtert, S., Harbin, M. M., Matznick, E., Yong, P., & Stein, K. M. (2025). Real-world outcomes in cardiac resynchronization therapy patients: Primary results of the SMART registry. *ESC Heart Failure, 12*(3), 1832–1847. Available from https://doi.org/10.1002/ehf2.15190, onlinelibrary.wiley.com/journal/20555822.

George, I., Rao, D. P., Jain, A., Ascione, G., Sharma, M., Meharwal, Z. S., Sarkar, B., Kochar, N., Shastri, N., Runt, J., Whisenant, B., Wilson, B., Kiser, A., Leon, M. B., & Pandey, K. (2025). 1-year results from a multicenter trial of a polymer surgical mitral valve. *Journal of the American College of Cardiology*. https://doi.org/10.1016/j.jacc.2025.06.017.

Giaretta, J., Crago, M., Hoang, T. P., Liu, X., Lee, A., Wang, Y., Farajikhah, S., Fletcher, D. F., Dehghani, F., Winlaw, D. S., & Naficy, S. (2024). Structural reinforcements as a strategy toward durable polymeric heart valves. *Cell Reports Physical Science, 5*(3), Available from https://doi.org/10.1016/j.xcrp.2024.101870, https://www.sciencedirect.com/science/journal/26663864.

FDA EFS guidance. (2013).

Gunn, R., Watkins, S. L., Boston, D., Rosales, A. G., Massimino, S., Navale, S., Fitzpatrick, S. L., Dickerson, J., Gold, R., Lee, G., & McMullen, C. K. (2024). Evaluation of a remote patient monitoring program during the COVID-19 pandemic: Retrospective case study with a mixed methods explanatory sequential design. *JMIR Formative Research, 8*, e55732. https://doi.org/10.2196/55732.

Gurevich, E., El Hassan, B., & El Morr, C. (2023). Equity within AI systems: What can health leaders expect? *Healthcare Management Forum, 36*(2), 119–124. Available from https://doi.org/10.1177/08404704221125368, https://journals.sagepub.com/home/HMF.

Han, J. J. (2021). Aeson—The Carmat total artificial heart is approved for enrollment in the United States. *Artificial Organs, 45*(5), 445–446. Available from https://doi.org/10.1111/aor.13959, http://onlinelibrary.wiley.com/journal/10.1111/(ISSN)1525-1594.

Hrymniak, B., Skoczyński, P., Skonieczny, B., Biel, B., Josiak, K., Aktanorowicz, P., Wieczorek, T., Zyśko, D., Banasiak, W., & Jagielski, D. (2025). Proper QRS for EMBLEM S-ICD across micra recipients—pilot study. *Journal of Clinical Medicine, 14*(5), 1420. https://doi.org/10.3390/jcm14051420.

Hu, P., Li, L., Sun, Y., Liu, Z., Wang, J., & Zhou, X. (2024). Single-cell multiomics guided mechanistic understanding of Fontan-associated liver disease. *Nature Medicine, 30*(6), 1347–1359. https://doi.org/10.1038/s41591-024-02993-7.

Kahwash, R., Butler, J., Khan, M. S., Chalasani, P., Bertolet, B., Gravelin, L., Lambert, C., Sarkar, S., Van Dorn, B., Laechelt, A., Wehking, J., Patel, N., Gerritse, B., Laager, V., & Zile, M. R. (2025). Incidence of cardiac arrhythmias identified by insertable cardiac monitors in patients with symptomatic heart failure. *JACC: Heart Failure, 13*(8), 102527. https://doi.org/10.1016/j.jchf.2025.102527.

Karatela, M. F., Fudim, M., Mathew, J. P., & Piccini, J. P. (2023). Neuromodulation therapy for atrial fibrillation. *Heart Rhythm the Official Journal of the Heart Rhythm Society, 20*(1), 100–111. Available from https://doi.org/10.1016/j.hrthm.2022.08.011, http://www.elsevier.com/inca/publications/store/7/0/2/3/3/3/index.htt.

Khush, K. K., Cherikh, W. S., Chambers, D. C., Goldfarb, S., Hayes, D., Kucheryavaya, A. Y., Levvey, B. J., Meiser, B., Rossano, J. W., & Stehlik, J. (2018). The International Thoracic Organ Transplant Registry of the International Society for Heart and Lung Transplantation: Thirty-fifth adult heart transplantation report—2018; focus theme: multiorgan transplantation. *The Journal of Heart and Lung Transplantation, 37*(10), 1155–1168. https://doi.org/10.1016/j.healun.2018.07.022.

Kirklin, J. K., Pagani, F. D., Kormos, R. L., Stevenson, L. W., Blume, E. D., Myers, S. L., Miller, M. A., Baldwin, J. T., Young, J. B., & Naftel, D. C. (2017). Eighth annual INTERMACS report: Special focus on framing the impact of adverse events. *Journal of Heart and Lung Transplantation, 36*(10), 1080–1086. Available from https://doi.org/10.1016/j.healun.2017.07.005, www.elsevier.com/locate/healun.

Knop, M., Weber, S., Mueller, M., & Niehaves, B. (2022). Human factors and technological characteristics influencing the interaction of medical professionals with artificial intelligence–enabled clinical decision support systems: Literature review. *JMIR Human Factors, 9*(1), e28639. https://doi.org/10.2196/28639.

Koçak, B., Ponsiglione, A., Stanzione, A., Bluethgen, C., Santinha, J., Ugga, L., Huisman, M., Klontzas, M. E., Cannella, R., & Cuocolo, R. (2025). Bias in artificial intelligence for medical imaging: Fundamentals, detection, avoidance, mitigation, challenges, ethics, and prospects. *Diagnostic and Interventional Radiology, 31*(2), 75–88. Available from https://doi.org/10.4274/dir.2024.242854, https://www.dirjournal.org/pdf/beb8919b-f013-4ea1-b1c8-40332e840fe1/articles/dir.2024.242854/75-88.pdf.

Kolfschooten (2023). , AI Act and MDR integration challenges. *European Journal of Risk Regulation, 14*(2), 145–159.

Kolfschooten, & EU (2021). Regulation of artificial intelligence: Challenges for patients' rights. *SSRN Electronic Journal.*

Kołodziejczak, M., Andreotti, F., Kowalewski, M., Buffon, A., Ciccone, M. M., Parati, G., Scicchitano, P., Umińska, J. M., De Servi, S., Bliden, K. P., Kubica, J., Bortone, A., Crea, F., Gurbel, P., & Navarese, E. P. (2017). Implantable cardioverter-defibrillators for primary prevention in patients with ischemic or nonischemic cardiomyopathy: A systematic review and meta-analysis. *Annals of Internal Medicine, 167*(2), 103–111. Available from https://doi.org/10.7326/M17-0120, http://annals.org/aim/article/2633844/

implantable-cardioverter-defibrillators-primary-prevention-patients-ischemic-nonischemic-cardiomyopathy-systematic.

Kormos, R. L., Cowger, J., Pagani, F. D., Teuteberg, J. J., Goldstein, D. J., Jacobs, J. P., Higgins, R. S., Stevenson, L. W., Stehlik, J., Atluri, P., Grady, K. L., & Kirklin, J. K. (2019). The society of thoracic surgeons intermacs database annual report: Evolving indications, outcomes, and scientific partnerships. *Annals of Thoracic Surgery, 107*(2), 341–353. Available from https://doi.org/10.1016/j.athoracsur.2018.11.011, www.elsevier.com/locate/athoracsur.

Koulouris, & Cascella (2025). *Electrophysiologic Study Interpretation Treasure Island (FL).* StatPearls Publishing.

Krabatsch, T., Netuka, I., Schmitto, J. D., Zimpfer, D., Garbade, J., Rao, V., Morshuis, M., Beyersdorf, F., Marasco, S., Damme, L., & Pya, Y. (2017). Heartmate 3 fully magnetically levitated left ventricular assist device for the treatment of advanced heart failure -1 year results from the Ce mark trial. *Journal of Cardiothoracic Surgery, 12*(1), Available from https://doi.org/10.1186/s13019-017-0587-3, http://www.cardiothoracicsurgery.org/.

Krishna, V., & Fasano, A. (2024). Neuromodulation: Update on current practice and future developments. *Neurotherapeutics the Journal of the American Society for Experimental NeuroTherapeutics, 21*(3), e00371. https://doi.org/10.1016/j.neurot.2024.e00371.

Lansac, E., Veen, K. M., Joseph, A., Blancarte Jaber, P., Sossi, F., Das-Gupta, Z., Aktaa, S., Sádaba, J. R., Thourani, V. H., Dahle, G., Szeto, W. Y., Bakaeen, F., Aikawa, E., Schoen, F. J., Girdauskas, E., Almeida, A., Zuckermann, A., Meuris, B., Stott, J., ... Takkenberg, J. J. M. (2025). The First International Consortium for Health Outcomes Measurement (ICHOM) standard dataset for reporting outcomes in heart valve disease: Moving From device- to patient-centered outcomes. *SInnovations: Technology and Techniques in Cardiothoracic and Vascular Surgery, 20*(2), 133–147. Available from https://doi.org/10.1177/15569845241269309, https://journals.sagepub.com/home/INV.

Lau, D. H., Pierre, B., Cabanas, P., Martens, E., Bisignani, G., Hofer, D., Berruezo, A., Eschalier, R., Mansourati, J., Gaspar, T., Sanfins, V. M., Erglis, A., Hain, A., Papaioannou, G., Cuneo, A., Tscholl, V., Schrader, J., & Deneke, T. (2023). Diagnostic yield of an insertable cardiac monitor in a large patient population. *Heart Rhythm O2, 4*(2), 97–102. Available from https://doi.org/10.1016/j.hroo.2022.11.005, https://www.journals.elsevier.com/heart-rhythm-o2.

Lekadir, K., Frangi, A. F., Porras, A. R., Glocker, B., Cintas, C., Langlotz, C. P., Weicken, E., Asselbergs, F. W., Prior, F., Collins, G. S., Kaissis, G., Tsakou, G., Buvat, I., Kalpathy-Cramer, J., Mongan, J., Schnabel, J. A., Kushibar, K., Riklund, K., Marias, K., ... Starmans, M. P. A. (2025). FUTURE-AI: International consensus guideline for trustworthy and deployable artificial intelligence in healthcare. *BMJ (Clinical Research ed.), 388*, e081554. https://doi.org/10.1136/bmj-2024-081554.

Lesyuk, W., Kriza, C., & Kolominsky-Rabas, P. (2018). Cost-of-illness studies in heart failure: A systematic review 2004–2016. *BMC Cardiovascular Disorders, 18*(1). https://doi.org/10.1186/s12872-018-0815-3.

Liebo, M. J., Israel, R. L., Lillie, E. O., Smith, M. R., Rubenson, D. S., & Topol, E. J. (2011). Is pocket mobile echocardiography the next-generation stethoscope? a cross-sectional comparison of rapidly acquired images with standard transthoracic echocardiography. *Annals of Internal Medicine, 155*(1), 33–39. Available from https://doi.org/10.7326/0003-4819-155-1-201107050-00005, http://www.annals.org/content/155/1/33.full.pdf+html.

Lille, A.H.C. (n.d.). Georges Hôpital Européen, Pompidou, Chu Ghu Pitié Salpêtrière, Dijon.

Lindman, B. R., Asch, F. M., Grayburn, P. A., Mack, M. J., Bax, J. J., Gonzales, H., Goel, K., Barker, C. M., Zalawadiya, S. K., Zhou, Z., Alu, M. C., Weissman, N. J., Abraham, W. T., Lindenfeld, J. A., & Stone, G. W. (2023). Ventricular remodeling and outcomes after mitral transcatheter edge-to-edge repair in heart failure: The COAPT trial. *JACC: Cardiovascular Interventions, 16*(10), 1160–1172. Available from https://doi.org/10.1016/j.jcin.2023.02.031, http://www.elsevier.com.

Liu, X., Song, Zhao, Z., Zhang, Y., & Liu, Y. (2022). Robust optimization of total cavopulmonary connections. *Journal of Biomechanical Engineering, 144*(11), 111004. https://doi.org/10.1115/1.4054709.

Luciani, S., Nederveen, L., Martinez, R., Caixeta, R., Chavez, C., Sandoval, R. C., Severini, L., Cerón, D., Gomes, A. B., Malik, S., Gomez, F., Ordunez, P., Maza, M., Monteiro, M., & Hennis, A. (2023). Noncommunicable diseases in the Americas: A review of the Pan American Health Organization's 25-year program of work. *Revista Panamericana de Salud Pública, 47*, 1. https://doi.org/10.26633/rpsp.2023.13.

Lund, L. H., Edwards, L. B., Dipchand, A. I., Goldfarb, S., Kucheryavaya, A. Y., Levvey, B. J., Meiser, B., Rossano, J. W., Yusen, R. D., & Stehlik, J. (2016). The Registry of the International Society for Heart and Lung Transplantation: Thirty-third adult heart transplantation report—2016; focus theme: primary diagnostic indications for transplant. *Journal of Heart and Lung Transplantation, 35*(10), 1158–1169. Available from https://doi.org/10.1016/j.healun.2016.08.017, www.elsevier.com/locate/healun.

Luo, Y., Zhang, H., & Zhou, Y. (2025). MRI-based radiomics to predict liver-related events in Fontan patients. *Radiology*. https://doi.org/10.1148/radiol.253244.

Malins, J. G., Anisuzzaman, D. M., Jackson, Lee, E., Naser, J. A., Bird, J. G., Friedman, P. A., Ngo, C. C., Oh, J. K., Tsaban, G., Pellikka, P. A., Thaden, J. J., Lopez-Jimenez, Attia, Z. I., Pislaru, S. V., & Kane, G. C. (2025). A deep learning model for classifying left ventricular enlargement for both transthoracic echocardiograms and handheld cardiac ultrasound. *European Heart Journal - Imaging Methods and Practice, 3.*

Manickam, P., Mariappan, S. A., Murugesan, S. M., Hansda, S., Kaushik, A., Shinde, R., & Thipperudraswamy, S. P. (2022). Artificial intelligence (AI) and internet of medical things (IoMT) assisted biomedical systems for intelligent healthcare. *Biosensors, 12*(8), 562. https://doi.org/10.3390/bios12080562.

Manyam, H., Burri, H., Casado-Arroyo, R., Varma, N., Lennerz, C., Klug, D., Carr-White, G., Kolli, K., Reyes, I., Nabutovsky, Y., & Boriani, G. (2023). Smartphone-based cardiac implantable electronic device remote monitoring: Improved compliance and connectivity. *European Heart Journal - Digital Health, 4*(1), 43–52. https://doi.org/10.1093/ehjdh/ztac071.

Mas-Peiro, S., Lhermusier, T., Urena, M., Nombela-Franco, L., Vilalta, V., Muñoz-Garcia, A., Amat-Santos, I., Atienza, F., Kleiman, N., Chamandi, C., Serra, V., Deyell, M. W., Campelo-Parada, F., Mondoly, P., Suc, G., Canadas-Godoy, V., Fernandez-Nofrerias, E., Castrodeza, J., Elizaga, J., ... Rodés-Cabau, J. (2025). Late arrhythmic burden in patients with left bundle branch block after TAVR with the Evolut valve. *Europace European Pacing, Arrhythmias, and Cardiac Electrophysiology Journal of the Working Groups on Cardiac Pacing, Arrhythmias, and Cardiac Cellular Electrophysiology of the European Society of Cardiology, 27*(4), Available from https://doi.org/10.1093/europace/euaf057, http://europace.oxfordjournals.org/.

Mayourian, J., Gearhart, A., La Cava, W. G., Vaid, A., Nadkarni, G. N., Triedman, J. K., Powell, A. J., Wald, R. M., Valente, A. M., Geva, T., Duong, S. Q., & Ghelani, S. J. (2024). Deep learning-based electrocardiogram analysis predicts biventricular dysfunction and dilation in congenital heart disease. *Journal of the American College of Cardiology, 84*(9), 815–828. Available from https://doi.org/10.1016/j.jacc.2024.05.062, https://www.sciencedirect.com/science/journal/07351097.

Mayourian, J., Asztalos, I. B., El-Bokl, A., Lukyanenko, P., Kobayashi, R. L., La Cava, W. G., Ghelani, S. J., Vetter, V. L., & Triedman, J. K. (2025). Electrocardiogram-based deep learning to predict left ventricular systolic dysfunction in paediatric and adult congenital heart disease in the USA: A multicentre modelling study. *The Lancet Digital Health, 7*(4), e264. Available from https://doi.org/10.1016/j.landig.2025.01.001, https://www.sciencedirect.com/science/journal/25897500.

Mayourian, J., van Boxtel, J. P. A., Sleeper, L. A., Diwanji, V., Geva, A., O'Leary, E. T., Triedman, J. K., Ghelani, S. J., Wald, R. M., Valente, A. M., & Geva, T. (2024). Electrocardiogram-based deep learning to predict mortality in repaired tetralogy of fallot. *JACC: Clinical Electrophysiology, 10*(12), 2600–2612. Available from https://doi.org/10.1016/j.jacep.2024.07.015, https://www.sciencedirect.com/science/journal/2405500X.

Mayourian, J., Geggel, R., La Cava, W. G., Ghelani, S. J., & Triedman, J. K. (2025). Pediatric electrocardiogram-based deep learning to predict secundum atrial septal defects. *Pediatric Cardiology, 46*(5), 1235–1240. Available from https://doi.org/10.1007/s00246-024-03540-7, https://www.springer.com/journal/246.

McDonagh, T. A., Metra, M., Adamo, M., Gardner, R. S., Baumbach, A., Böhm, M., Burri, H., Butler, J., Čelutkienė, J., Chioncel, O., Cleland, J. G. F., Coats, A. J. S., Crespo-Leiro, M. G., Farmakis, D., Gilard, M., Heymans, S., Hoes, A. W., Jaarsma, T., Jankowska, E. A., ... Kathrine Skibelund, A. (2021). 2021 ESC

Guidelines for the diagnosis and treatment of acute and chronic heart failure. *European Heart Journal, 42*(36), 3599–3726. https://doi.org/10.1093/eurheartj/ehab368.

Mehra, M. R., Goldstein, D. J., Cleveland, J. C., Cowger, J. A., Hall, S., Salerno, C. T., Naka, Y., Horstmanshof, D., Chuang, J., Wang, A., & Uriel, N. (2022). Five-year outcomes in patients with fully magnetically levitated vs axial-flow left ventricular assist devices in the MOMENTUM 3 randomized trial. *JAMA the Journal of the American Medical Association, 328*(12), 1233–1242. Available from https://doi.org/10.1001/jama.2022.16197, http://jama.jamanetwork.com/journal.aspx.

Mehra, M. R., Nayak, A., Morris, A. A., Lanfear, D. E., Nemeh, H., Desai, S., Bansal, A., Guerrero-Miranda, C., Hall, S., Cleveland, J. C., Goldstein, D. J., Uriel, N., Chen, L., Bailey, S., Anyanwu, A., Heatley, G., Chuang, J., & Estep, J. D. (2022). Prediction of survival after implantation of a fully magnetically levitated left ventricular assist device. *JACC: Heart Failure, 10*(12), 948–959. Available from https://doi.org/10.1016/j.jchf.2022.08.002, http://www.journals.elsevier.com/jacc-heart-failure.

Mohacsi, P., & Leprince, P. (2014). The CARMAT total artificial heart. *European Journal of Cardio-Thoracic Surgery, 46*(6), 933–934. Available from https://doi.org/10.1093/ejcts/ezu333, http://ejcts.oxfordjournals.org/.

Molina, E. J., Shah, P., Kiernan, M. S., Cornwell, W. K., Copeland, H., Takeda, K., Fernandez, F. G., Badhwar, V., Habib, R. H., Jacobs, J. P., Koehl, D., Kirklin, J. K., Pagani, F. D., & Cowger, J. A. (2021). The society of thoracic surgeons intermacs 2020 annual report. *Annals of Thoracic Surgery, 111*(3), 778–792. Available from https://doi.org/10.1016/j.athoracsur.2020.12.038, www.elsevier.com/locate/athoracsur.

Moscato, F., Gross, C., Maw, M., Schlöglhofer, T., Granegger, M., Zimpfer, D., & Schima, H. (2021). The left ventricular assist device as a patient monitoring system. *Annals of Cardiothoracic Surgery, 10*(2), 221–232. Available from https://doi.org/10.21037/acs-2020-cfmcs-218, www.annalscts.com/index.

Nair, N. (2022). Use of machine learning techniques to identify risk factors for RV failure in LVAD patients. *Frontiers in Cardiovascular Medicine, 9*. https://doi.org/10.3389/fcvm.2022.848789.

Nakano, M., Kondo, Y., Hongo, R. H., Takaoka, H., & Kobayashi, Y. (2025). Opening the door to a new era: A dual-chamber leadless pacemaker. *Journal of Arrhythmia, 41*(3). https://doi.org/10.1002/joa3.70100.

Narang, A., Bae, R., Hong, H., Thomas, Y., Surette, S., Cadieu, C., Chaudhry, A., Martin, R. P., McCarthy, P. M., Rubenson, D. S., Goldstein, S., Little, S. H., Lang, R. M., Weissman, N. J., & Thomas, J. D. (2021). Utility of a deep-learning algorithm to guide novices to acquire echocardiograms for limited diagnostic use. *JAMA Cardiology, 6*(6), 624–632. Available from https://doi.org/10.1001/jamacardio.2021.0185, http://jamanetwork.com/journals/jamacardiology.

Ødegaard, K. M., Hallén, J., Lirhus, S. S., Melberg, H. O., & Halvorsen, S. (2020). Incidence, prevalence, and mortality of heart failure: A nationwide registry study from 2013 to 2016. *ESC Heart Failure, 7*(4), 1917–1926. Available from https://doi.org/10.1002/ehf2.12773, onlinelibrary.wiley.com/journal/20555822.

Okwuosa, T. M., Greenland, P., Ning, H., Liu, K., Bild, D. E., Burke, G. L., Eng, J., & Lloyd-Jones, D. M. (2011). Distribution of coronary artery calcium scores by framingham 10-year risk strata in the MESA (multi-ethnic study of atherosclerosis). *Journal of the American College of Cardiology, 57*(18), 1838–1845. https://doi.org/10.1016/j.jacc.2010.11.053.

Otto, C. M., Nishimura, R. A., Bonow, Carabello, B. A., Erwin, J. P., Gentile, F., Jneid, H., Krieger, E. V., Mack, M., McLeod, Gara, Rigolin, P. T., & H, V. (2021). Sundt TM 3rd, Thompson A, Toly C. 2020 ACC/AHA guideline for the management of patients with valvular heart disease: A report of the American College of Cardiology/American Heart Association Joint Committee on Clinical Practice Guidelines. *Circulation, 143*, 72.

Overgaard, S. M., Graham, M. G., Brereton, T., Pencina, M. J., Halamka, J. D., Vidal, D. E., & Economou-Zavlanos, N. J. (2023). Implementing quality management systems to close the AI translation gap and facilitate safe, ethical, and effective health AI solutions. *Npj Digital Medicine, 6*(1), Available from https://doi.org/10.1038/s41746-023-00968-8, https://www.nature.com/npjdigitalmed/.

Palaniappan, K., Lin, E. Y. T., & Vogel, S. (2024). Global regulatory frameworks for the use of artificial intelligence (AI) in the healthcare services sector. *Healthcare, 12*(5), 562. https://doi.org/10.3390/healthcare12050562.

Park, A. (2023). Sooma Medical's neurostim device for at-home depression treatment lands FDA breakthrough tag. *Medtech*.

Perez, M. V., Mahaffey, K. W., Hedlin, H., Rumsfeld, J. S., Garcia, A., Ferris, T., Balasubramanian, V., Russo, A. M., Rajmane, A., Cheung, L., Hung, G., Lee, J., Kowey, P., Talati, N., Nag, D., Gummidipundi, S. E., Beatty, A., Hills, M. T., Desai, S., ... Turakhia, M. P. (2019). Large-scale assessment of a smartwatch to identify atrial fibrillation. *New England Journal of Medicine, 381*(20), 1909–1917. Available from https://doi.org/10.1056/NEJMoa1901183, http://www.nejm.org/medical-index.

Potapov, E. V., Antonides, C., Crespo-Leiro, M. G., Combes, A., Färber, G., Hannan, M. M., Kukucka, M., De Jonge, N., Loforte, A., Lund, L. H., Mohacsi, P., Morshuis, M., Netuka, I., Özbaran, M., Pappalardo, F., Scandroglio, A. M., Schweiger, M., Tsui, S., Zimpfer, D., & Gustafsson, F. (2019). 2019 EACTS Expert Consensus on long-term mechanical circulatory support. *European Journal of Cardio-thoracic Surgery, 56*(2), 230–270. Available from https://doi.org/10.1093/ejcts/ezz098, http://ejcts.oxfordjournals.org/.

Proposal for a Regulation of the European parliament and of the council laying down harmonised rules on artificial intelligence (artificial intelligence act) and amending certain union legislative acts. 2021.

Pundi, K. N., Johnson, J. N., Dearani, J. A., Pundi, K. N., Li, Z., Hinck, C. A., Dahl, S. H., Cannon, B. C., O'Leary, P. W., Driscoll, D. J., & Cetta, F. (2015). 40-year follow-up after the fontan operation long-term outcomes of 1,052 patients. *Journal of the American College of Cardiology, 66*(15), 1700–1710. Available from https://doi.org/10.1016/j.jacc.2015.07.065, www.elsevier.com/locate/jacc.

Pya, Y., Maly, J., Bekbossynova, M., Salov, R., Schueler, S., Meyns, B., Kassif, Y., Massetti, M., Zilbershlag, M., & Netuka, I. (2019). First human use of a wireless coplanar energy transfer coupled with a continuous-flow left ventricular assist device. *The Journal of Heart and Lung Transplantation, 38*(4), 339–343. https://doi.org/10.1016/j.healun.2019.01.1316.

Quartieri, F., Harish, M., Calò, L., Ebrahim, I., Fusco, A., Mester, S., Cauti, F., Park, S. J., Francia, P., Giovagnoni, M., Adragao, P., Vezi, B., Lin, W., Hutson, C. S., & Grammatico, A. (2023). New insertable cardiac monitors show high diagnostic yield and good safety profile in real-world clinical practice: Results from the international prospective observational SMART Registry. *Europace European Pacing, Arrhythmias, and Cardiac Electrophysiology Journal of the Working Groups on Cardiac Pacing, Arrhythmias, and Cardiac Cellular Electrophysiology of the European Society of Cardiology, 25*(5), Available from https://doi.org/10.1093/europace/euad068, http://europace.oxfordjournals.org/.

Rattka, I., Mastella, G., Martens, E., Laugwitz, K. L., & Rattka, M. (2025). Pulsed field ablation of refractory alternating atrial fibrillation and atrial flutter using Impella CP in a patient with cardiogenic shock: A case report. *European Heart Journal - Case Reports, 9*(5), Available from https://doi.org/10.1093/ehjcr/ytaf216, academic.oup.com/ehjcr.

Reddy, S., Bernstein, D., Taylor, A. L., Ogden, M., Chin, C., & Goldstein, B. H. (2020). Proceedings from the 2019 stanford single ventricle scientific summit. *Pediatric Research, 87*(5), 986–993. https://doi.org/10.1038/s41390-020-0796-0.

Reed, G. W., Harmon, E. K., Harb, S., Yun, J., Krishnaswamy, A., Abraham, W. T., & Kapadia, S. (2024). Design and rationale of the V-wave shunt mitraclip study. *American Journal of Cardiology, 227*, 29–36. Available from https://doi.org/10.1016/j.amjcard.2024.06.023, https://www.sciencedirect.com/science/journal/00029149.

Reiffel, J. A., Verma, A., Kowey, P. R., Halperin, J. L., Gersh, B. J., Elkind, M. S. V., Ziegler, P. D., Kaplon, R. E., Sherfesee, L., & Wachter, R. (2020). Rhythm monitoring strategies in patients at high risk for atrial fibrillation and stroke: A comparative analysis from the REVEAL AF study. *Heart Journal, 219*, 128–136. Available from https://doi.org/10.1016/j.ahj.2019.07.016, http://www.elsevier.com/inca/publications/store/6/2/3/2/7/2/index.htt.

Ren, H., Jing, F., Ma, Y., Wang, R., He, C., Wang, Y., Zhou, J., & Sun, Y. (2025). Harnessing artificial intelligence of things for cardiac sensing: Current advances and network-based perspectives. *Frontiers in Public Health, 13*. Available from https://doi.org/10.3389/fpubh.2025.1569887, http://journal.frontiersin.org/journal/public-health/section/public-health-education-and-promotion#archive.

Rodés-Cabau, J., Lindenfeld, J. A., Abraham, W. T., Zile, M. R., Kar, S., Bayés-Genís, A., Eigler, N., Holcomb, R., Núñez, J., Lee, E., Perl, M. L., Moravsky, G., Pfeiffer, M., Boehmer, J., Gorcsan, J., Bax, J. J., Anker, S., & Stone, G. W. (2024). Interatrial shunt therapy in advanced heart failure: Outcomes from the open-label cohort of the RELIEVE-HF trial. *European Journal of Heart Failure, 26*(4), 1078–1089. Available from https://doi.org/10.1002/ejhf.3215, http://onlinelibrary.wiley.com/journal/10.1002/(ISSN)1879-0844.

Rogers, J. G., Pagani, F. D., Tatooles, A. J., Bhat, G., Slaughter, M. S., Birks, E. J., Boyce, S. W., Najjar, S. S., Jeevanandam, V., Anderson, A. S., Gregoric, I. D., Mallidi, H., Leadley, K., Aaronson, K. D., Frazier, O. H., & Milano, C. A. (2017). Intrapericardial left ventricular assist device for advanced heart failure. *New England Journal of Medicine, 376*(5), 451–460. Available from https://doi.org/10.1056/NEJMoa1602954, http://www.nejm.org/doi/pdf/10.1056/NEJMoa1602954.

Rychik, J., Atz, A. M., Celermajer, D. S., Deal, B. J., Gatzoulis, M. A., Gewillig, M. H., Hsia, T. Y., Hsu, D. T., Kovacs, A. H., McCrindle, B. W., Newburger, J. W., Pike, N. A., Rodefeld, M., Rosenthal, D. N., Schumacher, K. R., Marino, B. S., Stout, K., Veldtman, G., Younoszai, A. K., & D'Udekem, Y. (2019). Evaluation and management of the child and adult with fontan circulation: A scientific statement from the american heart association. *Circulation, 140*(6), E234. Available from https://doi.org/10.1161/CIR.0000000000000696, http://circ.ahajournals.org.

Sadeghi, Z., Alizadehsani, R., CIFCI, M. A., Kausar, S., Rehman, R., Mahanta, P., Bora, P. K., Almasri, A., Alkhawaldeh, R. S., Hussain, S., Alatas, B., Shoeibi, A., Moosaei, H., Hladík, M., Nahavandi, S., & Pardalos, P. M. (2024). A review of explainable artificial intelligence in healthcare. *Computers and Electrical Engineering, 118*, 109370. https://doi.org/10.1016/j.compeleceng.2024.109370.

Sangha, V., Nargesi, A. A., Dhingra, L. S., Khunte, A., Mortazavi, B. J., Ribeiro, A. H., Banina, E., Adeola, O., Garg, N., Brandt, C. A., Miller, E. J., Ribeiro, A. L. P., Velazquez, E. J., Giatti, L., Barreto, S. M., Foppa, M., Yuan, N., Ouyang, D., Krumholz, H. M., & Khera, R. (2023). Detection of left ventricular systolic dysfunction from electrocardiographic images. *Circulation, 148*(9), 765–777. Available from https://doi.org/10.1161/CIRCULATIONAHA.122.062646, http://circ.ahajournals.org.

Santini, L., D'Onofrio, A., Dello Russo, A., Calò, L., Pecora, D., Favale, S., Petracci, B., Molon, G., Bianchi, V., De Ruvo, E., Ammirati, F., La Greca, C., Campari, M., Valsecchi, S., & Capucci, A. (2020). Prospective evaluation of the multisensor HeartLogic algorithm for heart failure monitoring. *Clinical Cardiology, 43*(7), 691–697. Available from https://doi.org/10.1002/clc.23366, http://onlinelibrary.wiley.com/journal/10.1002/(ISSN)1932-8737.

Schmitto, J. D., Pya, Y., Zimpfer, D., Krabatsch, T., Garbade, J., Rao, V., Morshuis, M., Beyersdorf, F., Marasco, S., Sood, P., Damme, L., & Netuka, I. (2017). HeartMate 3 fully magnetically levitated left ventricular assist device for the treatment of advanced heart failure - CE mark study 2-year results. *The Journal of Heart and Lung Transplantation, 36*(4), S66. https://doi.org/10.1016/j.healun.2017.01.162.

Schroder, J. N., McCartney, S. L., Jansen, P., Plichta, R., Katz, J. N., Smadja, D. M., Dewan, K. C., & Milano, C. A. (2023). The first autoregulated total artificial heart implant in the United States. *Annals of Thoracic Surgery Short Reports, 1*(1), 185–187. https://doi.org/10.1016/j.atssr.2022.09.007.

Schwennesen, H. T., Li, Z., Hammill, B. G., Clark, A. G., Pokorney, S., Hytopoulos, E., Turakhia, M. P., Cambra, J., & Piccini, J. P. (2024). Performance of ambulatory electrocardiographic data for prediction of stroke and heart failure events. *JACC: Advances, 3*(11), Available from https://doi.org/10.1016/j.jacadv.2024.101340, https://www.sciencedirect.com/journal/jacc-advances.

Sellers, K. K., Cohen, J. L., Khambhati, A. N., Fan, J. M., Lee, A. M., Chang, E. F., & Krystal, A. D. (2024). Closed-loop neurostimulation for the treatment of psychiatric disorders. *Neuropsychopharmacology Official Publication of the American College of Neuropsychopharmacology, 49*(1), 163–178. Available from https://doi.org/10.1038/s41386-023-01631-2, https://www.nature.com/npp/.

Sen, S., & Ramakrishnan, S. (2024). Artificial intelligence in pediatric cardiology: Where do we stand in 2024? *Annals of Pediatric Cardiology, 17*(2), 93–96. https://doi.org/10.4103/apc.apc_72_24.

Smith, H., Birchley, G., & Ives, J. (2024). Artificial intelligence in clinical decision-making: Rethinking personal moral responsibility. *Bioethics, 38*(1), 78–86. Available from https://doi.org/10.1111/bioe.13222, http://onlinelibrary.wiley.com/journal/10.1111/(ISSN)1467-8519.

Stone, G. W., Abraham, W. T., Lindenfeld, J. A., Kar, S., Grayburn, P. A., Lim, D. S., Mishell, J. M., Whisenant, B., Rinaldi, M., Kapadia, S. R., Rajagopal, V., Sarembock, I. J., Brieke, A., Marx, S. O., Cohen, D. J., Asch, F. M., & Mack, M. J. (2023). Five-year follow-up after transcatheter repair of secondary mitral regurgitation. *New England Journal of Medicine, 388*(22), 2037–2048. Available from https://doi.org/10.1056/NEJMoa2300213, http://www.nejm.org/medical-index.

Stone, G. W., Lindenfeld, J. A., Rodés-Cabau, J., Anker, S. D., Zile, M. R., Kar, S., Holcomb, R., Pfeiffer, M. P., Bayes-Genis, A., Bax, J. J., Bank, A. J., Costanzo, M. R., Verheye, S., Roguin, A., Filippatos, G., Núñez, J., Lee, E. C., Laufer-Perl, M., Moravsky, G., ... Abraham, W. T. (2024). Interatrial shunt treatment for heart failure: The randomized RELIEVE-HF trial. *Circulation, 150*(24), 1931–1943. Available from https://doi.org/10.1161/CIRCULATIONAHA.124.070870, http://circ.ahajournals.org.

Strik, M., Sacristan, B., Bordachar, P., Duchateau, J., Eschalier, R., Mondoly, P., Laborderie, J., Gassa, N., Zemzemi, N., Laborde, M., Garrido, J., Matencio Perabla, C., Jimenez-Perez, G., Camara, O., Haïssaguerre, M., Dubois, R., & Ploux, S. (2023). Artificial intelligence for detection of ventricular oversensing: Machine learning approaches for noise detection within nonsustained ventricular tachycardia episodes remotely transmitted by pacemakers and implantable cardioverter-defibrillators. *Heart Rhythm the Official Journal of the Heart Rhythm Society, 20*(10), 1378–1384. https://doi.org/10.1016/j.hrthm.2023.06.019.

Svennberg, E., Han, J. K., Caiani, E. G., Engelhardt, S., Ernst, S., Friedman, P., Garcia, R., Ghanbari, H., Hindricks, G., Man, S. H., Millet, J., Narayan, S. M., Ng, G. A., Noseworthy, P. A., Tjong, F. V. Y., Ramírez, J., Singh, J. P., Trayanova, N., Duncker, D., ... Zorzi, A. (2025). State of the art of artificial intelligence in clinical electrophysiology in 2025: A scientific statement of the European Heart Rhythm Association (EHRA) of the ESC, the Heart Rhythm Society (HRS), and the ESC Working Group on E-Cardiology. *Europace European Pacing, Arrhythmias, and Cardiac Electrophysiology Journal of the Working Groups on Cardiac Pacing, Arrhythmias, and Cardiac Cellular Electrophysiology of the European Society of Cardiology, 27*(5), Available from https://doi.org/10.1093/europace/euaf071, http://europace.oxfordjournals.org/.

Tettey-Engmann, F., Parupelli, S. K., Bauer, S. R., Bhattarai, N., & Desai, S. (2025). Advances in artificial intelligence-based medical devices for healthcare applications. *Biomedical Materials and Devices.* Available from https://doi.org/10.1007/s44174-025-00379-1, link.springer.com/journal/44174.

Teuteberg, J. J., Stewart, G. C., Jessup, M., Kormos, R. L., Sun, B., Frazier, O. H., Naftel, D. C., & Stevenson, L. W. (2013). Implant strategies change over time and impact outcomes: Insights from the INTERMACS (interagency registry for mechanically assisted circulatory support). *JACC: Heart Failure, 1*(5), 369–378. https://doi.org/10.1016/j.jchf.2013.05.006.

Tjong, F. V. Y., & Koop, B. E. (2018). The modular cardiac rhythm management system: The EMPOWER leadless pacemaker and the EMBLEM subcutaneous ICD. *Herzschrittmachertherapie und Elektrophysiologie, 29*(4), 355–361. Available from https://doi.org/10.1007/s00399-018-0602-y, http://www.springerlink.com/content/0938-7412/.

Upton, R., & Strom, J. B. (2025). Guidelines for the digital era: A vision for artificial intelligence in HFpEF. *Journal of the American Society of Echocardiography, 38*(7), 636. Available from https://doi.org/10.1016/j.echo.2025.03.014, https://www.sciencedirect.com/science/journal/08947317.

Vahanian, A., Beyersdorf, F., Praz, F., Milojevic, M., Baldus, S., Bauersachs, J., Capodanno, D., Conradi, L., De Bonis, M., De Paulis, R., Delgado, V., Freemantle, N., Gilard, M., Haugaa, K. H., Jeppsson, A., Jüni, P., Pierard, L., Prendergast, B. D., Sádaba, J. R., ... Bouleti, C. (2022). 2021 ESC/EACTS Guidelines for the management of valvular heart disease. *European Heart Journal, 43*(7), 561–632. https://doi.org/10.1093/eurheartj/ehab395.

Weirich, W. L., Gott, V. L., & Lillehei, C. W. (1957). The treatment of complete heart block by the combined use of a myocardial electrode and an artificial pacemaker. *Surgical Forum, 8*, 360–363.

Westaby (2022). Evolution of a circulatory support system with full implantability: Personal perspectives on a long journey. *The British journal of cardiology, 29*(3).

WHO (2021). Ethics and Governance of Artificial Intelligence for Health.

Williams, K. A., Kim, J. T., & Holohan, K. M. (2013). Frequency of unrecognized, unreported, or underreported coronary artery and cardiovascular calcification on noncardiac chest CT. *Journal of Cardiovascular Computed Tomography, 7*(3), 167–172. https://doi.org/10.1016/j.jcct.2013.05.003.

Yokota, J., Fujiu, K., Doi, K., & Takeda, N. (2025). Ventricular tachycardia ablation using map merge capable of integrating multiple sessions. *International Heart Journal, 66*(2), 327–328. https://doi.org/10.1536/ihj.24-685.

Yokota, S., Uemura, K., Unoki, T., Matsushita, H., Kakuuchi, M., Yoshida, Y., Sasaki, K., Kawada, T., Nishikawa, T., Kataoka, Y., Peterson, J., Sunagawa, K., Alexander, J., & Saku, K. (2024). Novel closed-loop control system of dual rotary blood pumps in total artificial heart based on the circulatory equilibrium framework: A proof-of-concept in vivo study. *IEEE Transactions on Biomedical Engineering, 71*(12), 3358–3369. https://doi.org/10.1109/tbme.2024.3420907.

Zhou, K., & Gattinger, G. (2024). The evolving regulatory paradigm of AI in MedTech: A review of perspectives and where we are today. *Therapeutic Innovation and Regulatory Science, 58*(3), 456–464. Available from https://doi.org/10.1007/s43441-024-00628-3, https://www.springer.com/journal/43441.

Further reading

https://www.fda.gov/medical-devices/investigational-device-exemption-ide/early-feasibility-studies-efs-program.

CHAPTER 10

Healthcare access in the changing world: Global challenges, inequiities and future directions

Huda Aldhanhani[1] **and Sofia Konstantinopoulou**[2,3]

[1]Pediatric Infectious Diseases Consultant, Sheikh Khalifa Medical City, SEHA, PureHealth, Abu Dhabi, United Arab Emirates, [2]Pulmonary Medicine, Division of Pediatrics, Sheikh Khalifa Medical City, PureHealth, Abu Dhabi, United Arab Emirates, [3]Adjunct Assistant Professor of Pediatrics, Khalifa University, Abu Dhabi, United Arab Emirates

10.1 Introduction

Access to healthcare can be defined as the opportunity and ease with which communities and individuals can utilize necessary healthcare services according to their specific needs (Levesque et al., 2013). It has beenrecognized as a fundamental human right by the World Health Organization (WHO) since 1984. Over time, global efforts have contributed to measurable improvements in healthcare access. The Global Burden of Disease Study, for example, reports a steady increase in the Healthcare Access and Quality (HAQ) Index, with global scores rising from 37.6 in 1990 to 54.4 in 2016.

Despite this progress, significant gaps in healthcare access persist worldwide. Many populations continue to face barriers related to availability, affordability, and quality of care, highlighting ongoing global inequalities. These disparities are evident not only between countries but also within them, underscoring the complexity of achieving equitable healthcare access (Cu et al., 2021; World Health Organization, WHO, Universal).

In response to these challenges, universal health coverage (UHC) has emerged as a central framework for improving healthcare systems. It is a multidimensional concept encompassing population coverage, services coverage, and financial protection as its core components alongside equality and quality as its integral elements. It is widely regarded by policymakers as a fundamental approach to improving population health, driving economic development, and promoting social justice. Furthermore, UHC plays a critical role in minimizing disparities, strengthening effective and comprehensive health governance, and fostering resilient health systems (Endalamaw et al., 2022). However, even with the adoption of UHC by many

The Future of Pharma Across All Sectors in the Artificial Intelligence Era. DOI: https://doi.org/10.1016/B978-0-443-40572-3.00023-X

countries, disparities in healthcare access remain substantial (Cu et al., 2021; World Health Organization, WHO, Universal). According to the HAQ Index (2016), substantial subnational disparities in healthcare access persist across many countries. These inequalities are evident not only in developing nations such as China and India, but also within developed countries. For example, Blackpool recorded the lowest scores ((79·7 [76·6–82·8])) in England, while Mississippi ((81·5 [78·6–84·2])) demonstrated the lowest performance in the United States, highlighting significant variations in healthcare access within countries (Fullman et al., 2018).

According to the 2017 Global Monitoring Report, approximately 7.3 billion people are unable to access all the essential health services they need. Additionally, it is estimated that 8.6 million deaths in 2016 were attributed to inadequacies in either access or quality of healthcare, particularly in low- and middle-income countries (LMICs), as indicated by a systematic analysis from 137 countries (Cu et al., 2021). Currently, nearly one-third of the world's population lacks regular access to essential medicines, a figure that may underestimate the situation in impoverished areas of Africa and Asia, where this lack may rise to as much as 50% of the population (World Health Organization, WHO, 2023). In contrast, the impact in developed nations, such as those in the European region, reveals that unmet medical care needs are estimated to be around 2%, with some countries reporting higher figures exceeding 5% (Abatemarco et al., 2024), financial barriers continue to be a predominant obstacle to care access, in US 14% of adults report difficulty accessing healthcare with higher prevenance among those with sociodemographic risk factors reaching 27% therefore the cost related barriers affected not only the non insured population but even one fifth of those insured (Rifai et al., 2021).

In 2015, the United Nations Sustainable Development Goals (SDGs) were adopted to establish and navigate a global collaboration aiming to achieve health equity and sustainable development by 2030. While health is a priority for this agenda, particularly through Goal 3, which aims to ensure healthy lives and promote well-being for all ages (Levesque et al., 2013).

To track progress toward UHC, two specific metrics are utilized: SDG Target 3.8.1, focusing on healthcare services coverage (Fig. 10.1), and SDG Target 3.8.2, concentrating on catastrophic health spending. A systematic review of 58 articles and 23 presenting findings from LMICs and 35 from high-income countries (HICs) emphasizes the differing barriers to healthcare access. In LMICs, the absence of services is more pronounced, while in HICs, the primary concerns tend to revolve around patient experience and quality rather than availability alone (Dawkins et al., 2021; World Health Organization, WHO, SDG).

10.2 The dimensions of healthcare access

Access to healthcare is the result of the interaction between personal characteristics, household dynamics, social and physical environments, and the attributes of health systems, organizations, and providers. There are five main dimensions of healthcare access:

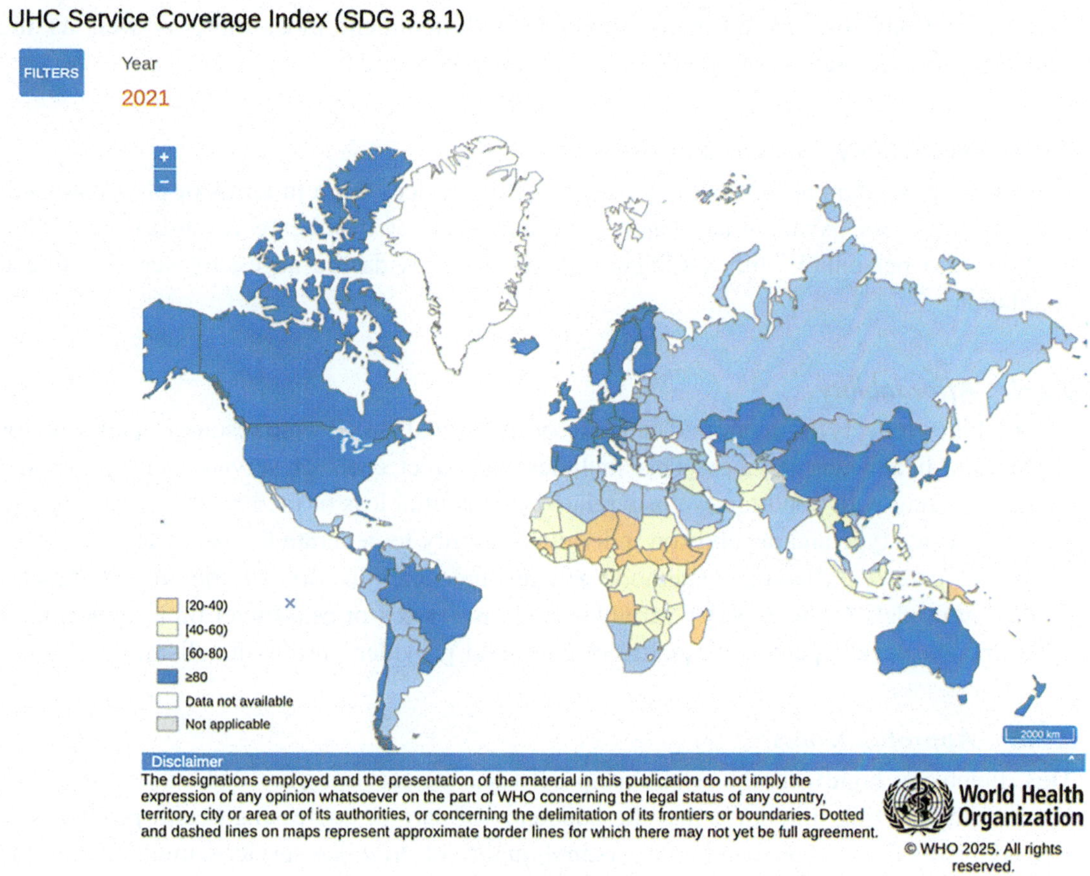

Figure 10.1
The global service coverage index, SDG 3.8.1 (World Health Organization, WHO, SDG) (https://www.who.int/data/gho/data/themes/topics/service-coverage). Map lines delineate study areas and do not necessarily depict accepted national boundaries.

10.2.1 Approachability

- This dimension pertains to the awareness of existing services and their accessibility to individuals, and has an impact on the health of the individual, in which the approach to these services can be affected by information sharing and transparency, and may be less recognized in various social or geographical population groups, thus making them less approachable.

10.2.2 Acceptability

- Similar to approachability, it may also be affected by the cultural and social influences that affect individuals' acceptance of healthcare services. It emphasizes the importance of societal attitudes towards different providers and treatment modalities, as well as the perceived appropriateness of engaging with healthcare systems.

10.2.3 Availability and accommodation

- This dimension refers to the accessibility of health services, both in terms of physical reach and timely access. Availability denotes the existence of healthcare resources, including facilities and personnel, with sufficient capacity to provide the necessary services to the population.

10.2.4 Affordability

- Affordability reflects the economic capacity of individuals to allocate resources and time for appropriate healthcare services. This includes the direct costs of services and associated expenses, along with opportunity costs related to potential loss of income. Affordability can vary by service type and depends on individuals' ability to generate the necessary resources to pay for care (e.g., payment methods and resource mobilization). Economic studies on utilization models often consider variables such as service prices, travel time, opportunity costs, income levels, perceived quality of care, and providers' professionalism.

10.2.5 Appropriateness

- This dimension highlights the relationship between the services provided and the needs of clients, emphasizing timeliness and the adequacy of care in addressing health problems. It also addresses the technical and interpersonal quality of provided services, underscoring the importance of both what services are offered and how these are delivered.

The interplay among these dimensions is dynamic, as they can impact one another in various ways. Additionally, individuals engage with these dimensions through five key abilities: the ability to perceive, seek, reach, pay, and engage. Understanding these dimensions and abilities is crucial for assessing and improving healthcare access on a global scale (see Fig. 10.2) (Levesque et al., 2013).

10.2.6 Global health challenges

The global health landscape is characterized by the compounding interactions of longstanding and emerging challenges that place significant strain on healthcare systems worldwide. These challenges include the escalating prevalence of noncommunicable diseases (NCDs), frequent outbreaks of infectious diseases, and increasing environmental health risks. The recent COVID-19 pandemic has illuminated the substantial vulnerabilities of even the most well-resourced health systems, exposing critical weaknesses in healthcare infrastructure and exacerbating existing health inequities.

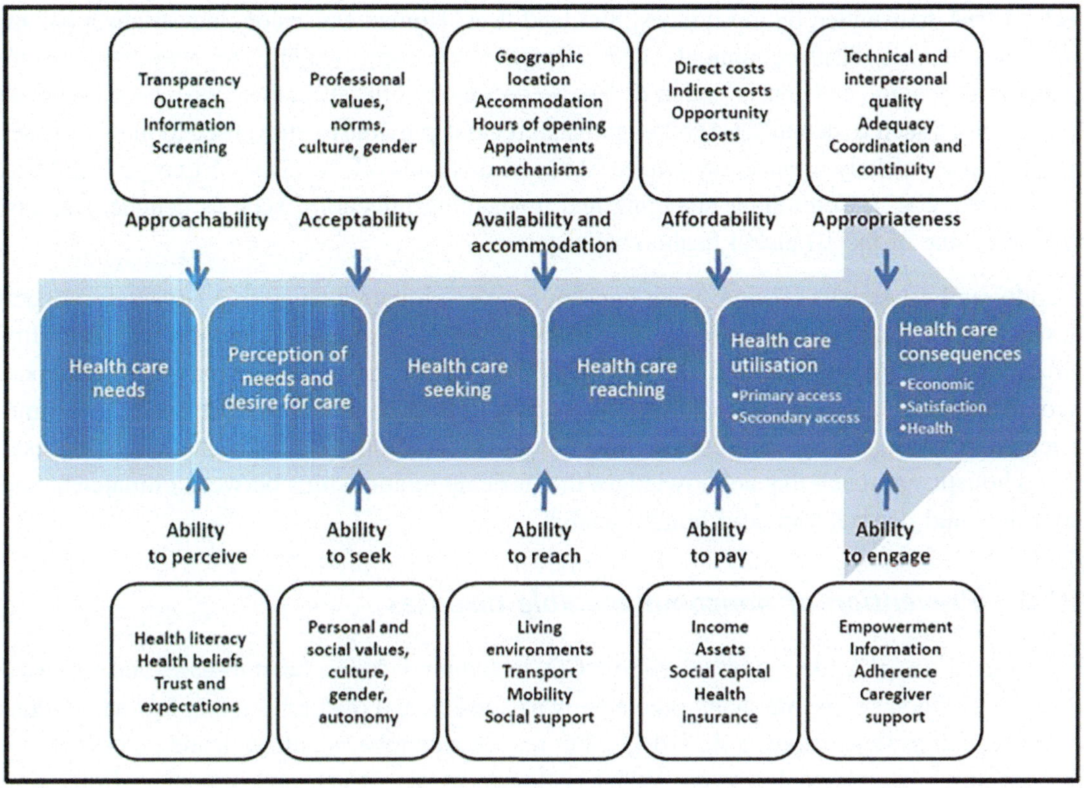

Figure 10.2
Conceptual framework of access to healthcare (Levesque et al., 2013).

The top 10 challenges to global public health were proposed by the WHO for actions as follows:

10.3 Climate change and pollution's impact on global health

It is estimated that nearly 7 million premature deaths annually are linked to inhalation of polluted air, affecting approximately 90% of the world's population (Annual Reviews, World). Poor air quality not only leads to respiratory and cardiovascular diseases (CVDs) but also exacerbates existing health disparities, particularly in vulnerable populations.

Climate change is associated with direct effect on health such as heat related disorders, allergies, lung diseases, and infectious diseases, as well as extreme weather changes injuries while indirectly may also affect access to food, forced demobilization of communities, and other social consequences such as mental illness and collective violence (Levy et al., 2017) Moreover, dynamic changes in ecology and climate are closely tied to the emergence of infectious diseases, thereby posing significant risks to humans, animals, and wildlife. Most emerging diseases are vector-borne, transmitted by mosquitoes, flies, and fleas. Human expansion, industrialization, and land use changes displace animals and disrupt ecosystems, leading to alterations in the distribution, activity, and concentration of disease vectors. For instance, there have been outbreaks of arboviruses such as dengue and chikungunya in regions previously unexposed to these diseases, including parts of Italy, France, the United States, and islands off the coast of Europe and Africa (Nova et al., 2022). Controlling emerging and reemerging infections, such as dengue, was also considered one of the 10 global health challenges.

In addition, heat stress is a significant consequence of climate change that adversely impacts human health. Rising temperatures can lead to higher rates of hospitalization and mortality, particularly among workers and the elderly. Furthermore, heat stress negatively influences income potential and access to nutrition, thereby influencing the overall health outcomes (Kjellstrom et al., 2016). Addressing these interconnected public health challenges necessitates a holistic approach that acknowledges the intricate relationships between climate change, environmental degradation, and human health.

10.4 Prevention of noncommunicable diseases

70% of deaths worldwide can be traced to NCD, including diabetes, heart disease, and cancer. A total of 15 million people are dying prematurely as a result, and over 85% are in low and middle-income countries (Kjellstrom et al., 2016). After recognizing tobacco, alcohol, and processed food as a leading cause of NCD by the WHO (Palmedo et al., 2017), and although efforts were consolidated in promoting healthy living, eating, and physical activities have been adopted for so many years, which did have some positive impact, such as reduction in cigarette smoking from 42% in 1965 to 14% in 2019. On the contrary, CVDs, cancer, diabetes, and obstructive lung diseases continue to be the top 4 most common causes of death among NCDs and continue to affect nearly 2/3 of the American's in their life course (Mazzucca et al., 2021). Therefore, more recently, the WHO launched a new initiative by urging all countries to increase real prices of sugary drinks, alcohol, and tobacco by 50% by 2035 in an effort to combat the rise of NCDs (World Health Organization (WHO), Antimicrobial).

With the rise of media and the advent of the social media era, innovative communication strategies, particularly counter-marketing, have emerged as effective interventions to reduce the consumption of unhealthy products. Counter-marketing aims to expose the motives behind, and denormalize the marketing activities of, producers of these unhealthy products. By highlighting the misleading tactics used by these industries, counter-marketing not only informs consumers but also empowers them to make healthier choices. These strategies can be particularly functional when tailored to target specific populations. For instance, campaigns can focus on vulnerable groups who may be more susceptible to the persuasive tactics of unhealthy product marketing (Kjellstrom et al., 2016). And one of the important NCDs that also carries a threat to global health is cancer, for which Global Cancer Trends and Contributing Factors is recognized as a threat.

Taking a global perspective, the number of cancer deaths is projected to escalate significantly, from approximately 12 million new cases and 7 million deaths in 2008 to an estimated 26 million new cases and 11.4 million deaths by 2030.

In 2007, around 72% of cancer deaths occurred in low- and middle-income countries, highlighting a growing disparity in cancer burden across different regions. Lung cancer remains the leading cause of cancer mortality worldwide, followed by stomach, colorectal, and breast cancers. Several contributing factors to this rise in cancer incidence and mortality include an aging population and tobacco smoking. While smoking is widely recognized as a carcinogen, particularly in developed countries, cancer has multifactorial causes that encompass biological, social, and environmental factors. In addition to lifestyle choices, infections with various pathogens contribute significantly to cancer risk. Notable infectious agents include:

- Human Immunodeficiency Virus (HIV)
- Hepatitis B Virus (HBV)
- Hepatitis C Virus (HCV)
- Human Papillomavirus (HPV)
- Epstein-Barr Virus (EBV)
- Human Herpes Virus 8 (HHV-8)
- *Helicobacter pylori*
- *Schistosoma haematobium*

Collectively, infections account for nearly 18% of cancer cases globally, underscoring the need for comprehensive cancer prevention strategies that address both communicable and noncommunicable disease risk factors. Lifestyle modifications, particularly regular physical exercise and the cessation of smoking, along with early screening and prompt diagnosis, have been linked to reduced mortality from cancer.

Despite these insights, there remains a significant gap in research and interest related to preventive strategies when compared to the advances made in cancer treatment. This disparity calls for an increased focus on prevention in public health policy and cancer research, emphasizing the need for integrated approaches that promote healthy lifestyles, timely interventions, and the implementation of effective screening programs (World Health Organization, WHO, 2024).

10.5 Preventing global pandemics

10.5.1 Combating drug resistance and understanding and monitoring high-risk pathogens

Antimicrobial resistance (AMR) is recognized as one of the top global threats to public health. In 2019, nearly 1.27 million deaths worldwide were directly linked to AMR, with an additional 4.95 million deaths associated with it. Furthermore, AMR poses significant risks to animals, plants, and agricultural production, creating a considerable threat to food security. In addition to its link to mortality, AMR is associated with substantial economic costs, with estimates suggesting it could be responsible for an additional US$ 1 trillion in healthcare costs by 2050 and GDP losses ranging from US$ 1 trillion to US$ 3.4 trillion per year by 2030, according to the World Bank (World Health Organization (WHO), Antimicrobial).

AMR is not exclusively linked to bacterial infections; it also affects parasitic, tropical, viral, and fungal infections. Moreover, AMR is associated with a lack of access to clean water for both humans and animals, highlighting its complexity and connection to environmental factors (World Health Organization, WHO, 2024).

Given these interconnections, a "One Health" approach is essential. This integrated strategy facilitates collaboration among stakeholders from various sectors such as human health, food production, animal health, and environmental sustainability to ensure the effective implementation and monitoring of necessary interventions. The goal is to achieve optimal and sustainable health outcomes for people, animals, and ecosystems (Chowdhury & Ravi, 2022).

Tackling AMR in the human health sector necessitates global efforts focusing on the key areas to control the emergence of these pathogens through robust infection prevention and control measures, ensuring equitable access, early diagnosis and treatment, vigilant surveillance to detect emerging trends in AMR, and further investment in research and development (R&D) for the creation of new medicines, diagnostics, and prevention tools (Mazzucca et al., 2021).

The Global Action Plans were established in 2015 by the WHO, which was a major step forward to overcome the AMR threat while focusing on the following five objectives:

- Improving awareness and understanding of AMR through effective communication, education, and training
- Strengthening the knowledge and evidence base through research and surveillance programs
- Reducing the infection rate through enhancing effective sanitation, hygiene, and infection prevention measures
- Optimizing the use of antimicrobial medicines in both human and animal health sectors
- Developing the economic case for sustainable investment that takes account of the needs of all countries and to increase investment in new medicines, diagnostic tools, vaccines, and other interventions (World Health Organization (WHO), WHO).

In 2017, the WHO published the Bacterial Priority Pathogens List (BPPL) to guide investments in research and development and to inform the strategies for surveillance and control of antibacterial resistance. Despite ongoing efforts, the global antibiotic pipeline remains a significant challenge, hampered by limited worldwide investment. This list was further updated in 2024 to reflect changes due to recent global events, such as the COVID-19 pandemic, and to address identified gaps. The revision aims to direct the focus of leaders, researchers, and industry stakeholders towards high-priority pathogens selected based on factors such as mortality rates, incidence, nonfatal health burdens, resistance trends, transmissibility, preventability within healthcare settings and communities, treatability, and the availability of pipeline medications. The pathogens are further subclassified into "critical pathogens," "high priority," and "medium priority" categories graph-1 (Colditz & Wei, 2012) (Fig. 10.3).

While immunization is recognized as a vital global tool in combating infectious diseases, including those linked to AMR, vaccine hesitancy and availability have emerged as significant threats. The increase in vaccine hesitancy undermines efforts to achieve widespread immunization. Vaccination is estimated to prevent approximately 2.5 million deaths among children under five years of age; however, vaccine-preventable diseases continue to claim the life of one child every 20 seconds (Chowdhury & Ravi, 2022; Galagali et al., 2022).

Despite ongoing initiatives to improve access to immunizations, the mortality rate among children under five remains a pressing concern in developing countries, where it accounts for 93% of child mortality in regions of Africa and Asia. It is estimated that 20% of newborns each year do not receive the vaccinations they need. Typically, these immunization services are delivered through primary healthcare systems, which constitute the first point of contact for patients. Unfortunately, individuals living in rural areas continue to face significant challenges in accessing these essential services (World Health Organization, WHO, 2024).

While vaccine hesitancy is not a new phenomenon, it has existed for over 200 years since the first vaccine was administered. Social media and open communication platforms have brought it renewed attention. Although global vaccination coverage has significantly increased since the 1980s, immunization rates for vaccines against tuberculosis, diphtheria, tetanus, pertussis, measles, and polio have been declining since 2012. This trend poses a serious threat to the elimination of preventable diseases. The reasons individuals in HICs and LMICs choose not to vaccinate are complex and multifaceted. A vaccine advisory group to the WHO has identified complacency, inconvenient access to vaccines, and lack of confidence as key factors contributing to vaccine hesitancy. Additionally, vaccine hesitancy can stem from various influences, such as a lack of knowledge, misguided religious beliefs, and exposure to antivaccine misinformation (Chowdhury & Ravi, 2022; Galagali et al., 2022).

Healthcare equity, particularly in vulnerable settings, is an important global health challenge, yet disparities in the healthcare system and action plans need to be addressed.

10.6 Healthcare disparities and action plans

Health disparities refer to the differences and gaps in the quality of health and healthcare experienced by various racial, ethnic, and socio-economic groups (Riley, 2012). They can also

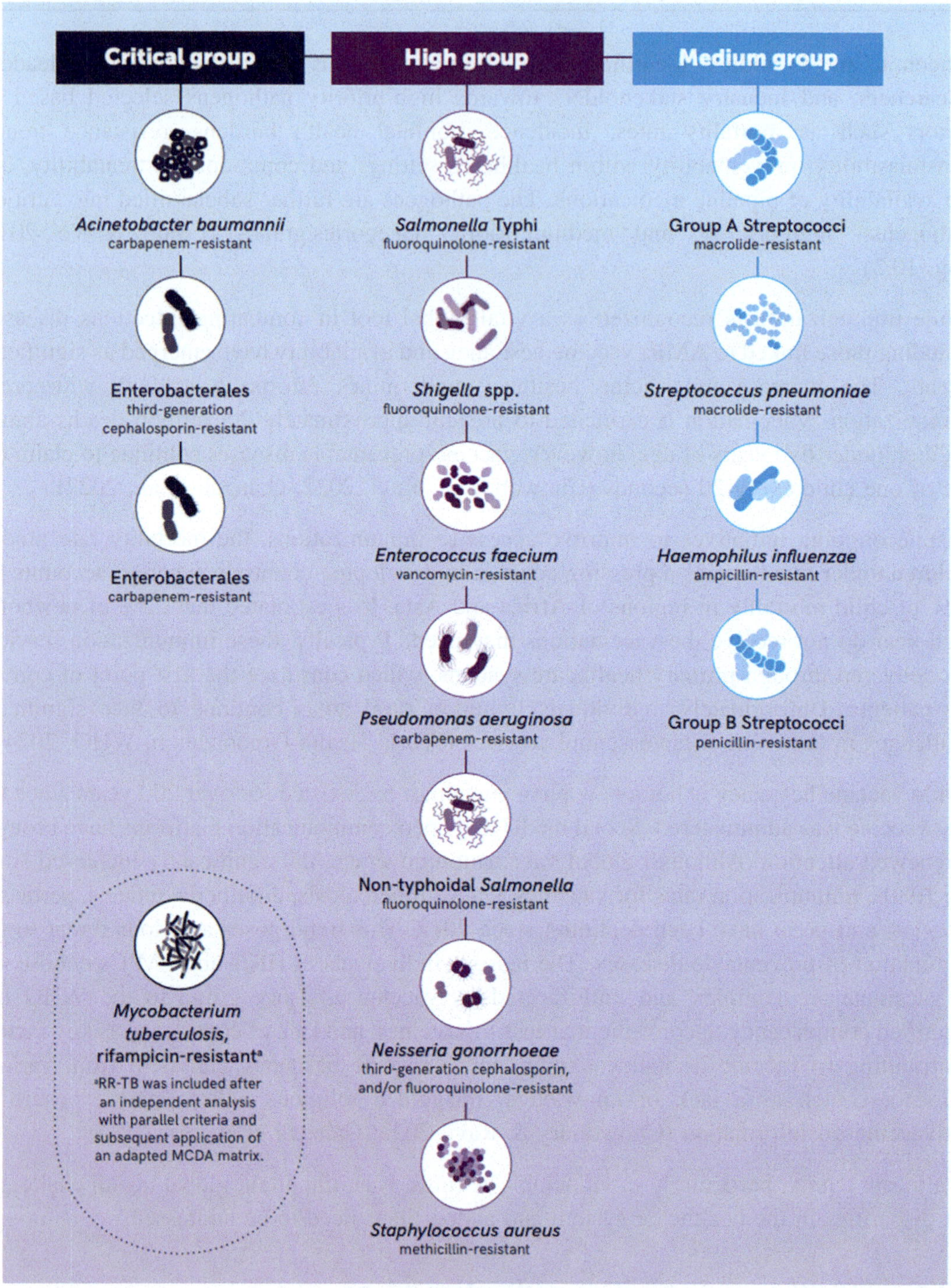

Figure 10.3

WHO bacterial priority pathogens list, 2024: Bacterial pathogens of public health importance to guide research, development, and strategies to prevent and control antimicrobial resistance, https://www.who.int/publications/i/item/9789240093461 (World Health Organization, WHO, 2024).

be understood as population-specific variations in the prevalence of disease, health outcomes, or access to healthcare services.

Several illustrative examples underscore the severity of these disparities as follows:

- Infant mortality rates for Black babies are nearly 2.5 times higher than those for White babies
- Life expectancy for Black men and women is nearly a decade shorter compared to their White counterparts
- Diabetes rates are over 30% higher among Native Americans and Latinos than among Whites; and mortality rates from heart disease, stroke, and prostate and breast cancers are significantly elevated in Black populations (Short & Zacher, 2022).

10.7 Women health and healthcare disparity

Women's health is defined as the physical, mental, and social well-being of women, and it is a broad category of population health. Women's health is socially patterned like other human health. As a group, women has been marginalized for many centuries across different regions not only for healthcare access but also for other rights such as education and political rights such as voting or even bodily autonomy, this has affected poorer and disabled women more than others while currently women have more economic and political power than they did in the past yet they remain underrepresented at the highest levels of business and government. Women'slife expectancy may vary from 80 years in nearly 46 high- income countries to less than 58 years in Africa, with a higher death rate among younger-aged women (Mariani et al., 2017).

Globally, ischemic heart disease, stroke, and chronic obstructive pulmonary disease account for 45% of deaths among women over the age of 60, compared to 15% attributed to cancer in the same age group. Breast cancer, which is the leading cause of cancer-related deaths among women, saw approximately 1.7 million new cases and 0.5 million deaths in 2012. In low- and middle-income countries, breast cancer is often diagnosed at advanced stages, leaving limited curative options. As a result, the five-year survival rate can be as low as 40% in low-income countries, compared to approximately 80% in HICs such as those in North America and Sweden.

In addition to cancer care, reproductive and maternal health remains a significant cause of mortality in Africa. According to the WHO Millennium Development Goals Progress Report, 1 in 30 women in Africa die during childbirth, in stark contrast to 1 in 5600 in developed countries. This disparity is closely linked to a lack of education and inadequate maternal care.

Furthermore, in 2013, 60% of new HIV infections among individuals younger than 25 occurred in girls and young women. Untreated sexually transmitted infections are often associated with adverse pregnancy outcomes and can increase the risk of malignancies. HPV-related cervical cancer constitutes 70% of cervical cancer cases worldwide, making it the second most common cancer among women, with approximately 530,000 new cases and more than 270,000 deaths annually (Sharma et al., 2025).

There are multiple factors contributing to healthcare access disparities among different populations, particularly in LMICs. Key barriers include:

1. Availability of healthcare services: Many communities, especially in rural areas, face a shortage of healthcare facilities and providers, limiting access to essential services.
2. Transportation needs: The lack of reliable transportation can hinder individuals from reaching healthcare services, particularly in remote regions where facilities are sparse.
3. Economic barriers: Out-of-pocket expenses and inadequate insurance coverage create significant financial barriers to accessing care. Individuals often forgo necessary treatment due to the costs associated with healthcare services.
4. Healthcare education and awareness: A lack of education about healthcare and the importance of preventive services contributes to the underutilization of available resources. This gap in understanding often results in late diagnoses and poor health outcomes.
5. Stigma and employment: Health issues can carry stigma, impacting a person's self-esteem and fitness to work. This, in turn, affects their income and ability to seek care.
6. Investment deficits: Insufficient investment in healthcare infrastructure leads to a lack of medications, medical equipment, and other vital resources needed for effective care delivery.

While the utilization of digital health and telehealth services presents opportunities to improve access for certain populations in more developed regions, these solutions may not be as effective in poorer countries that lack the necessary infrastructure for implementing such innovative interventions. Without robust internet connectivity, digital literacy, and supportive health systems, the potential benefits of telehealth cannot be realized fully (Chowdhury & Ravi, 2022).

10.8 Harnessing technologies in healthcare access, artificial intelligence, and global health challenges

Millions of people’s health and well-being are at risk of several factors and multiple overlapping crises, including but not limited to infectious disease outbreaks, rising malnutrition rates, and lack of sufficient medical access; all hit the vulnerable the most

Global public health priorities play a crucial role in addressing the most pressing health challenges faced by populations worldwide. They are dynamic and evolve in response to emerging health challenges and crises, which need effective collaboration among countries to secure global health. Mental health, the Impact of climate change, CVDs, diabetes, infectious diseases, health system, and population aging are examples of challenges that are examples of these challenges that are known to pose a vast burden worldwide.

Table 10.1 Global health challenges and strategic solutions (Levesque et al., 2013).

Section	Key topics	Challenges	Solutions/global actions
Challenges of climate change	Causes and effects of climate change, air quality, smog	Fossil fuel use, deforestation, extreme weather, food insecurity, health risks (e.g., respiratory diseases, cancer)	Renewable energy, sustainable agriculture, reforestation, Paris Agreement, public awareness, community engagement
Emerging diseases	COVID-19, HIV, Lyme disease, *E. coli*, Hantavirus, Dengue, Zika, West Nile	Rapid spread, zoonotic origins, diagnostic challenges, vaccine development, vector control	Early detection, surveillance, community-based reporting, public awareness, vector control strategies
Reemerging diseases	Malaria, TB, cholera, pertussis, influenza, AMR, gonorrhea	Drug resistance, low vaccination rates, disrupted healthcare systems, environmental changes	Improved surveillance, genomic sequencing, vaccination programs, antibiotic stewardship, public health policies
Noncommunicable diseases	Cardiovascular diseases, diabetes, cancer, chronic respiratory diseases	Lifestyle factors (smoking, poor diet, inactivity), environmental pollution, healthcare access disparities	Health education, lifestyle modification programs, equitable healthcare access, pollution control
Natural disasters	Floods, earthquakes, tsunamis, cyclones	Waterborne diseases, overcrowded shelters, disrupted healthcare systems, economic losses	Integrated health systems, community education, multihazard preparedness plans, research, policy integration
Wars, terrorism, crises	Ukraine war, Gaza conflict, bioterrorism, humanitarian crises	Healthcare system destruction, mental health issues, displacement, vaccine-preventable disease resurgence	Humanitarian aid, mental health support, healthcare system rebuilding, conflict resolution, global cooperation
Global partnerships	UN, WHO, SDGs, global health governance	Fragmented coordination, funding shortages, political prioritization of national interests over global health	Strengthening WHO capacity, equitable resource distribution, global health security frameworks, universal health coverage

Utilization of the artificial intelligence (AI) functions, such as deep learning, machine learning, and natural language development in addressing the global health challenges and mitigating and prioritizing health needs, such as disease surveillance improvement, diagnosis, treatment selection, and clinical laboratory testing.

Crucial ethics, privacy, and bias issues were raised to ensure AI's responsible and equitable integration in the global public health landscape. Additionally, the human inability to see how ML systems make their decisions, a "black box," brought uncertainty and threatened trust among the users regarding its application (Zaidan, 2023) (Table 10.1).

10.9 Conclusion

Access to healthcare is a multifaceted issue that remains a pressing global challenge. As highlighted in this chapter, the disparities in healthcare access are influenced by a range of social, economic, and systemic factors that affect individuals and communities differently. Despite improvements in healthcare access over the decades, with reported increases in the Global HAQ Index, significant gaps persist. The dimensions of healthcare access approachability, acceptability, availability and accommodation, affordability, and appropriateness interact dynamically to shape the healthcare experiences of individuals. Understanding these dimensions is crucial for identifying barriers to healthcare and implementing effective solutions.

In addressing these challenges, it is crucial to align global health initiatives, such as the SDGs, with efforts to strengthen healthcare systems. By fostering international cooperation, investing in healthcare infrastructure, and implementing innovative solutions, including the responsible use of technologies like AI.

It is evident that sustained commitment, cross-sector collaboration, and active community engagement are necessary to transform healthcare access into a universal reality. With a concerted effort, we can move closer to achieving health equity and ensuring that quality healthcare is accessible for all individuals, regardless of their circumstances.

References

Abatemarco, A., Aria, M., Beraldo, S., & Collaro, M. (2024). Measuring health care access and its inequality: A decomposition approach. *Economic Modelling, 132*, 106659. https://doi.org/10.1016/j.econmod.2024.106659.

Annual Reviews. World health threats. https://www.annualreviews.org/page/worldhealththreats

Chowdhury, J., & Ravi, R. P. (2022). Healthcare accessibility in developing countries: A global healthcare challenge. *Journal of Clinical and Biomedical Research.*

Colditz, G. A., & Wei, E. K. (2012). Preventability of cancer: The relative contributions of biologic and social and physical environmental determinants of cancer mortality. *Annual Review of Public Health, 33*, 137–156. https://doi.org/10.1146/annurev-publhealth-031811-124627.

Cu, A., Meister, S., Lefebvre, B., et al. (2021). Assessing healthcare access using Levesque's conceptual framework: A scoping review. *International Journal for Equity in Health, 20*, 116. https://doi.org/10.1186/s12939-021-01416-3.

Dawkins, B., Renwick, C., Ensor, T., Shinkins, B., Jayne, D., & Meads, D. (2021). What factors affect patients' ability to access healthcare? An overview of systematic reviews. *Tropical Medicine & International Health: TM & IH, 26*, 1177–1188. https://doi.org/10.1111/tmi.13651.

Endalamaw, A., Gilks, C. F., Ambaw, F., & Assefa, Y. (2022). Universality of universal health coverage: A scoping review. *PLoS One, 17*(8), e0269507. https://doi.org/10.1371/journal.pone.0269507.

Fullman, N., Yearwood, J., Abay, S. M., et al. (2018). Measuring performance on the healthcare access and quality index for 195 countries and territories and selected subnational locations: A systematic analysis from the Global Burden of Disease Study 2016. *Lancet, 391*, 2236–2271.

Galagali, P. M., Kinikar, A. A., & Kumar, V. S. (2022). Vaccine hesitancy: Obstacles and challenges. *Current Pediatrics Reports, 10*(4), 241–248. https://doi.org/10.1007/s40124-022-00278-9.

Kjellstrom, T., Briggs, D., Freyberg, C., Lemke, B., Otto, M., & Hyatt, O. (2016). Heat, human performance, and occupational health. *Annual Review of Public Health, 37*, 97–112. https://doi.org/10.1146/annurev-publhealth-032315-021740.

Levesque, J. F., Harris, M. F., & Russell, G. (2013). Patient-centred access to health care: Conceptualising access at the interface of health systems and populations. *International Journal for Equity in Health, 12*, 18. https://doi.org/10.1186/1475-9276-12-18.

Levy, B. S., Sidel, V. W., & Patz, J. A. (2017). Climate change and public health. *Annual Review of Public Health, 38*, 241–257. https://doi.org/10.1146/annurev-publhealth-031816-044232.

Mariani, G., Kasznia-Brown, J., Paez, D., et al. (2017). Improving women's health in low- and middle-income countries: challenges and priorities. *Nuclear Medicine Communications, 38*(12), 1019–1023. https://doi.org/10.1097/MNM.0000000000000751.

Mazzucca, S., Arredondo, E. M., Hoelscher, D. M., Haire-Joshu, D., Tabak, R. G., Kumanyika, S. K., & Brownson, R. C. (2021). Expanding implementation research to prevent chronic diseases in community settings. *Annual Review of Public Health, 42*, 135–158. https://doi.org/10.1146/annurev-publhealth-090419-102547.

Nova, N., Athni, T. S., Childs, M. L., Mandle, L., & Mordecai, E. A. (2022). Global change and emerging infectious diseases. *Annual Review of Resource Economics, 14*, 333–354. https://doi.org/10.1146/annurev-resource-111820-024214.

Palmedo, P. C., Dorfman, L., Garza, S., Murphy, E., & Freudenberg, N. (2017). Countermarketing alcohol and unhealthy food: An effective strategy for preventing noncommunicable diseases. *Annual Review of Public Health, 38*, 119–144. https://doi.org/10.1146/annurev-publhealth-031816-044303.

Rifai, M., Mahtta, D., Kherallah, R., et al. (2021). Prevalence and determinants of difficulty in accessing medical care in U.S. adults. *American Journal of Preventive Medicine, 61*(4), 492–500. https://doi.org/10.1016/j.amepre.2021.03.026.

Riley, W. J. (2012). Health disparities: Gaps in access, quality and affordability of medical care. *Transactions of the American Clinical and Climatological Association, 123*, 167–172.

Sharma, M., Akhter, M. S., Roy, S., & Srejon, R. (2025). Future issues in global health: Challenges and conundrums. *International Journal of Environmental Research and Public Health, 22*(3), 325. https://doi.org/10.3390/ijerph22030325.

Short, S. E., & Zacher, M. (2022). Women's health: Population patterns and social determinants. *Annual Review of Sociology, 48*, 277–298. https://doi.org/10.1146/annurev-soc-030320-034200.

World Health Organization (WHO). Antimicrobial resistance. https://www.who.int/news-room/fact-sheets/detail/antimicrobial-resistance

World Health Organization (WHO). (2023). *Issues and Challenges in Access to Medicines Faced by Small Countries in the WHO European Region: Policy Brief.* Copenhagen: WHO Regional Office for Europe. https://iris.who.int.

World Health Organization (WHO). SDG target 3.8: achieve universal health coverage. https://www.who.int/data/gho/data/themes/topics/service-coverage (accessed June 25, 2025).

World Health Organization (WHO). Universal health coverage (UHC). https://www.who.int/health-topics/universal-health-coverage (accessed June 20, 2025).

World Health Organization (WHO). WHO bacterial priority pathogens list, 2024. https://iris.who.int

World Health Organization (WHO). WHO launches bold push to raise health taxes and save millions of lives. https://www.who.int/news/item/02-07-2025-who-launches-bold-push-to-raise-health-taxes-and-save-millions-of-lives

Zaidan, A. M. (2023). The leading global health challenges in the artificial intelligence era. *Frontiers in Public Health, 11*. https://doi.org/10.3389/fpubh.2023.1328918.

CHAPTER 11

Precision medicine: personalizing treatments for improved outcomes

Paraskevi Papadopoulou[1] and Constantine A. Stratakis[2,3,4,5,6]

[1]Department of Natural Sciences, Deree-The American College of Greece, Athens, Greece, [2]Research Institute, HCA Hospital for Endocrine Surgery, Tampa, FL, United States, [3]ASTREA Health, Athens, Greece, [4]Medical Genetics, H. Dunant Hospital, Athens, Greece, [5]IMBB, FORTH, Human Genetics and Precision Medicine, Heraklion, Greece, [6]Pediatrics, University of Athens Medical School, Athens, Greece

11.1 Introduction

11.1.1 Precision medicine versus personalized medicine (EU vs US use of terms)

Precision medicine (PM) is an innovative approach to health and healthcare that tailors medical treatments to the individual characteristics of each patient (Akhoon, 2021; Baltagiannis et al., 2020; Collins & Varmus, 2015). While the terms "precision medicine" and "personalized medicine" are often used interchangeably, there are subtle distinctions between the two (Baltagiannis et al., 2020; Behl et al., 2022; Papadopoulou & Lytras, 2023). Precision medicine emphasizes the integration of genetic, environmental, and lifestyle factors to deliver precise interventions, whereas personalized medicine takes a broader approach, focusing on the holistic customization of care (Akhoon, 2021; Baltagiannis et al., 2020; Behl et al., 2022).

The terminology surrounding this field varies across regions, especially in the United States (US) versus Europe (EU). In the US, "precision medicine" is more commonly used, reflecting a focus on using genomic and molecular data to deliver targeted treatments. The National Institutes of Health (The National Institutes of Health:The Promise of Precision Medicine, 2025) defines PM as "an innovative approach that takes into account individual differences in genes, environment, and lifestyles." This term gained prominence after the launch of the US Precision Medicine Initiative in 2015, which aimed to accelerate biomedical research and develop tailored therapies (Collins & Varmus, 2015). This approach contrasts with conventional medicine, which typically develops treatments based on the average patient response within a population without considering individual and sex differences. Instead, PM seeks to identify subgroups of patients who share similar molecular or clinical characteristics, enabling more targeted and effective therapeutic interventions.

The Future of Pharma Across All Sectors in the Artificial Intelligence Era. DOI: https://doi.org/10.1016/B978-0-443-40572-3.00015-0

In Europe, however, "personalized medicine" is more prevalent, focusing on customized healthcare approaches (Abul-Husn & Kenny, 2019; Baltagiannis et al., 2020; Papadopoulou & Lytras, 2023; Personalized Medicine Coalition (PMC), 2017). This preferred term emphasizes a broader scope that includes prevention, diagnosis, and treatment strategies tailored to individual patient needs. European organizations, such as the European Alliance for Personalized Medicine, advocate for this term to highlight the holistic approach to healthcare customization (Abul-Husn & Kenny, 2019; Papadopoulou & Lytras, 2023). Despite these differences in terminology, both concepts share the common goal of optimizing health and healthcare through individualization. The European Health Information Portal (EHIP) facilitates access to population health and healthcare data, information, and expertise across Europe. It provides a forum for the rapid exchange of information across countries to learn from each other's challenges and implement best practices. The EHIP contains catalogs for data sources, National and European projects, research infrastructures, capacity-building activities, and COVID-19-related resources that help researchers, policymakers, data providers, developers, and the general public to find and access population health information promptly (What is the Health Information Portal?, 2025).

The effects our unique genetic makeup and life experiences have on our health, our susceptibility to illness, and our reactions to medical interventions are questions that PM aims to answer (Baltagiannis et al., 2020; Collins & Varmus, 2015; Popescu et al., 2024; Naithani et al., 2021). We can theoretically prescribe the best treatments for each individual, improve policymaking by better predicting population health, and possibly even solve some of the mysteries surrounding the workings of life itself if we understand how genes and the environment interact to define pathophysiological traits (Akhoon, 2021; Baltagiannis et al., 2020; Li & Warner, 2020). Although this goal has not yet been achieved, we now possess the investigative tools to accomplish it. The central tenet of PM lies in understanding how an individual's genetic makeup interacts with environmental and lifestyle factors to influence health, disease susceptibility, and response to treatments (Akhoon, 2021; Bonkhoff & Grefkes, 2022). This understanding holds transformative potential for healthcare, enabling clinicians to prescribe the most effective treatments for each patient, predict population health trends, and unravel complex biological mechanisms underlying diseases (Collins & Varmus, 2015). The advent of advanced genomic, transcriptomic, and proteomic tools now provides unprecedented opportunities to achieve these goals, marking a significant departure from traditional one-size-fits-all approaches (Behl et al., 2022; Calabretta et al., 2020; Calinski et al., 2021).

11.1.2 The shift from one-size-fits-all to personalized treatments

Traditional medical practices often relied on standardized treatments applied broadly across populations, with little regard for individual variability and sex-related differences. While effective in some cases, this approach has significant limitations, particularly for patients whose unique genetic and environmental factors influence disease progression and treatment outcomes (Behl et al., 2022).

Precision medicine revolutionizes this paradigm by leveraging advanced technologies, such as next-generation sequencing (NGS), the use of clustered regularly interspaced short palindromic repeats (CRISPR), which is a gene editing technology that allows scientists to modify DNA sequences in living organisms, and big data analytics, to identify biomarkers and predict treatment efficacy at an individual level. For instance, pharmacogenomic studies have demonstrated how genetic variations can significantly influence drug metabolism, paving the way for tailored therapies that minimize adverse effects and maximize efficacy (Behl et al., 2022).

Overall, PM aims to improve health and healthcare by predicting the best course of action for complex diseases like cancer, diabetes, and COVID-19. By understanding a patient's metabolomics and genetic makeup, PM can determine predisposition, diagnostic, prognostic, and predictive biomarkers, providing optimal care for chronic and acute diseases. In clinical settings, timely modeling of clinical and multiomics data is crucial for identifying underlying biologic pathways, modifiable risk factors, and early detection and prevention of complex disorders. AI and machine learning (ML) algorithms enhance precision medicine by extending information and modeling patient-specific data against annotation data (Ahmed, 2022). Indeed, high-throughput technologies and cost reduction have enabled the generation of large amounts of multiomics data, enabling clinical applications. Combination therapy, a method for treating diseases like cancer, can be identified and developed using patient-specific multiomics data integration (John et al., 2020). Similarly, the following review paper states that AI is being increasingly used in oncology to understand cancer biology. Deep learning and ML are being used for the detection, prognosis, and administration of treatments. Large language models like ChatGPT are being used in clinics. Multiomics data types are being combined to create decision-support tools. The authors point to the challenges and constraints that need to be evaluated for future use in clinical settings (Gao et al., 2024). Multiomics analyses, utilizing technologies in genomics, transcriptomics, epigenomics, proteomics, and metabolomics, are crucial for PM. However, integrated multiomics analyses have not been widely applied, hindering further progress in PM. More efforts are needed to develop an effective analytical infrastructure (John et al., 2020; Olivier et al., 2019).

Even though AI in oncology, as an example, has grown rapidly, aiming to improve clinical decision-making, access to care, and efficiency, the adoption remains limited due to barriers like biased data, data management, and outdated regulations. To overcome these, stakeholders should train the workforce, standardize data, fund research, and collaborate on multidisciplinary AI tools. According to this review paper, this will lead to safer, high-value oncology care (Chua et al., 2021).

Prevention is the key to a healthy life. Diabetes, as another example, imposes a significant healthcare burden, and uniform treatment approaches often lead to progressive failure and complications. Advances in genomic research have laid the foundation for PM in diabetes prevention and management. The following review explores the genetic basis of diabetes, the role of genomic medicine in treatment, and the need for integrating genetic information into risk prediction models and drug discovery. Further research is essential to translate these findings into clinical practice, enabling personalized treatment strategies for improved patient outcomes not only in diabetes but for most diseases (Xie et al., 2018).

11.1.3 Overview of the chapter's objectives

This chapter provides a comprehensive examination of PM across multiple dimensions. We explore the foundational technologies that enable personalized healthcare, examine clinical applications across various medical specialties, and discuss the challenges and opportunities that lie ahead. The chapter aims to:

1. Provide healthcare professionals with a thorough understanding of PM principles
2. Examine current clinical applications and emerging technologies
3. Address implementation challenges and ethical considerations
4. Outline future directions and potential breakthroughs
5. Offer practical insights for healthcare system integration

This chapter, therefore, examines the multifaceted domain of PM, tracing its historical evolution, exploring its methodological underpinnings, and highlighting its transformative applications in various fields, including oncology, cardiology, endocrinology, genetic disorders, brain diseases, and pharmacology. It examines the technological innovations, such as the use of multiomics and AI, CRISPR (Barrangou, 2020; Das et al., 2022; Davies et al., 2024; Derry, 2021; Severi & Akbari, 2024), and AlphaFold2 & 3 (Abramson et al., 2024; Jumper et al., 2021), that enable these advancements and addresses the ethical, regulatory, and accessibility challenges that must be overcome to realize the full potential of PM. Finally, the chapter outlines strategic pathways for integrating PM into global healthcare systems, ensuring equitable access and improved patient outcomes.

11.2 Background: the foundations of precision medicine

11.2.1 Historical development of precision medicine

The journey of PM began with the discovery of the DNA double helix in 1953 by Watson and Crick, followed by advancements like Sanger sequencing in 1977, and the Human Genome Project, launched in 1990 and completed in 2003, which marked a pivotal moment by providing the first complete map of human genetic information. This achievement catalyzed the development of genomic medicine and set the stage for the PM revolution. Key milestones in precision medicine development include: 1953: Discovery of DNA double helix structure, 1990–2003: Human Genome Project completion, 1998: First FDA-approved pharmacogenomic test (HercepTest), 2011: Launch of the Cancer Genome Atlas (TCGA), 2015: President Obama's Precision Medicine Initiative, **2018:** FDA approval of first tissue-agnostic cancer treatment, 2020: CRISPR-Cas9 gene editing receives Nobel Prize, 2021: AlphaFold protein structure prediction breakthrough (Naithani, Atal et al., 2021; Naithani, Sinha et al., 2021). Precision oncology, as an example, has led to a need for predictive assays for patient treatment selection. The complexity of signaling and transcriptional networks complicates the development of biomarkers. Artificial intelligence (AI) and ML tools have enabled the digitization of tissue images, improving patient management. The following review paper evaluated AI-based computational approaches for digital pathology, focusing on deep neural networks and providing feature-based methodologies. The authors point to the challenges that include validation datasets, regulatory approval, and fair reimbursement strategies (Bera et al., 2019).

11.2.2 The role of genomics, transcriptomics, proteomics, and metabolomics

The "omics" sciences have been pivotal in understanding the molecular basis of diseases, enabling the development of targeted therapies and diagnostics (Adashi & Stratakis, 2024; Aronson & Rehm, 2015; Cecchin & Stocco, 2020; Coler et al., 2024; Genomics England, 2021; Li & Warner, 2020; Lau & Wu, 2018; Wang et al., 2023).

The last three decades marked a transformative era in mammalian cloning, driven by pioneers Sir Ian Wilmut, Ryuzo Yanagimachi, and Mark Westhusin. Wilmut's cloning of Dolly revolutionized biotechnology, while Yanagimachi's nuclear transfer research led to the first cloned mouse, Cumulina. Westhusin expanded cloning to various species, including the first cloned cat, Copycat (CC). Their groundbreaking work has established somatic nuclear transfer as a crucial tool for advances in regenerative medicine and in vitro gametogenesis (Adashi & Stratakis, 2024).

11.2.3 Integration of big data and advanced analytics in personalizing care

The gap between the potential of genomics in PM and its current implementation is evident due to outdated workflows, regulatory barriers, and incompatible healthcare infrastructures. Achieving its full potential requires systemic changes in billing, reimbursement, and technical architectures, with evolving roles for clinical geneticists and genetic counselors. Integrating genomic data at the point of care can significantly improve patient outcomes, but overcoming these obstacles is essential to prevent avoidable deaths and fulfill the promise of PM (Walton & Christensen, 2023).

More importantly, it is the convergence of big data analytics and ML that has revolutionized PM, allowing for the analysis of vast datasets to inform patient-specific treatment strategies

(Hassan et al., 2022). As an example, the integration of genomic data with electronic health records (EHRs) has been key to advancing PM. Growing EHR adoption and population-based biobanks enable translational and implementation research, driving its progress. This review explores advancements in health data digitization, genomic research in healthcare systems, and emerging strategies for widespread PM implementation (Abul-Husn & Kenny, 2019).

11.2.4 Examples of multiomics technologies

A cornerstone of PM is the ability to comprehensively profile patients at the molecular level. Multiomics approaches integrate various biological data layers—such as genomics, transcriptomics, proteomics, and metabolomics to generate a holistic view of disease mechanisms and treatment responses. These systems and personalized interventions ultimately improve patient outcomes.

See Fig. 11.1 for how the Precision Medicine Ecosystem has evolved over the past years.

Genomics: The blueprint of life—Genomics provides the foundational layer of multiomics by analyzing the complete set of DNA within an organism, including genes and noncoding regions. In the context of PM, genomic data are critical for identifying disease-causing mutations, predicting drug responses, and assessing individual susceptibility to various conditions. The advent of whole genome sequencing (WGS) and whole exome sequencing (WES) has dramatically improved access to genomic insights, with sequencing costs dropping from billions of dollars in the early 2000s to under $1000 per genome today. Clinical applications of genomics are vast. Pharmacogenomics enables the prediction of how patients metabolize and respond to medications based on genetic variants, while cancer genomics facilitates the identification of driver mutations that inform targeted therapies. Additionally, genomics plays a key role in diagnosing rare genetic disorders and supporting carrier screening to assess reproductive risks (Collins & Varmus, 2015).

Transcriptomics: gene expression and regulation—Transcriptomics builds upon genomics by analyzing RNA transcripts to understand which genes are actively expressed in specific tissues under particular physiological or pathological conditions. This layer provides dynamic insight into gene regulation and cellular function. RNA sequencing (RNA-seq) has become a standard tool for transcriptome analysis, offering high-resolution profiles of gene expression. Notably, single-cell RNA sequencing (scRNA-seq) has transformed our understanding of cellular heterogeneity within tissues and tumors, enabling the identification of rare cell populations, lineage tracing, and mapping of treatment responses at the cellular level. These technologies offer valuable opportunities for discovering novel therapeutic targets and understanding disease progression mechanisms (Ortega-Batista et al., 2025; Su et al., 2022).

Proteomics: functional molecular insights—While genomics and transcriptomics reveal potential biological functions, proteomics provides a direct view of functional molecular

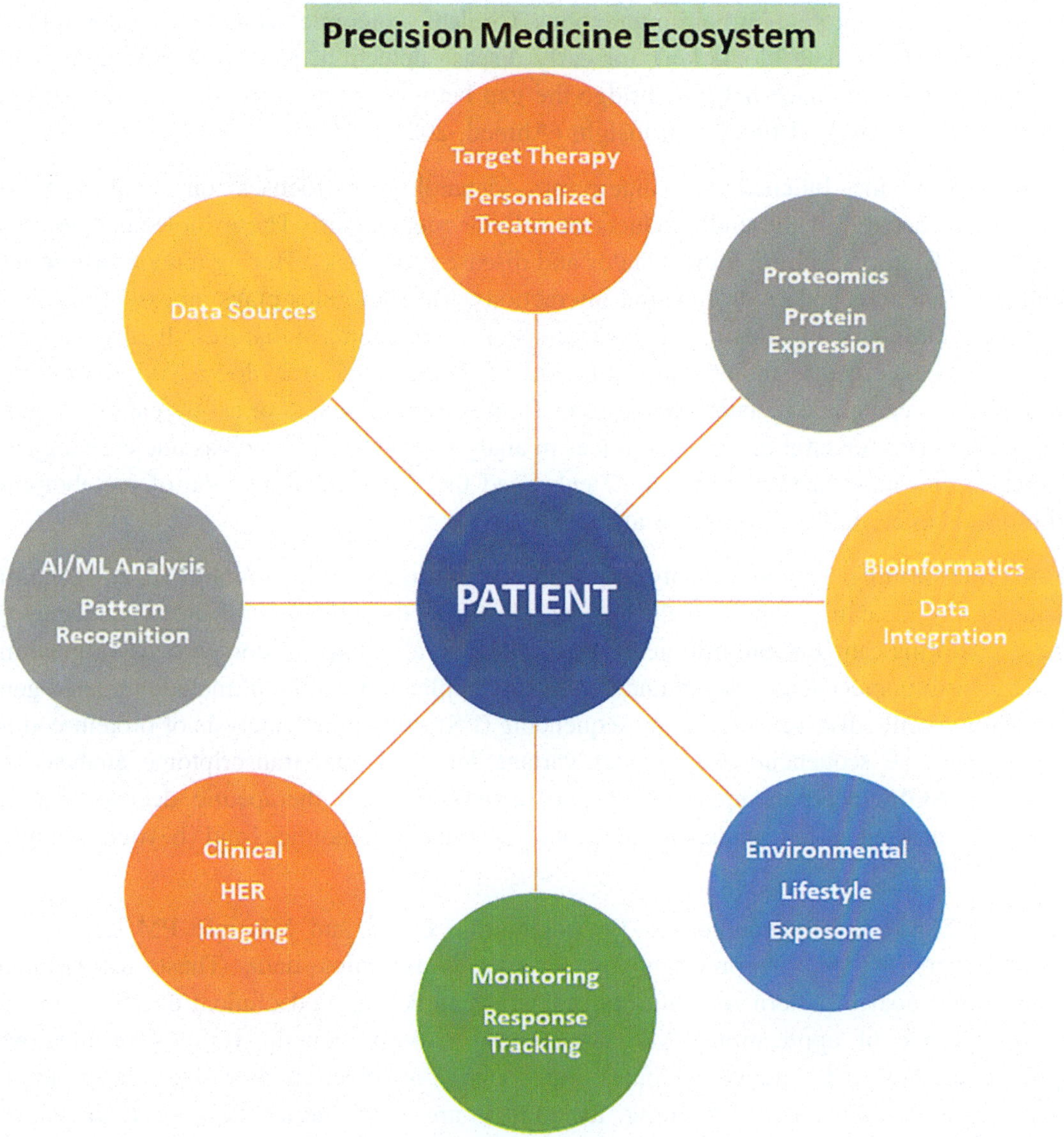

Figure 11.1
Precision Medicine Ecosystem. The PM ecosystem places the patient at the center. This is a well-accepted best practice, but not fully implemented across the various healthcare systems. *PM*, Personalized Medicine.

machinery. Proteomics involves the large-scale study of proteins as the effectors of cellular processes, making it a vital tool in understanding disease mechanisms and identifying therapeutic targets. Modern mass spectrometry technologies support high-throughput proteomic analyses, enabling quantitative assessments of protein abundance, posttranslational modifications, and protein–protein interactions. Clinical proteomics is increasingly employed to discover and validate biomarkers for early disease detection, prognosis, and therapeutic monitoring. This approach helps to bridge the gap between gene expression and phenotype, adding a critical layer of functional insight (Ahmed, 2022).

Metabolomics: the biochemical fingerprint—Metabolomics focuses on small-molecule metabolites that reflect the end products of cellular metabolism. These molecules serve as sensitive indicators of physiological states and disease processes, offering unique insight into biological functions and environmental interactions. Metabolomics plays an essential role in biomarker discovery by identifying disease-specific metabolic signatures. It also supports personalized therapeutic monitoring, nutrition medicine, and toxicology. As an example, metabolomics can guide dietary interventions for metabolic diseases or assess patient-specific drug metabolism for safer dosing. Advances in analytical platforms, such as nuclear magnetic resonance and mass spectrometry, have enhanced the accuracy and scope of metabolomic profiling (Gao et al., 2024; Singh et al., 2023).

NGS: transforming genomic analysis—NGS technologies have revolutionized genomic medicine by enabling rapid, scalable, and cost-effective DNA and RNA sequencing. These platforms can generate billions of reads per run, allowing for comprehensive genomic profiling with unprecedented speed and depth. Key applications of NGS include targeted gene panels for specific disease loci, exome sequencing (ES) for detailed analysis of protein-coding regions, genome sequencing for broader variant detection, and transcriptome analysis via RNA-seq. NGS underpins many diagnostic, prognostic, and therapeutic decision-making processes, making it an indispensable tool in clinical genomics and beyond (Sultova et al., 2021).

AI and ML in precision medicine—The integration of AI and ML into PM has opened new frontiers in the interpretation of complex multiomics data. These technologies enable sophisticated pattern recognition, predictive modeling, and clinical decision support across a range of applications. ML models can classify genetic variants of unknown significance, predict treatment outcomes, and identify novel biomarkers from large, multi-dimensional datasets. Deep learning techniques are also increasingly used in digital pathology, radiogenomics, and personalized treatment recommendation systems. However, challenges remain regarding model transparency, data bias, clinical validation, and regulatory acceptance.

Cloud computing and data infrastructure—The enormous volume of data generated by PM initiatives necessitates a scalable and secure computational infrastructure. Cloud computing platforms enable researchers and clinicians to store, analyze, and share large datasets across institutions while maintaining compliance with data protection regulations. These platforms support collaborative research, facilitate real-time data integration, and provide access to advanced computational tools and AI pipelines. Cloud-based solutions are especially critical in multicenter studies and global health initiatives where data harmonization and interoperability are essential (Nguyen et al., 2024).

Data integration challenges in precision medicine—Despite the promise of multiomics, integrating data from diverse molecular layers remains a complex challenge. Differences in data formats, measurement scales, noise levels, and missing values can hinder meaningful integration. Robust normalization techniques, dimensionality reduction, and advanced statistical frameworks are needed to harmonize data across omics platforms. Moreover, issues such as data heterogeneity, scalability, and standardization must be addressed to ensure reproducibility and clinical utility. Ethical concerns about data privacy and security, especially concerning patient information, are also critical. Achieving true interoperability across systems will require coordinated efforts in developing common data models, open-source tools, and international data-sharing agreements (Hassan et al., 2022; Mukherjee et al., 2025; Papadopoulou & Lytras, 2023; Su et al., 2022).

Overall, the foundation of PM rests on our ability to comprehensively characterize individual patients at the molecular level. Multiomics approaches integrate data from various biological layers to create a holistic view of disease mechanisms and treatment responses.

11.2.5 Key progress in drug design and drug development

Pharmaceutical products are crucial for doctors to prevent, cure, control, or modify disease processes. With increasing knowledge of human diseases, the design of pharmaceutical compounds has evolved. The FDA approved human insulin in 1982, leading to rapid growth in biologics in various disease areas. Unlike chemically synthesized single molecules, biologics are pharmaceutical compounds with complex structures derived from biological sources, such as mammalian cell lines, microbial agents, plants, and fungi. Manufacturing processes involve living systems and complex processes, requiring high technological expertise for consistency and quality. These compounds often have additional moieties, requiring special formulations such as stabilizers and preservatives for storage and influencing their properties (Chan & Chan, 2017).

Around 25% of marketed drugs are mixtures of agents, often racemates of synthetic chiral drugs. These mixtures often differ in pharmacodynamic and pharmacokinetic profiles due to stereochemical discrimination. The "racemate-versus-enantiomer" debate since the mid-1980s highlights the advantages of single-isomer products, such as improved selectivity and therapeutic index. Regulatory authorities have issued guidelines for dealing with chiral molecules, and racemic mixtures may still be developed but require justification. Some "old" mixtures are being reexamined as potential single-isomer products (Hutt, 2002; Hutt & Tan, 1996; Mc.Conathy & Owens, 2003).

In addition, the rapid growth of the biopharmaceutical market is attributed to increasing demand, particularly for innovative products like generics, biobetters, and biosimilars

(Declerck et al., 2017; Guideline on similar biological medicinal products, 2025)(a), which enhance efficacy and reduce treatment costs. As far as generics are concerned, a study comparing the definition and classification of generic medications by regulatory agencies worldwide, focusing on emerging markets and WHO regions, found significant variability in the definition and classification of these drugs (Alfonso-Cristancho et al., 2015). About half of the 21 countries had an official country-level definition, while two-thirds had specific requirements. Most countries require bioequivalence, but a few require bioavailability studies. The study suggests that standardization of definitions is necessary for international comparisons.

Several additional studies and reviews provide a comprehensive outlook on the field's growth potential and its significance in modern medicine, highlighting the transformative role of biopharmaceutical drugs in treating a broad range of diseases, including cancer and metabolic disorders (Chan & Chan, 2017; Kesik-Brodacka, 2018). As an example, the review article (Kesik-Brodacka, 2018) discusses the growth and impact of biopharmaceuticals since 1982, highlighting their transformative role in treating diseases like cancer and metabolic disorders. It highlights recent advancements, challenges in registration and regulation, and evolving market trends, including monoclonal antibodies, recombinant vaccines, and molecular biology techniques.

Various gene expression systems have been used for the development of drugs, such as (i) mammalian expression systems (Roshani et al., 2023), (ii) bacterial expression systems, (iii) yeast expression systems, and (iv) insect cell line systems. Transgenic animals, plant expression systems, cell-free protein synthesis, gene therapy, CRISPR for genome editing, monoclonal antibodies (mAbs), bispecific antibodies (bsAbs), and antibody-drug conjugates are additional methods used to produce pharmaceuticals and biopharmaceuticals, as further described in the review article (Kesik-Brodacka, 2018).

More recently, important advances have taken place in vaccine production. Vaccines have been crucial in preventing infectious diseases for over two centuries, preventing 3.5–5 million deaths annually. They have eradicated pathogens like smallpox and wild poliovirus. The history of vaccine development spans from the 17th century to the present day. Immunological principles, vaccine types, and mRNA vaccine technology are discussed in the following review article. The study focuses on the benefits, which include reducing morbidity and mortality, fostering socioeconomic development, and addressing vaccine hesitancy. Research, collaboration, and widespread vaccine use are essential for successful health outcomes.

Furthermore, the use of AI for drug discovery, AI for PM, and Generative AI for drug design has already made significant advances, mainly due to AI systems released such as AlphaFold2 and 3, which are further elaborated under findings (Abramson et al., 2024; Jumper et al., 2021).

11.3 Methodology

11.3.1 Literature review on present and future use of precision medicine

A comprehensive review of current applications and future directions in PM was done, focusing on its impact across various medical specialties.

11.3.2 Research questions

1. To what extent do genomic and proteomic advancements contribute to the success of personalized treatments in mainly oncology, cardiology, endocrinology, rare genetic disorders, infectious diseases, neurodegenerative conditions, and pharmacology?
2. How can emerging technologies like CRISPR, AlphaFold3, and digital twins expand the applications of precision medicine across diverse patient populations and in drug design and development?

11.3.3 Review protocol

Literature review strategy: This comprehensive review of PM was conducted using a systematic approach to ensure thoroughness and accuracy. The methodology followed established guidelines for narrative reviews while incorporating elements of systematic review best practices.

Databases searched: PubMed/MEDLINE, Web of Science, Embase, Cochrane Library, Google Scholar, ClinicalTrials.gov (ongoing trials).

Search terms used: Primary terms: "precision medicine," "personalized medicine," "individualized medicine," "targeted therapy," "pharmacogenomics," "genomic medicine" Secondary terms: "biomarkers," "multiomics," "artificial intelligence," "machine learning," "gene therapy," "CRISPR," "digital health," "wearable devices" Specialty-specific terms: "precision oncology," "cardiovascular genetics," "diabetes precision medicine," "neurodegenerative diseases," and "rare diseases (RDs)."

Search filters: Language: English publication, type: original research, reviews, clinical trials, guidelines, date range: January 2020–July 2025 (with selected historical references)

11.3.4 Selection criteria

Inclusion criteria: Peer-reviewed publications in English. Original research studies were examined, as well as systematic reviews, metaanalyses, clinical trials, observational studies, guidelines, and consensus statements from professional organizations, regulatory guidance documents, economic evaluations, and health technology assessments. **Exclusion criteria used:** Non-English publications without English abstracts, conference abstracts and posters, editorial comments and letters (unless particularly relevant), studies with insufficient methodological detail, animal studies without clear human relevance, and duplicate publications. Quality assessment performed: Each included article or study was evaluated using appropriate quality assessment tools. Data extraction performed: Data were systematically extracted using standardized forms. Study characteristics: Authors, year, country, study design, sample size. Population: Demographics, disease characteristics, and genetic background. Interventions: Precision medicine approaches and technologies used. Outcomes: Primary and secondary endpoints and safety measures. Results: Integration and synthesis of the results were followed to address the research questions. Limitations: Study limitations and potential biases were addressed. Evidence synthesis: Given the heterogeneity of PM applications, a narrative synthesis approach was used. Thematic analysis: Organized findings by medical specialty and technology. Temporal analysis: Examined the evolution of PM approaches. Geographic analysis: Identified regional differences in implementation. Quality assessment: Weighted evidence based on study quality and relevance. Limitations of the review: Methodological limitations, and rapid pace of change. Some information may become outdated quickly. Publication bias: Positive results may be overrepresented. Language bias: English-only publications may miss important international work. Database limitations: Some specialized databases may not have been searched. Grey literature: Limited inclusion of non-peer-reviewed sources. Content limitations technology focus: Emphasis on established technologies versus emerging ones. Clinical translation: Identified gaps between research findings and clinical implementation. Population diversity: Limited representation of diverse populations in studies. Long-term outcomes: Insufficient follow-up data for many interventions. Cost-effectiveness: Limited economic data for many PM applications. Temporal limitations: snapshot in time: Review reflects current state of knowledge. Regulatory changes: The evolving regulatory landscape may affect conclusions. Technology evolution: Rapid technological advancement may outpace review. Clinical adoption: Variable implementation across healthcare systems. Future review considerations: Living systematic review. Continuous updating as new evidence emerges. International collaboration: Including more diverse geographical perspectives. Patient perspectives: Greater emphasis on patient-reported outcomes. Implementation science: An effort was made to focus on real-world implementation challenges. Economic modeling: More comprehensive cost-effectiveness analyses are needed. A Prisma diagram is not included as this is not a full systematic review.

11.4 Findings

Precision medicine has demonstrated significant potential across diverse medical disciplines, driven by advancements in genomics, proteomics, and cutting-edge technologies like CRISPR and AI-based predictive models. The key findings focus on the practical and successful applications and technological enablers of PM in mainly oncology, cardiology, endocrinology, rare genetic disorders, infectious diseases, neurodegenerative conditions, and pharmacology. Through case studies and indicative research, the transformative impact of PM on patient outcomes and its role in driving personalized healthcare are highlighted.

From oncology's genomic profiling for tailored cancer therapies to cardiology's use of genetic testing for risk assessment, PM is bridging the gap between theoretical promise and clinical implementation. Moreover, in rare genetic disorders (Gabay, 2019; The Lancet Global Health, 2024), gene therapies have revolutionized treatment approaches, while precision diagnostics and personalized vaccines have bolstered efforts against antimicrobial resistance and emerging infectious diseases.

11.4.1 Personalized treatments in practice

Table 11.1 depicts a summary of PM applications across various disciplines and indicative studies. More case examples are provided in Section 11.4.2.

Table 11.1 Precision medicine applications across disciplines.

Discipline	Example	Application	Indicative studies
Oncology	Use of trastuzumab for HER2-positive breast cancer.	Genomic profiling to tailor cancer therapies.	Wang et al. (2024)
Cardiology	Pharmacogenomics-based cholesterol-lowering therapies.	Genetic testing to assess risk factors and guide treatment.	Krittanawong et al. (2022)
Endocrinology	Personalized interventions for Type 2 diabetes using pharmacogenomic insights.	Precision treatment for metabolic disorders and adrenal issues.	Kalra et al. (2020)
Rare genetic disorders	Luxturna for RPE65 mutation-associated Leber congenital amaurosis.	Gene therapy targeting specific genetic mutations.	Chiu et al. (2021)
Neurodegenerative diseases	Amyloid-targeting therapies for Alzheimer's disease (e.g., aducanumab).	Biomarker-driven approaches to improve diagnostic accuracy and treatment.	Bargar et al. (2021), Berry et al. (2018), Chatterjee et al. (2024), Cho et al. (2023), Domingo et al. (2021), Gallo Marin et al. (2021), Jack et al. (2013), Morenas-Rodríguez et al. (2022), Rasmussen & Langerman (2019), Huang et al. (2023)
Infectious diseases_vaccines	Development of personalized vaccines for emerging pathogens like COVID-19.	Genomic insights into combating antimicrobial resistance (AMR).	Montin et al. (2024)

11.4.2 Clinical applications by specialty case studies: precision medicine in action

11.4.2.1 Oncology applications

Cancer represents the most advanced application of PM, with numerous targeted therapies approved based on molecular biomarkers. The transition from histology-based to molecular-based cancer classification has revolutionized treatment approaches.

11.4.2.1.1 Molecular profiling and targeted therapy

Comprehensive genomic profiling of tumors identifies actionable mutations that can be targeted with specific therapies. The concept of "precision oncology" involves matching patients to treatments based on their tumor's molecular characteristics rather than solely on tumor location.

Notable examples include: HER2-positive breast cancer: Trastuzumab (Herceptin) targets HER2 overexpression (Swain, Shastry & Hamilton, 2023). EGFR-mutated lung cancer: Erlotinib and other EGFR inhibitors (Naveed Ahmad et al., 2022; Two Distinct Primary EGFR-Mutated Lung Adenocarcinoma Within the Same Patient: A Case Report, n.d.). BRAF-mutated melanoma: Vemurafenib and combination therapies (Imani et al., 2024). PD-L1 expression: Immune checkpoint inhibitors (Tang et al., 2022).

11.4.2.1.2 Liquid biopsies and circulating tumor DNA

Liquid biopsies analyze circulating tumor DNA (ctDNA) in blood samples, providing a noninvasive method for tumor monitoring and treatment selection. This approach enables real-time tracking of tumor evolution and resistance mechanisms.

Applications include: Early detection: Identifying cancer before clinical symptoms. Treatment monitoring: Tracking treatment response and resistance. Minimal residual disease: Detecting microscopic tumor remnants. Resistance mechanisms: Understanding treatment failure.

Genomic profiling in tailoring cancer therapies: Genomic profiling has enabled the development of targeted therapies for various cancers, improving patient outcomes (Cecchin & Stocco, 2020; Gao et al., 2024; Goričar et al., 2021; Heath et al., 2024; Neagu et al., 2024; Sadee, 2017; Sadee et al., 2023).

Success stories of targeted drugs for breast and lung cancer: Targeted therapies have shown significant success in treating specific subtypes of breast and lung cancer (Asgharzade et al., 2020; Bulotta et al., 2011; Elamin et al., 2013; Hossain et al., 2021; Neagu et al., 2023; Sultova et al., 2021; Thakur & Kutty, 2019; Xiao et al., 2022).

In another study, a Bayesian network metaanalysis (NMA) was conducted to compare the efficacy and safety of various first-line treatment regimens for human epidermal growth factor receptor 2 (HER2)-positive advanced breast cancer (ABC). Progression-free survival (PFS), overall survival (OS), objective response rate (ORR), and adverse events of grade 3 or higher (≥ 3 AEs) were calculated and analyzed with NMA. Out of 10,313 manuscripts, 28 randomized controlled trials involving 11,680 patients were analyzed. Results showed that the combination of trastuzumab with tyrosine kinase inhibitors was more favorable than dual-targeted therapy. The study concluded that monochemotherapy (Docetaxel) combined with dual-targeted therapy (Trastuzumab and Pertuzumab) remains the optimal choice for ABC treatment. The combination of trastuzumab with tyrosine kinase inhibitors, (Pyrotinib) demonstrated a significant improvement in PFS and ORR, yet not conclusive (Wang et al., 2024).

The following papers explore genomic medicine, utilizing DNA variation to improve human health. They discuss the mechanisms of drug action variability, pharmacokinetics, and pharmacodynamics, clinical trial data, and ongoing pharmacogenetics implementation (Cecchin & Stocco, 2020; Goričar et al., 2021; Sadee, 2017; Sadee et al., 2023).

Another study found clinically relevant pharmacogenetic (PGx) variants in 62.7% of participants, potentially benefiting 14,540 patients per year in England. Validating these variants in real-world data, the study found a significant association between PGx variants in four genes (DPYD, NUDT15, TPMT, UGT1A1) associated with toxicity induced by five drugs used in patient cancer treatment (capecitabine, fluorouracil, mercaptopurine, thioguanine, irinotecan). Reporting gene variants can inform prescribing and reduce ADR risk (Leong et al., 2024).

Breast cancer (BC), as another example, is highly heterogeneous, requiring integrated omics approaches ("onco-breastomics") for precise diagnosis and treatment. Advances in genomics, proteomics, metabolomics, and epiomics reveal insights into BC progression and tumor microenvironments. Novel liquid biopsy techniques, including blood-, saliva-, and milk-based omics, enable noninvasive diagnostics. Future directions focus on multiomics integration and single-cell analyses for personalized oncology. Omics-based BC research supports accurate classification, subtype characterization, and single-cell analyses, paving the way for predictive, precision, and personalized oncology (Neagu et al., 2023). Onco-breastomics identifies biomarkers reflecting differences linked to ethnicity, age, gender, environment, and socioeconomic factors, including genomic, immune, metabolic, and microbiomic variations. This approach deepens understanding of BC disparities, clarifying variations in incidence, mortality, and treatment response. By integrating genomics, proteomics, and exposomics, it enables targeted interventions for diverse patient groups (Neagu et al., 2024).

A recent review article identifies the prostate-specific membrane antigen (PSMA) as a crucial biomarker and therapeutic target in prostate cancer. Theranostic 177Lu-PSMA-617 was approved in 2022 for men with PSMA-PET-positive metastatic castration-resistant prostate cancer. However, not all patients respond to PSMA-radioligand therapy due to heterogeneity in tumor expression. Understanding PSMA regulation and heterogeneity can inform PM approaches to PSMA theranostics and other emerging therapies.

Health disparities pose barriers to effective oncology treatment, but precision oncology offers the potential to reduce them. A study of 12,627 patients from six cancer centers (2010–20) found minimal racial disparities, geographic location, or poverty level among molecularly tested patients, though disparities persisted for young non-White women and broader populations when they analyzed the interactions of age, race, and sex. Mutations in genes like TP53 and KRAS influenced survival and varied by race. Expanded access to molecular testing can improve health equity by addressing genomic-driven disparities and enhancing outcomes across diverse patient groups (Heath et al., 2024).

11.4.2.1.3 Chimeric antigen receptor T therapy

Immunotherapy, once considered a new treatment for advanced cancers, is now a cornerstone of cancer treatment. Chimeric antigen receptor (CAR T)-cell therapies, made from a patient's own T cells, have shown promise in some cases. FDA approved the first CAR T-cell therapy in 2017 for children with acute lymphoblastic leukemia (ALL) (Mullard, 2017), and others for adults with blood cancers. T cells are crucial for cell-mediated immunity, and genetically modified therapies like CAR-T and T-cell receptor (TCR) have shown promise in treating malignant tumors. These therapies have shown promising clinical outcomes, and it is predicted that genetically engineered T-cell immunotherapies will become effective treatments (Zhao & Cao, 2019). CAR-T therapy is another promising treatment for hematological cancers as well due to its precise targeting and long-term protection. It is also being explored for noncancerous diseases like autoimmune disorders, fibrosis, senescence-associated diseases, and infectious diseases, with recent advancements highlighting its potential for further refinement. While CAR-T immune cell therapies have revolutionized oncology, their efficacy against solid tumors remains limited due to challenges like dense stromal barriers and immunosuppressive microenvironments. Advancements in nanobiotechnology have developed strategies to enhance CAR-T cell efficacy in solid tumor treatment. Biomaterials can optimize treatments by improving the tumor microenvironment, controlling CAR-T cell release, and promoting cell infiltration (Song et al., 2025).

11.4.2.2 Cardiovascular medicine

Cardiovascular PM focuses on risk stratification, drug selection, and treatment optimization based on genetic and molecular factors.

11.4.2.2.1 Pharmacogenomics in cardiology

Genetic variants significantly influence cardiovascular drug responses, affecting both efficacy and safety.

Key applications include: Warfarin dosing: CYP2C9 and VKORC1 variants affect warfarin metabolism (Natarajan et al., 2013). Clopidogrel response: CYP2C19 variants influence antiplatelet effects (Dean & Kane, 2012). Statin-induced myopathy: SLCO1B1 variants predict muscle toxicity (Stewart, 2013). ACE inhibitor response: Genetic variants affect blood pressure response (El Cheikh et al., 2025).

11.4.2.2.2 Polygenic risk scores

Polygenic risk scores (PRS) combine information from multiple genetic variants to predict disease risk. In cardiovascular medicine, PRS can identify individuals at high risk for coronary artery disease, enabling early intervention.

11.4.2.2.3 Precision approaches to heart failure

Heart failure treatment increasingly incorporates molecular biomarkers and genetic information to guide therapy selection and dosing. Examples include: Natriuretic peptide testing: Guiding diagnosis and treatment monitoring (Çelik et al., 2025). Genetic testing for cardiomyopathies: Identifying familial forms and treatment options (Vogiatzi et al., 2022). Biomarker-guided therapy: Using troponin and other markers for risk stratification (Parhi et al., 2025).

Advances in genetic testing for cardiovascular conditions: Genetic testing has facilitated the identification of individuals at risk for cardiovascular diseases, enabling early interventions. Long-term use of statins has been linked to increased hyperglycemic adverse events (HAEs). Proprotein convertase subtilisin/kexin type 9 (PCSK9-mAbs), a new lipid-lowering drug, has been widely used to reduce cholesterol levels in patients with coronary heart disease. However, recent studies suggest no significant relationship between PCSK9-mAbs and HAEs, and no relationship between PCSK9-mAbs and nonalcoholic fatty liver disease. Longer-term follow-up studies need to confirm it. Genetic polymorphisms and variants may affect HAEs, but no genetic testing is necessary (Zhang et al., 2023).

Personalized cholesterol-lowering treatments through pharmacogenomics: Pharmacogenomics has informed personalized approaches to managing cholesterol levels, enhancing treatment efficacy.

As evident in the following study (Krittanawong et al., 2022), genetic polymorphisms in a population can cause drug-gene response variations, potentially contributing to specific disease processes. Mendelian randomization is used to identify genetic variants in candidate genes that impact low-density lipoprotein cholesterol (LDL-C) regulating pathways and cardiovascular disease outcomes. The LDL receptor-degrading protein, PCSK9, is a candidate for pharmacological inhibition. PCSK9 inhibitors (PCSK9i) are cholesterol-lowering medications that reduce LDL by inhibiting LDL receptor (LDLR) degradation. PM offers the promise of developing a more efficacious approach that considers genetic variation and targets different patient populations. Understanding the pharmacogenomics of PCSK9 is crucial for developing effective and cost-effective PCSK9i therapy.

The following study investigates the impact of statin therapy on the risk of atherosclerotic cardiovascular disease and its major complication, acute heart failure (AHF). It found that previous statin therapy was associated with a significantly decreased rate of AHF on admission, regardless of age, sex, or younger or older age. Additionally, previous statin therapy predicted a lower risk of 30-day mortality in patients presenting with AHF on admission. The study concludes that previous statin therapy is associated with a reduced risk of AHF and improved survival from AHF (Bugiardini et al., 2022).

Advances in genetic and environmental factors have helped understand morbidity and mortality in pediatric cardiology as well. Genomics and pharmacogenetics focus on risk prediction and drug safety. However, challenges exist in implementing personalized medicine in pediatric cardiology (Kikano & Kannankeril, 2022).

Personalization in cardiac medicine involves analyzing a patient's clinical presentation, risk factors, and biomarkers. PM uses innovative imaging for myocardial structure and electrophysiology. Genome analyses and digital technologies have potential in cardiovascular PM, based on disease frequency and bio-signals. However, these approaches have not yet been widely implemented in complex cardiovascular diseases (Hasenfuß et al., 2024).

Cardiovascular disease (CVD) includes conditions like coronary artery disease, stroke, and deep vein thrombosis. AI is transforming CVD diagnosis and management by enhancing clinical decision-making, improving imaging accuracy, and enabling personalized treatment plans. AI also expands access to diagnostics in remote areas and influences medical training, research, and practice. This review explores AI's growing role in revolutionizing cardiovascular medicine (Bouris & Avgerinos, 2024).

Dilated cardiomyopathy (DCM) is a condition causing left ventricular dysfunction and dilatation. Over the past two decades, there has been significant progress in understanding DCM's genetic basis. Advanced imaging techniques, clinical work-ups, and family screening have improved diagnosis and treatment. Genotype-directed therapies are emerging in precision medicine, and recent developments focus on updating the genetic background, identifying pathogenic variants, and distinguishing athletic heart syndrome from subclinical DCM (Orphanou et al., 2022).

In a related study by Antonopoulos et al., it is stated that DCM, a heart muscle disorder with nonischemic etiology, causes heart failure and risk of malignant ventricular arrhythmias and sudden cardiac death. Advances in cardiogenetics and imaging have improved disease recognition and identification of DCM phenotypes. Genotype-phenotype associations have been established for specific subtypes, but remain elusive. Imagenetics, combining imaging and genetics, is expected to advance research and contribute to PM in DCM management and treatment (Antonopoulos et al., 2024).

This review discusses the rationale, evidence, and current and future directions for personalizing antiplatelet treatment regimens in cardiovascular patients undergoing percutaneous coronary intervention, despite increased bleeding risk (Galli et al., 2022).

Chronic obstructive pulmonary disease (COPD) is a global epidemic affecting 10% of subjects over 45 years. It is characterized by eosinophilic inflammation, which is a subgroup of patients. Recent studies have explored the role of type 2 inflammation and epithelial-derived alarmins (TSLP and IL-33) in COPD. Results suggest that blocking a wider spectrum of cytokines, such as IL-4 and IL-13, is more promising than targeting a single cytokine. Targeting T2 inflammation or IL-33 could represent a step forward in PM for COPD treatment (Varricchi & Poto, 2024).

11.4.2.3 Endocrinology and metabolic disorders

Precision medicine in endocrinology focuses on diabetes management, obesity treatment, and rare metabolic disorders.

11.4.2.3.1 Diabetes precision medicine

Type 2 diabetes represents a heterogeneous group of disorders with different underlying mechanisms. Precision approaches aim to classify patients into subtypes based on pathophysiology. Emerging classifications include: Severe insulin-deficient diabetes : Requiring insulin therapy (Herder & Roden, 2022). Severe insulin-resistant diabetes: Associated with fatty liver and kidney disease (Dewidar et al., 2020). Mild obesity-related diabetes: Linked to obesity and metabolic syndrome (Raverdy et al., 2022). Mild age-related diabetes: Gradual onset in older adults (Bando, 2021).

11.4.2.3.2 Monogenic diabetes

Approximately 2%–3% of diabetes cases result from single gene mutations. Molecular diagnosis enables specific treatment approaches: MODY (Maturity-Onset Diabetes of the Young): Sulfonylurea-responsive forms (Hoffman et al., 2023). Neonatal diabetes: Specific genetic subtypes requiring different treatments (Dahl & Kumar, 2020). Syndromic diabetes: Associated with additional clinical features (Colclough et al., 2022).

11.4.2.3.3 Obesity and metabolic syndrome

Precision approaches to obesity consider genetic susceptibility, metabolic profiling, and microbiome composition to develop personalized treatment strategies.

Personalized treatment for Type 2 diabetes: PM approaches have led to personalized treatment strategies for Type 2 diabetes, improving glycemic control. Numerous studies point to the direction of PM in endocrinology (Adashi & Stratakis, 2024; Ham et al., 2024; Joshi et al., 2024; Nguyen et al., 2024; Stratakis, 2024a, 2024b; Yildiz et al., 2024). (Adler et al., 2000; Bastepe et al., 2000; Carreira et al., 2000; Davis et al., 2000; Dhatariya et al., 2000; Farooqi et al., 2000; Feingold, Anawalt, et al., 2000; Feingold et al. (2000a); Feingold et al., 2000b; Feingold, Feingold, Anawalt, Blackman, Boyce, Chrousos, Corpas, De Herder, Dhatariya, Dungan, Hofland, Kalra, Kaltsas, Kapoor, Koch, Kopp et al., 2000; Juszczak et al., 2000; Tchang et al., 2000; Warden et al., 2000; Zhou et al., 2000).

A common denominator of metabolic disorders is stress. Stress is a state of threatened homeostasis countered by physiological and behavioral responses aimed at restoring balance. The stress system, primarily involving the hypothalamic-pituitary-adrenal (HPA) axis and autonomic nervous system (ANS), coordinates adaptive responses through interactions with the central nervous system and peripheral organs. Dysregulation of this system, especially under chronic stress, can disrupt homeostasis and contribute to endocrine, metabolic, gastrointestinal, and immune disorders. This chapter explores the physiology of the stress system and its role in stress-related diseases, bringing our attention to the importance of prevention (Tsigos et al., 2000).

Obesity is both a chronic disease and a major contributor to conditions like type 2 diabetes, hypertension, and CVDs. While BMI and waist circumference remain primary diagnostic tools, emerging imaging technologies may improve risk assessment. Obesity rates have risen globally, with U.S. adult prevalence at 40% and higher rates among minority groups. The increasing prevalence among children and adolescents signals long-term challenges, making prevention and innovative solutions essential to reversing current trends and alleviating burdens on the healthcare system (Purnell et al., 2000).

Intermittent fasting, particularly time-restricted eating such as the 8/16 protocol, offers potential benefits for metabolism and weight management. Endocrinologists can integrate this approach into personalized treatment plans, taking into account each patient's unique medical history. However, caution is needed to prevent the promotion of eating disorders due to their restrictive nature (Chavanne & Jacobi, 2024).

Metabolic disorders: The following study in 2009 revealed a previously unknown function for autophagy in regulating intracellular lipid stores, macrolipophagy. It found that inhibition of autophagy in cultured hepatocytes and mouse liver increased triglyceride storage in lipid droplets. This critical function in lipid metabolism could have implications for human diseases with lipid over-accumulation, such as metabolic syndrome (Singh et al., 2009). Recently, the same lab researchers concluded that fasting stimulates physiological adaptations like increased circulating fatty acids and mitochondrial respiration for survival. However, the mechanisms behind these adaptations and respiratory sufficiency during fasting remain unclear. This study reveals that fasting or lipid availability stimulates mTORC2 activity, which sustains mitochondrial fission and respiratory sufficiency. This unexpected reactivation of mTORC2 during fasting unexpectedly drives these adaptations (Martinez-Lopez et al., 2023; Singh et al., 2023).

11.4.3 Genetic disorders and rare genetic disorders

Development of therapies addressing specific mutations: Gene therapies, such as Luxturna for Leber congenital amaurosis (LCA)and Zolgensma for spinal muscular atrophy, have provided groundbreaking treatments for rare genetic disorders. Rare eye diseases, such as inherited retinal dystrophies (IRDs), are caused by gene mutations that lead to irreversible retinal degradation. Gene therapies are needed to restore functional retinal proteins. Advances in gene identification and delivery systems have led to gene therapies for IRDs. In 2017, voretigene neparvovec-rzyl (Luxturna), an adeno-associated virus vector-based drug, was approved for treating LCA (Chiu et al., 2021).

The following study elaborates on the fact that precision public health presents a major opportunity to diagnose every RD patient by leveraging clinical ES and emerging technologies. Advancements in computational approaches and large-scale data integration will drive RD discovery, but global collaboration, research participation, and systemic healthcare integration are essential. Expanding access to genome-wide testing, supporting RD researchers, and fostering international cooperation to provide each RD patient with a diagnosis and possible treatment within one year (Boycott et al., 2019).

Examples: Duchenne muscular dystrophy: Development of exon-skipping therapies like eteplirsen (Boycott et al., 2019; Duan et al., 2021; Takeda et al., 2021).

Thalassemias: Gene-editing technologies like CRISPR have enabled corrective therapies (Frangoul et al., 2021; Global Thalassaemia Review, 2023; Kattamis et al., 2022; Musallam et al., 2024; Parums, 2024).

Sickle cell anemia: (Colombatti & Sainati, 2016; Frangoul et al., 2021; McManus et al., 2024).

11.4.3.1 Rare diseases

RDs, affecting 300 million people globally, have a significant genetic cause, and about 95% lack approved treatments, while the average diagnosis time is 4–8 years. With over 7000 types of RDs, the burden worldwide is significant (European Commission, 2025; Eurordis, EURORDIS, 2025). The UN has called for access to safe, affordable health services, while advances in whole-genome sequencing have reduced costs. However, accessibility remains a challenge. Parents and carers face psychological distress, financial concerns, and stigmatization (Gabay, 2019; Larizza & Cubellis, 2023; The Lancet Global Health, 2024).

Diagnostic approaches: Genomic testing has revolutionized RD diagnosis: WES**:** Identifying disease-causing variants (Bartha & Győrffy, 2019). WGS: Comprehensive genomic analysis

(Brlek et al., 2024). Chromosomal microarray: Detecting copy number variants (Hollenbeck et al., 2017). Targeted gene panels: Focused analysis of disease-specific genes M, B., (2025) Targeted Gene Panels: Revolutionizing Genomic Testing for Precision Oncology—Crown Bioscience.

Gene therapy applications: Gene therapy represents the ultimate PM approach for genetic disorders: Luxturna: Gene therapy for inherited blindness (European Medicines Agency, 2025a). Zolgensma: Treatment for spinal muscular atrophy (European Medicines Agency, 2025b). Hemophilia gene therapies: Addressing bleeding disorders (European Medicines Agency, 2025c). Sickle cell disease: CRISPR-based gene editing approaches (FDA, 2025).

Public health overall increasingly relies on technologies like genomics and data science to improve early diagnosis and care, particularly for RD caused by previously hard-to-identify genetic mutations. Advances in precision public health integrate insights on affected populations, timing, and locations of disease occurrence, informing national frameworks like the Western Australian Rare Diseases Strategic Framework. Knowledge sharing across international networks has driven policy development and transformative clinical service delivery. This paper informs us of the paradigm shift that enhances diagnostic accuracy and care for RD patients, guided by their individual and population health needs (Baynam et al., 2017; Larizza & Cubellis, 2023).

11.4.3.2 Neurodegenerative diseases

Neurological PM addresses the genetic and molecular basis of various brain disorders, focusing on early detection and targeted interventions.

11.4.3.2.1 Alzheimer's disease

Genetic factors significantly influence Alzheimer's disease (AD) risk and progression. Precision medicine approaches include: APOE genotyping: Assessing genetic risk factors (Novotni et al., 2019). Amyloid PET imaging: Detecting brain amyloid deposits (Chapleau et al., 2022). Tau biomarkers: Monitoring disease progression (Ossenkoppele et al., 2022). Genetic screening: Identifying familial forms (Andrews et al., 1994).

11.4.3.2.2 Parkinson's disease

Precision medicine in Parkinson's disease (PD) focuses on genetic subtypes and personalized treatment approaches: Genetic testing: Identifying monogenic forms (LRRK2, SNCA, etc.) (Jia et al., 2022). Deep brain stimulation: Personalized targeting and programming (Hollunder et al., 2022). Biomarker development: Tracking disease progression and treatment response (Han, 2024).

The spectrum related to autism is another area of intense research, not covered in this chapter (Litman et al., 2025).

11.4.4 Rare neurological disorders

Gene therapy approaches for rare neurological disorders represent successful PM applications: Spinal muscular atrophy: Zolgensma gene therapy (European Medicines Agency, 2025b). Duchenne muscular dystrophy: Antisense oligonucleotides (Wilton-Clark & Yokota, 2023). Huntington's disease: Targeted RNA interference therapies (Chen et al., 2018).

Precision approaches in AD: Biomarker-driven diagnostics and amyloid-targeting therapies like aducanumab (AmeliMojarad, 2024; Delgado et al., 2021; Papadopoulou et al., 2024; Theoharides, 2020, 2021; Shippy et al., 2024).

AD is a common form of dementia characterized by amyloid-β plaques and neurofibrillary tangles. Microglia, the primary immune cells, provide neuroprotection but can also promote neuroinflammation. Recent studies show that microglial utilization of nutrients and trace metals, such as zinc, is crucial for controlling their activation and effector functions. Understanding how zinc homeostasis influences microglial-mediated neuroinflammation in AD is essential for new treatments (AmeliMojarad, 2024; Shippy et al., 2024).

Recent trials of anti-amyloid-β monoclonal antibodies in early AD have shown limited clinical benefits and a significant risk of adverse events. It is crucial to explore complementary therapeutic approaches and explore neuroinflammatory biomarkers to characterize the pathophysiology of AD. Neuroinflammation is a crucial component of AD pathogenesis, and a stage-dependent neuroinflammatory process in the AD brain is needed. The emergence of reliable blood-based neuroinflammatory biomarkers, particularly glial fibrillary acidic protein (GFAP), could help classify AD patients based on the ATI(N) biomarker framework. Longitudinal analyses are needed to accurately monitor cerebral inflammation dynamics. An effective anti-neuroinflammatory therapy should target microglia and astrocytes, considering individual ATI (N) status (Lista et al., 2024).

Neuroinflammation is a significant underlying cause of AD, with genetic variants-TREM2, CD33, PILRA, CR1, MS4A, CLU, ABCA7, EPHA1, and HLA-DRB5-HLA-DRB1 potentially linked to it. This inflammation is triggered by various molecular pathways regulated by TNF-α, TGF-β, IL-1β, and the receptor proteinTREM2. Microglia and astrocytes are key drivers and regulators of neuroinflammation, which synergize with amyloid-β and tau accumulation, leading to synaptotoxicity and neurodegeneration. Despite the potential therapeutic benefits, clinical trials involving antiinflammatory compounds have not achieved primary efficacy endpoints. Future research should focus on developing individualized therapeutic strategies targeting neuroinflammation using biomarker-drug candidates of neuroinflammation, such as TREM2, IL-1β, MCP-1, IL-6, TNF-α receptor complexes,

TGF-β, and YKL-40, coupled with systems biology approaches, as pointed out in the following review article (Hampel et al., 2020).

The following study analyzed cross-sectional tau-PET and longitudinal T1-weighted MRI scan data from 186 participants with AD. It found that factors such as excitatory-inhibitory ratio, myelination, synaptic density, glycolytic index, and functional connectivity influence the relationship between tau pathology and neurodegeneration. The study also found spatial similarity between tau pathology and glycolytic index, synaptic density, and functional connectivity across brain regions. The molecular and connectivity architecture of the human brain is linked to the different effects of tau pathology on neurodegeneration (Nabizadeh et al., 2025).

Advancements in in vivo biomarkers are revolutionizing the understanding and treatment of neurodegenerative diseases, such as AD. The deposition of amyloid-β plaques and neurofibrillary tangles, along with the activation of glial cells and neuroinflammatory response, contribute to neurodegeneration and cognitive dysfunction. The development of PET tracers has led to a growing interest in imaging reactive astrocytes in the AD continuum. The multitracer PET approach allows for the analysis of regional and temporal patterns of astrocytosis, fibrillar Aβ deposition, glucose metabolism, and brain structural changes. This approach may also contribute to understanding the role of novel plasma biomarkers of reactive astrocytes, particularly GFAP, at different stages of disease progression (Rodriguez-Vieitez et al., 2024).

Microglia, immune cells in the central nervous system, play a crucial role in AD development. The role of microglial activation and its neuroinflammatory response in AD pathogenesis is explored in the following study. Plant-derived natural compounds (PDNCs) can potentially modulate microglia-associated neuroinflammation in AD treatment. Dysregulated activation of microglial receptors and their downstream pathways can impair immune homeostasis. PDNCs can delay AD progression by inhibiting proinflammatory receptors, activating antiinflammatory ones, and regulating Aβ clearance (Shen et al., 2024).

The European olive tree (*Olea europaea L.*) and its polyphenols show therapeutic potential for treating neuroinflammation and cognitive impairment, particularly in conditions like long COVID, Alzheimer's, Parkinson's, and multiple sclerosis. Olive polyphenols exhibit antioxidant, antiinflammatory, neuroprotective, and antiviral properties, making them promising therapeutic candidates. Future research should focus on molecular mechanisms, supplementation effects, clinical trials, and synergistic formulations to enhance efficacy and safety. These findings highlight the translational value of olive polyphenols in managing cognitive dysfunction (Papadopoulou et al., 2024). Future research should focus on molecular pathways, clinical trials, and synergistic effects (Delgado et al., 2021; Papadopoulou et al., 2024; Theoharides, 2017; Theoharides & Leeman, 2019).

This review explores the potential health benefits of phenolic secoiridoids from olive oil by-products in preventing AD. These polyphenols show antioxidant, anti-inflammatory, and neuroprotective properties. The olive oil industry produces significant waste, which presents an untapped source of bioactive compounds. However, human clinical trials remain limited due to variability in extraction methods and AD complexity. Future studies should focus on standardizing protocols and conducting robust clinical trials (Gonçalves et al., 2024).

PD: Genetic profiling to identify LRRK2 mutations has enabled personalized treatment strategies (Bargar et al., 2021; Grétarsdóttir et al., 2021; Hernández-García et al., 2024; Papadopoulou et al., 2024; Theoharides, 2021; Samanthula et al., 2021; Brundin et al., 2020).

ALS: Advances in understanding genetic contributors (e.g., SOD1 mutations) have led to targeted therapeutic development. Amyotrophic lateral sclerosis (ALS) is a progressive neurodegenerative disorder causing muscle weakness and paralysis (Picher-Martel et al., 2016). Research focuses on understanding and treating monogenic familial forms, but few disease-modifying therapies exist. Advances in preclinical models are needed to better capture ALS's heterogeneous nature and guide translation and precision medicine development. Novel model systems can help guide translation and understanding. ALS is a neurodegenerative disorder affecting motor neurons, causing death from respiratory failure. Current treatments include Riluzole, Edaravone, and Sodium phenylbutyrate/Taurursodiol. Recent breakthroughs in targeting genetic disease forms offer hope for improved care and therapy. This review summarizes ALS therapy, including medication and supportive therapy, and discusses ongoing developments and prospects in the field (Tzeplaeff et al., 2023).

11.4.5 Microbiome

The following article provides an update and new features introduced over the last 2 years on the Genomes OnLine Database (GOLD) which is an online metadata repository at the Department of Energy Joint Genome Institute, designed to catalog and manage information related to (meta)genomic sequence projects, enabling researchers to access a wide range of metadata from its four levels: Study, Organism/Biosample, Sequencing Project, and Analysis Project. Since its inception in 1997, GOLD has expanded by adding diverse metadata fields, intuitive features, advanced search capabilities, and enhanced data visualization tools to meet the growing demand for genomic research metadata (Mukherjee et al., 2025).

Recent studies highlight the role of gut and oral microbiota in AD via the microbiota-gut-brain axis, linking dysbiosis to neuroinflammation. Altered bacterial taxa like Bacteroides, Firmicutes, and Porphyromonas gingivalis increase microglial activation, cytokine production, and intestinal permeability, facilitating endotoxin translocation and brain inflammation. Microbial metabolites, including SCFAs and amyloids, influence neuroinflammatory processes, with butyrate showing antiinflammatory potential. Modulating microbiota offers a promising therapeutic strategy to reduce neuroinflammation and slow AD progression (Popescu et al., 2024).

The following review article deals with pharmacomicrobiomics, a rapidly developing field that aims to contribute significantly to predictive, personalized, preventive, and participatory (P4) medicine, particularly in precision oncology. It helps clinicians predict treatment response, reduce side effects, and improve overall outcomes for cancer patients. The field also holds potential for personalized microbiome-based therapeutics, enhancing precision oncology and personalized medicine by using the right drug, dose, patient, and time (Arga et al., 2024).

This review article explores the relationship between microbiome and cancer, its impact on treatment outcomes, and the challenges in developing microbiome-based interventions. It highlights the potential of pharmacomicrobiomics in guiding cancer treatment decisions and improving patient outcomes, highlighting the transformative potential of this field (Le Ngoc et al., 2024).

This additional review article explores the molecular mechanisms affecting the gut microbiota's impact on antitumor immunity and cancer immunotherapy efficacy. It identifies four potential molecular mechanisms: immunomodulation, molecular mimicry, mumps, and microbial metabolites. The findings suggest that gut microbiota significantly influences antitumor immunity and cancer immunotherapy effectiveness (Yin et al., 2024).

Individual variability in drug response (IVDR) is a significant cause of adverse drug reactions (ADRs) and prolonged therapy. Genetic diversity only explains a small proportion of IVDR. The gut microbiota plays a crucial role in modulating therapeutic outcomes in human diseases. The field of pharmacomicrobiomics, which has almost a decade of history, aims to explore the correlation between microbiota variation and IVDR or ADRs. It highlights the need for innovative multiomics approaches, integrating genomic data, and translating lab data into clinical practice, as mentioned in the following review article (Zhao et al., 2023).

This review article examines the role of gut microbiota in AD, highlighting its role in modulating neuroinflammation and glial cell function. A systematic literature search reveals that dysbiosis, an imbalance in gut microbiota composition, may accelerate AD onset and progression. Therapeutic strategies targeting gut microbiota, such as probiotics, prebiotics, and fecal microbiota transplantation, show promise in modulating AD pathology. Understanding gut microbiota's role in AD pathogenesis could lead to innovative diagnostic, preventive, and therapeutic approaches (Yang et al., 2024).

11.4.6 Infectious diseases—vaccines

Precision medicine in infectious diseases focuses on pathogen characterization, resistance detection, and personalized treatment selection. Antimicrobial resistance Genomic approaches enable rapid identification of resistance mechanisms: WGS: Comprehensive resistance profiling. Rapid diagnostics: Point-of-care resistance testing. Personalized therapy: Tailored antibiotic selection. Outbreak investigation: Tracking transmission patterns. Viral infections: Precision approaches to viral infections include: HIV treatment: Genotypic resistance testing.

Hepatitis C: Genotype-specific treatment regimens. Influenza: Strain-specific vaccine development. COVID-19: Variant characterization and treatment optimization.

Precision approaches in combating antimicrobial resistance (AMR): Genomic surveillance has improved the identification of resistance genes, informing precision treatments. Examples, MRSA and tuberculosis.

Antibiotic resistance is rapidly spreading, challenging infection control efforts. While PCR-based nucleic acid testing is commonly used, it is time-consuming, highlighting the need for new strategies. The CRISPR-Cas system offers a promising approach to detect, target, and even reverse bacterial resistance. This review explores CRISPR-based detection methods, including nanoparticle-assisted approaches, and recent advances in using CRISPR-Cas for combating antimicrobial resistance and modulating bacterial virulence (Wu et al., 2021).

Personalized Vaccine Development: COVID-19 mRNA vaccines, like Pfizer-BioNTech, showcase how precision approaches expedite vaccine design for emerging pathogens.

This review examines the role of biomedical research in developing vaccines, highlighting the advancements in virology, immunology, molecular biology, and pharmaceutical technologies like CRISPR-Cas9. It also discusses challenges like regulatory hurdles, vaccine hesitancy, and new pathogens. The review advocates for interdisciplinary collaboration and innovative strategies, highlighting the importance of vaccines in combating health threats and the need for continued investment in biomedical science and technology (Weerarathna et al., 2024).

Restoring trust requires further research on the need for PM in infectious diseases, public health, and vaccines (Equils et al., 2023).

11.4.7 CRISPR and gene editing

CRISPR-Cas9 technology has revolutionized gene editing, enabling precise modifications to DNA sequences with unprecedented accuracy and efficiency (Doudna & Charpentier, 2014). This breakthrough technology has opened new possibilities for treating genetic diseases and developing personalized therapeutic approaches based on individual genetic profiles. CRISPR-Cas12a enzymes are versatile genome-editing tools used in viral diagnosis, agriculture, and human therapeutics. However, their limited targeting capability is limited to 1% of the genome. A recent bacterial-based directed evolution assay and rational engineering have identified variants with expanded protospacer adjacent motif (PAM) recognition, allowing access to previously inaccessible genomic loci (Ma et al., 2025).

11.4.8 Therapeutic applications

CRISPR-based therapies are advancing from laboratory to clinic, with several promising applications showing significant clinical potential. Sickle cell disease treatment involves editing patient cells to produce functional hemoglobin, offering hope for patients with this devastating genetic disorder (Laurent et al., 2024). Beta-thalassemia treatment focuses on correcting genetic defects in blood cell production, potentially eliminating the need for lifelong blood transfusions (Almotiri et al., 2025). LCA treatment represents a pioneering approach using direct in vivo gene editing for inherited blindness, demonstrating the potential for treating previously incurable genetic conditions (Zhang & Xu, 2025). Duchenne muscular dystrophy treatment aims to restore dystrophin protein function, potentially slowing or halting the progression of this debilitating muscle-wasting disease (Ingle et al., 2025).

11.4.9 Base editing and prime editing

Advanced gene editing technologies offer greater precision and expanded therapeutic possibilities beyond traditional CRISPR-Cas9 approaches. Base editing techniques enable the conversion of single DNA bases without creating double-strand breaks, reducing the risk of unintended genetic modifications while maintaining therapeutic efficacy (Vanhooydonck et al., 2025). Prime editing technology allows for precise insertions, deletions, and substitutions with minimal off-target effects, expanding the range of genetic corrections that can be achieved safely. Epigenome editing approaches modify gene expression without changing the underlying DNA sequence, offering potential for treating diseases caused by abnormal gene regulation rather than genetic mutations (Zang et al., 2025).

11.4.10 Delivery systems

Effective gene editing requires sophisticated delivery methods to ensure therapeutic genetic material reaches target cells safely and efficiently. Lipid nanoparticles serve as protective carriers for genetic material, shielding it from degradation while facilitating cellular uptake (Woodward et al., 2024). Viral vectors utilize modified viruses for gene delivery, taking advantage of natural viral mechanisms for efficient cellular entry and genetic material transfer. Electroporation techniques employ physical methods for cellular delivery, using electrical fields to create temporary pores in cell membranes for therapeutic uptake. Tissue-specific targeting approaches direct therapies to specific organs or cell types, minimizing off-target effects while maximizing therapeutic efficacy (Gibson et al., 2025).

11.5 Mini case study vignette (anonymized)

11.5.1 Mini case vignette: implementing precision medicine in a multispecialty health system

A large tertiary healthcare system serving both urban and semi-rural populations sought to integrate precision medicine into routine clinical care. While the organization had access to NGS, advanced imaging, and EHRs, precision approaches were applied inconsistently across departments.

Initial efforts focused on oncology, where tumor genomic profiling was used to guide targeted therapies. However, challenges quickly emerged. Molecular data were stored separately from clinical records, clinicians reported limited confidence in interpreting genomic results, and reimbursement pathways for companion diagnostics were unclear. At the same time, cardiology and endocrinology departments expressed interest in pharmacogenomics and risk stratification tools but lacked standardized workflows.

In response, the institution launched a phased precision medicine program. A centralized molecular diagnostics unit was established to harmonize genomic testing and reporting. AI-enabled clinical decision support tools were integrated into the EHR, offering treatment recommendations with transparent explanations. Targeted training programs were introduced for clinicians, emphasizing genomic literacy and ethical considerations. Importantly, patient consent processes were redesigned using a dynamic consent model, allowing individuals greater control over data use.

Within 18 months, targeted therapy utilization increased, ADRs decreased in pharmacogenomics-guided prescribing, and clinician confidence improved. Nevertheless, challenges persisted around long-term sustainability, data governance, and extending access to smaller regional clinics.

Discussion prompt: Which components of this implementation most directly support scalability and equity—and what additional policy or reimbursement changes would be required to sustain the model?

11.6 Technological enablers of personalized treatments

Artificial intelligence and ML technologies are revolutionizing PM by enabling sophisticated analysis of complex biomedical data and supporting clinical decision-making. These technological advances are transforming how healthcare providers diagnose diseases, predict treatment responses, and deliver personalized interventions to patients across diverse clinical settings.

11.6.1 Machine learning algorithms

Various ML approaches are applied to PM, each offering unique advantages for different types of clinical problems. Supervised learning algorithms predict outcomes from labeled training data, enabling the development of diagnostic and prognostic models based on historical patient data. Unsupervised learning techniques discover hidden patterns in data without predetermined outcomes, revealing new insights into disease mechanisms and patient subgroups. Reinforcement learning approaches optimize treatment strategies by learning from the consequences of clinical decisions, potentially improving therapeutic outcomes through iterative refinement. Ensemble methods combine multiple models for improved accuracy and robustness, reducing the risk of errors from any single algorithmic approach.

11.6.2 Deep learning in medical imaging

Deep learning (DL) algorithms have achieved remarkable success in medical image analysis, often matching or exceeding human expert performance across multiple medical specialties. In radiology, automated detection systems can identify tumors, fractures, and pathological changes with high accuracy, supporting radiologists in making faster and more precise diagnoses (Krawczuk et al., 2025). The field of pathology has been transformed through digital slide analysis and cancer diagnosis capabilities, enabling pathologists to process larger volumes of cases while maintaining diagnostic accuracy. Ophthalmology applications have shown particular promise, with DL systems demonstrating exceptional performance in diabetic retinopathy screening and age-related macular degeneration detection, potentially expanding access to specialized care in underserved areas. Dermatology has benefited from advanced skin cancer classification and melanoma detection algorithms that can analyze dermatological images with accuracy comparable to experienced dermatologists, offering potential for early detection and improved patient outcomes (Yousef et al., 2022).

11.6.3 Natural language processing

Natural language processing (NLP) technologies extract valuable information from unstructured clinical texts, unlocking the wealth of data contained in EHRs and medical literature. Clinical documentation applications enable automated coding and information extraction, reducing administrative burden while improving data quality and accessibility for research and clinical decision-making. Literature mining capabilities allow researchers to identify relevant research findings from vast databases of scientific publications, accelerating the translation of research discoveries into clinical practice. Phenotype extraction techniques characterize patient clinical features from narrative clinical notes, enabling more comprehensive patient profiling for PM applications. Adverse event detection systems monitor drug safety signals by analyzing clinical documentation and patient reports, contributing to pharmacovigilance and improving medication safety (Benrubi et al., 2025).

11.6.4 Predictive modeling

ML models predict clinical outcomes and treatment responses, enabling proactive healthcare management and personalized treatment selection. Risk stratification algorithms identify high-risk patients who may benefit from intensive monitoring or preventive interventions, allowing healthcare providers to allocate resources more effectively. Treatment optimization models assist clinicians in selecting optimal therapies based on patient characteristics, disease features, and predicted treatment responses, improving therapeutic outcomes while minimizing adverse effects. Adverse event prediction systems help prevent medication-related harm by identifying patients at increased risk for specific drug-related complications before they occur. Prognosis assessment models estimate disease trajectories and long-term outcomes, supporting informed decision-making for patients and families while guiding care planning. The following review examines surgical site infections (SSIs), which are a significant complication after spinal surgery, causing increased morbidity, hospital stays, and healthcare costs. Traditional statistical models have been used to predict SSI risk, but AI and ML methods have also been used. The review highlights the need for standardized model benchmarking and external validation to assess generalizability. Advancing beyond conventional tabular data with state-of-the-art AI models could significantly expand predictive analytics and guide clinical decision-making (Ndjonko et al., 2025).

11.6.5 The role of AI and machine learning in predictive modeling

AI facilitates predictive analytics for treatment efficacy, identifying at-risk populations, and drug repurposing. Examples include DeepMind's AlphaFold for protein structure prediction (Abramson et al., 2024; Jumper et al., 2021). The AlphaFold-21 model revolutionized protein modeling and design, enabling various applications. The AlphaFold3 model, updated with a diffusion-based architecture, predicts complexes like proteins, nucleic acids, small molecules (ligands), ions, and modified residues. Its improved accuracy demonstrates that high-accuracy modeling across biomolecular space can be achieved within a single deep-learning framework.

11.6.6 Multimodal data integration

Predictive models increasingly integrate diverse data types to provide comprehensive assessments of patient health and treatment needs. Clinical data from EHR and laboratory results provide foundational information about patient health status and disease progression. Genomic data including genetic variants and molecular profiles offer insights into disease susceptibility and treatment response potential. Imaging data from medical images and radiological findings contribute visual information that complements other data modalities. Behavioral data incorporating lifestyle factors and patient-reported outcomes provide context for understanding health behaviors and their impact on clinical outcomes.

11.6.7 Validation and implementation

Ensuring model reliability and clinical utility requires rigorous validation processes that demonstrate safety, efficacy, and generalizability across different populations and clinical settings. Cross-validation techniques assess model performance on independent datasets, providing confidence in predictive accuracy and generalizability. External validation involves testing models in different populations and clinical environments to ensure broad applicability. Clinical validation demonstrates clinical utility and patient outcomes, showing that predictive models actually improve care quality and patient health. Regulatory approval processes, including FDA, EMA, and other regulatory requirements, ensure that predictive models meet safety and efficacy standards before clinical implementation.

The technological enablers of personalized treatments represent a convergence of advanced computational methods, biotechnology innovations, and digital health tools that are transforming modern healthcare. These technologies work synergistically to create new possibilities for PM, enabling more accurate diagnoses, personalized treatment selection, and continuous health monitoring. As these technologies continue to evolve and mature, they promise to make PM more accessible, effective, and integrated into routine clinical practice, ultimately improving patient outcomes and transforming the delivery of healthcare services.

11.6.8 Multiomics applications and use of artificial intelligence

Innovative omics technologies are enabling researchers to access multilayer information from various molecular layers, providing a holistic view of tumor behavior. Personalized omics technologies have transformed healthcare by enabling personalized treatments based on individual genetic and metabolic profiles. AI, particularly DL significantly improved medical diagnosis and treatment in cancer research. DL's automated feature extraction and ability to handle large amounts of data have led to applications in early cancer detection, diagnosis, molecular characterization, patient outcomes prediction, personalized treatment, radiotherapy workflows, anti-cancer drug discovery, and clinical trials (Ahmed, 2020; Chen et al., 2021). However, extracting valuable insights from the increasing amount of data presents challenges. Advancements in NGS technologies have led to the accumulation of large amounts of multiomics data, providing a holistic view of cancer's biological networks and pathways. However, these data present challenges in processing, analyzing, and interpreting. Artificial intelligence has emerged as a powerful solution to these challenges, enabling the integration of complex patterns and valuable information from large-scale datasets. This synergy is revolutionizing cancer research and clinical practice, particularly in early detection, diagnosis, prognosis, treatment, and pathology as stated by (Li et al., 2024).

Artificial intelligence has shown the ability to analyze complementary multimodal data streams, fueling cancer PM. Advances in AI-based multiomics approaches include early cancer screening, diagnosis, response assessment, and prognosis prediction. Future trends in this field are expected to shift towards AI-based multiomics technologies as pointed out by (He et al., 2023).

High-dimensional characterization of genomics, epigenomics, transcriptomics, proteomics, and metabolomics has opened new horizons for understanding cancers and tumor heterogeneity (Ahmed, 2020; Bhinder et al., 2021; John et al., 2020; Neagu et al., 2023; Olivier et al., 2019). Breast cancer (BC) as an example, is a complex disease with a wide range of genotypic and phenotypic variations. To accurately diagnose, perform prognosis, and treat BC, in-depth investigations into its molecular basis are crucial.

The following review (Neagu et al., 2023) discusses both classic and novel omics fields, which can be integrated into onco-breastomics. Advances in molecular profiling strategies and analytical techniques have generated large-scale multiomics datasets, mainly from genomics, transcriptomics, and proteomics. Metabolomics-based approaches reflect the dynamic response of BC cells to genetic modifications. Interactomics promotes a holistic view of BC research by constructing and characterizing protein-protein interaction networks. New omics- and epiomics-based multidimensional approaches provide insights into BC heterogeneity and its underlying mechanisms. Salivaomics, urinomics, and milkomics are integrative omics that have potential for early and noninvasive diagnoses in BC.

Another example is esophageal cancer, which is a complex malignancy with significant tumor heterogeneity, affecting progression from onset to metastasis. However, manipulating this heterogeneity could be a new therapeutic strategy. Artificial intelligence, particularly ML, and DL algorithms, has emerged as a promising computational tool for analyzing and dissecting patient-specific, multiomics data. This review provides a comprehensive review of tumor heterogeneity from a multiomics perspective (Li et al., 2023).

AI has revolutionized vaccine development, enhancing efficiency and precision. It aids in antigen selection, epitope prediction, adjuvant identification, and optimization strategies. AI algorithms use genomic data, protein structures, and immune system interactions to predict antigenic epitopes and prioritize antigens. However, challenges like data heterogeneity and regulatory considerations need to be addressed. Integrating emerging technologies like single-cell omics and synthetic biology can improve vaccine design precision and scalability (Olawade et al., 2024).

AI-enabled computational tools have revolutionized vaccine design and development by creating predictive models and data-driven decision-making processes. Understanding these computational resources can help in selecting appropriate tools for each step of vaccine development, enhancing research efficiency, and reducing costs (Ananya et al., 2024).

See Fig. 11.2 for a detailed multiomics integration workflow currently utilized.

11.6.9 Digital health tools

Digital health technologies are transforming PM by enabling continuous monitoring, data collection, and personalized interventions. These tools create new opportunities for patient engagement, remote care delivery, and real-time health management.

11.6.9.1 Digital tools and wearable technologies

Wearable and biosensor technologies provide real-time physiological monitoring, generating continuous streams of health data that can inform personalized treatment decisions. Continuous glucose monitoring systems offer real-time blood sugar tracking for diabetes management, enabling patients to make immediate adjustments to their treatment regimens.

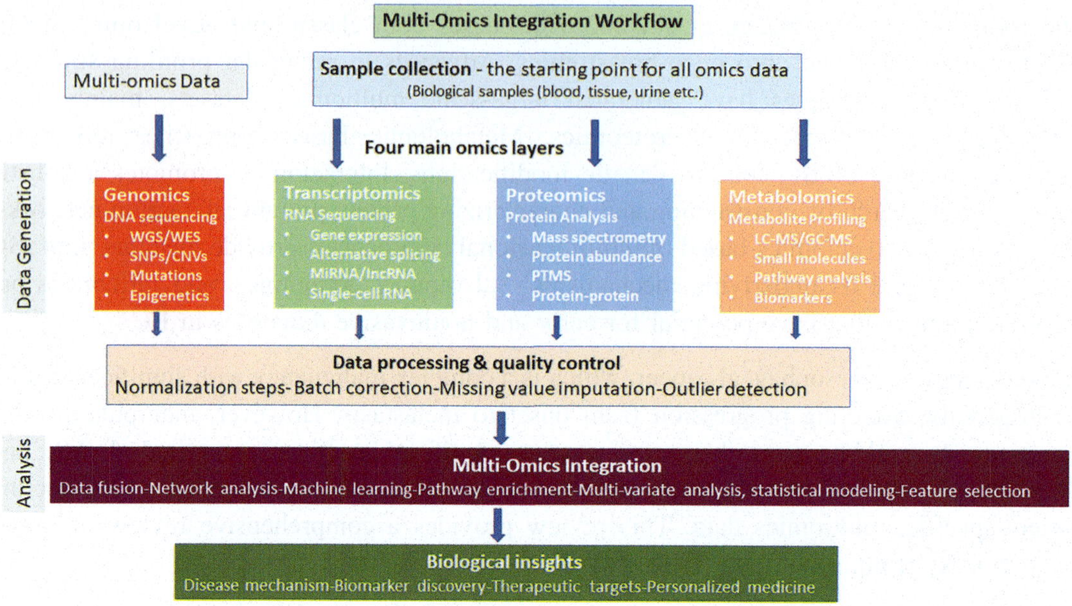

Figure 11.2
Multiomics integration workflow. The workflow steps need to be assessed throughout the process.

Heart rate variability monitoring provides valuable insights into cardiovascular health assessment, supporting early detection of cardiac abnormalities and guiding exercise prescriptions. Sleep monitoring capabilities analyze circadian rhythms and sleep quality, contributing to the understanding of sleep disorders and their impact on overall health. Activity tracking features measure physical activity and fitness parameters, supporting personalized exercise recommendations and lifestyle interventions. Good examples include wearables like Fitbit (Schyvens et al., 2024) and Apple Watch (Hajj-Boutros et al., 2023) which enable continuous monitoring, providing real-time data for personalized interventions. This systematic review finds that devices like the Fitbit Charge 4 and WHOOP show higher accuracy in estimating sleep parameters but still require improvements in sleep stage classification. Despite ongoing advancements in wearables, scientific research on their accuracy remains limited, hindering definitive conclusions. Future studies should adopt standardized protocols with larger sample sizes to improve comparability and strengthen research in this field (Schyvens et al., 2024). Table 11.2 lists several digital tools and wearable technologies.

11.6.9.2 Mobile health applications

Smartphone applications enable personalized health management by providing convenient tools for patient self-monitoring and care coordination. Medication adherence applications

Table 11.2 Digital health applications in healthcare.

Application name	Primary function	Source
MyChart	Provides patients with access to their personal health records, appointment scheduling, and direct communication with healthcare providers.	MyChart (2025)
FreeStyle Libre 3	Continuous glucose monitoring system for individuals with diabetes, offering real-time blood sugar readings.	FreeStyle Libre (2025)
BetterHelp	Offers virtual counseling and mental health services, including digital journals, goal trackers, and wellness webinars.	betterhelp (2025)
Click Therapeutics	Develops mobile software applications used as prescription medical treatments for various conditions.	clicktherapeutics (2025)
Evidation	Allows users to record healthy behaviors and earn points redeemable for cash, providing insights and health education resources.	Evidation (2025)
Sleepio	Digital insomnia treatment using cognitive behavioral therapy (CBT) techniques to improve sleep without medication.	Big Health (2025)
Ada Health	AI-powered app providing medical consultations based on personal medical history and common medical knowledge.	Ada (2025)
CardMedic	Facilitates communication between healthcare providers and patients with language barriers through a digital flashcard system.	CardMedic (2025)
Quest Prehab	Digital program helping patients prepare for surgeries, aiming to reduce recovery times and hospital readmissions.	QuestPrehab (2025)

include reminder systems and tracking capabilities that help patients maintain consistent treatment regimens. Symptom monitoring platforms collect patient-reported outcome measures, providing valuable data for clinical decision-making and treatment optimization. Lifestyle tracking applications monitor diet, exercise, and behavior modification efforts, supporting comprehensive approaches to health management. Clinical trial participation tools enable remote data collection and monitoring, expanding access to research opportunities while reducing participant burden. The number of mHealth application users and their frequency of usage will increase when commercially accessible mHealth applications are used in a health guidance setting (Onoue et al., 2025).

11.6.9.3 Telemedicine and remote monitoring

Digital platforms expand access to PM by overcoming geographical barriers and enabling continuous care delivery. Virtual consultation systems provide remote specialist access, particularly valuable for patients in underserved areas who may have limited access to specialized care. Remote patient monitoring platforms enable continuous health surveillance, allowing healthcare providers to track patient status and intervene proactively when needed (Kostopoulou et al., 2025). Digital therapeutics represent software-based interventions that can deliver evidence-based treatments directly to patients through digital platforms. Artificial intelligence chatbots provide automated health support, offering 24/7 availability for basic health questions and guidance (Testa et al., 2025).

Integration of EHRs for Real-Time Data Access: EHRs facilitate seamless integration of genomic data and clinical workflows, enabling faster decision-making.

In a recent review paper, the authors pointed to the need to integrate statistical algorithms with omics and nano-omics for enhanced diagnostic accuracy and treatment efficacy (Coskun et al., 2024). The authors point to the fact that medical laboratory services are crucial for healthcare, enabling precise biomolecule measurement and impacting global health outcomes. Personalized reference values are essential for accurate interpretation of omics data, and the convergence of nanotechnology and omics sciences is transforming personalized laboratory medicine by providing diagnostic precision and innovative therapeutic strategies (Coskun et al., 2024).

Metagenomics and Metatranscriptomics involve examining nucleotide sequences, gene identification, and biological function analysis. However, the complexity of sequence data presents challenges in processing analysis. Advanced visualization tools are crucial for effective exploration, querying, and analysis of these complex datasets, as stated in the following review article, which highlights the critical role of advanced visualization tools in enabling effective exploration, querying, and analysis of these complex datasets. The article categorizes various visualizers based on their intended applications and highlights their utility in empowering bioinformaticians and nonbioinformaticians to interpret and derive insights from meta-omics data effectively (Aplakidou et al., 2024).

Table 11.3 highlights various technologies driving PM and their applications, with supporting studies.

11.6.10 Overall summary findings and key highlights

Oncology: Genomic tools like NGS have redefined cancer care by enabling personalized therapies that improve survival rates. Trastuzumab, for example, has significantly extended the lifespan of HER2-positive breast cancer patients.

Infectious diseases: Genomic epidemiology has provided insights into AMR, while personalized vaccines, including mRNA technologies, have revolutionized prevention strategies for diseases like COVID-19.

Technological synergies: Advanced tools such as AI, CRISPR, and wearable devices are not only enhancing diagnostic accuracy but also enabling real-time treatment adaptation, thereby reducing healthcare costs and improving quality of life.

Table 11.3 Technological enablers of precision medicine.

Technology	Application	Example	Indicative studies
Genomic sequencing	Decoding individual genomes for targeted therapies.	Whole-genome sequencing in identifying BRCA mutations for breast cancer prevention.	Zhu et al. (2022)
CRISPR-Cas9	Gene editing to address inherited diseases.	CRISPR-based therapies for sickle cell anemia.	Jinek et al. (2012), McManus et al. (2024)
AlphaFold	Predicting protein structures to accelerate drug development.	Application in developing treatments for neurodegenerative diseases.	Abramson et al. (2024), Jumper et al. (2021)
Digital twins	Simulating patient-specific conditions for precise interventions.	Personalized modeling for managing heart failure.	Thangaraj et al. (2024)
AI and machine learning	Predictive modeling for treatment efficacy and patient stratification.	AI algorithms for early detection of lung cancer.	de Margerie-Mellon and Chassagnon (2023)
Wearable devices	Monitoring real-time health metrics for adaptive treatments.	Use of continuous glucose monitors in managing diabetes.	Cappon et al. (2019)

Targeted therapies: The development and implementation of targeted therapies, such as trastuzumab for HER2-positive breast cancer, have revolutionized treatment approaches by focusing on specific molecular targets.

Pharmacogenomics and its role in predicting treatment efficacy: Pharmacogenomics has advanced considerably. It examines how genes affect a person's response to drugs, enabling the prediction of treatment efficacy and the minimization of adverse effects.

Precision diagnostics and their influence on treatment strategies: Advancements in precision diagnostics, including genomic sequencing, have enhanced the ability to tailor treatments to individual patients.

Drug design and drug development: AlphaFold2 &3 revolutionized structural biology and protein structure prediction and function, and have enhanced the success rate in pharmacology.

11.7 Challenges, implications, and limitations of precision medicine

11.7.1 Technical challenges

11.7.1.1 Data integration and standardization

As already mentioned, PM generates vast amounts of heterogeneous data that must be integrated meaningfully, presenting significant technical challenges. The field faces substantial challenges with data format heterogeneity, as different platforms generate data in various formats that must be reconciled for effective analysis. Semantic interoperability remains a critical concern, requiring systems to ensure consistent data interpretation across different platforms and institutions. Quality control measures are essential for maintaining data accuracy and reliability, while missing data handling presents ongoing difficulties in addressing incomplete datasets. Additionally, temporal data integration poses challenges in combining data collected at different time points, requiring sophisticated analytical approaches to maintain data integrity and usability.

11.7.1.2 Computational scalability

Processing large-scale multiomics datasets requires significant computational resources that strain current infrastructure capabilities. Storage requirements have reached petabyte-scale genomic databases, demanding robust and scalable storage solutions. Processing power limitations affect the ability to analyze complex datasets within reasonable timeframes, while network bandwidth constraints impact the transfer of large datasets across institutions. Algorithm optimization remains crucial for developing efficient analysis methods that can handle the complexity and volume of precision medicine data. Cloud infrastructure has emerged as a potential solution for scaling computational resources dynamically, though implementation challenges persist in ensuring security and accessibility.

11.7.1.3 Analytical complexity

Multiomics data analysis presents numerous statistical and computational challenges that require sophisticated methodological approaches. Multiple testing correction becomes essential for controlling false discovery rates when analyzing thousands of genetic variants simultaneously. Batch effects must be carefully managed to remove technical variations between experiments that could confound results. Dimensionality reduction techniques are necessary for handling high-dimensional data while preserving meaningful biological signals. Network analysis adds complexity in understanding molecular interactions and their relationships to disease phenotypes. Perhaps most challenging is causal inference, which requires distinguishing correlation from causation in complex biological systems where multiple factors interact simultaneously.

11.7.2 Ethical considerations

11.7.2.1 Ethical considerations in genetic testing and data sharing

The rise of PM has brought ethical dilemmas, particularly in the areas of genetic testing and data privacy. As genomic data becomes a crucial component of personalized treatments, concerns about how this sensitive information is collected, stored, and shared have intensified.

Patients may be reluctant to undergo genetic testing due to fears of discrimination by insurers or employers, as well as potential misuse of their data.

To address these concerns, regulatory frameworks such as the General Data Protection Regulation (GDPR) (GDPR, 2025) and the AI Act in Europe (AI ACT, 2025) have established strict guidelines on genetic data protection, emphasizing informed consent, data anonymization, and security protocols. GDPR compliance reports highlight the importance of transparency in data handling and reinforce the need for patient-centric policies. Additionally, initiatives promoting secure data-sharing frameworks, such as blockchain-based health records, are being explored to enhance trust and security in precision medicine.

11.7.2.2 Privacy and confidentiality

Genomic and health data contain highly sensitive personal information that requires robust protection measures to maintain patient trust and comply with regulatory requirements. Data security protocols must protect against unauthorized access and breaches, implementing multilayered security approaches including encryption, access controls, and audit trails. Anonymization techniques must remove identifying information while preserving data utility for research purposes, balancing privacy protection with scientific value. Consent frameworks must ensure informed consent for data use, addressing the complexity of genomic data that may have implications for family members and future generations. Data sharing policies must balance research benefits with privacy risks, establishing clear guidelines for when and how sensitive genetic information can be shared among researchers and institutions. The prevention of genetic discrimination requires careful consideration of how genetic information might be misused in employment, insurance, or social contexts.

11.7.2.3 Informed consent

Traditional consent models may be inadequate for PM applications, necessitating new approaches that account for the evolving nature of genetic research and its implications. Dynamic consent models allow patients to modify their consent preferences over time as research progresses and new applications emerge. Broad consent approaches seek to obtain permission for future research uses that may not be fully defined at the time of initial data collection. Genetic testing in children presents unique ethical challenges, requiring careful consideration of pediatric consent issues and the child's future autonomy. Incidental findings management becomes complex when genetic testing reveals unexpected discoveries that may have health implications for patients and their families. The return of results policies must address decisions about what information should be shared with patients, balancing the potential benefits of genetic knowledge with the psychological and social implications of such information.

11.7.2.4 Genetic discrimination

Genetic information could potentially be used for discrimination across various sectors of society, requiring comprehensive protective measures and ongoing vigilance. Employment discrimination concerns focus on protecting individuals from genetic-based hiring decisions that could unfairly limit career opportunities based on genetic predispositions. Insurance discrimination prevention requires safeguards against genetic-based coverage denials, ensuring that genetic information cannot be used to exclude individuals from health, life, or disability insurance. Educational discrimination protections must ensure equal access to educational opportunities regardless of genetic status. Social stigma associated with genetic predisposition to disease requires careful management through education, policy, and cultural change initiatives to prevent discrimination based on genetic characteristics.

11.7.3 Regulatory frameworks

11.7.3.1 Regulatory policies and clinical validity

The regulatory landscape for PM presents another significant challenge. Approval pathways for targeted therapies and companion diagnostics vary across regions, leading to inconsistencies in implementation. For example, the U.S. Food and Drug Administration (FDA, 2025) and the European Medicines Agency (European Medicines Agency, 2025d) have different evaluation criteria and approval timelines for precision-based treatments. This divergence can delay the global availability of novel therapies and create barriers for pharmaceutical companies seeking international approval.

Standardizing regulatory policies and establishing harmonized guidelines for clinical validation are essential for accelerating the adoption of precision medicine. FDA guidance documents outline the agency's approach to evaluating genomic-based therapies, including companion diagnostics and real-world evidence integration. Expanding such frameworks to align with international regulatory bodies would streamline approvals and enhance global access to precision treatments.

While PM has the potential to revolutionize healthcare, its implementation is filled with challenges related to cost, ethical considerations, and regulatory barriers. Overcoming these obstacles requires a multifaceted approach, including financial assistance programs, robust data protection policies, and streamlined regulatory frameworks like the European AI Act (AI ACT, 2025). By fostering global collaboration and adopting inclusive healthcare strategies, precision medicine can transition from being an exclusive innovation to a widely accessible and transformative medical practice.

11.7.3.2 FDA versus EMA approval processes

Precision medicine products require specialized regulatory pathways that address their unique characteristics and complexity. Companion diagnostics, which identify patients suitable for specific treatments, require coordinated review processes that evaluate both the diagnostic test and the associated therapeutic intervention. Software as medical devices, particularly AI-based diagnostic and treatment tools, present novel regulatory challenges requiring new evaluation frameworks that can assess algorithm performance, safety, and clinical utility. Gene therapies represent complex biological products requiring specialized review processes that address manufacturing, safety, and efficacy concerns unique to genetic interventions. Combination products that integrate devices and drugs used together require coordinated regulatory review to ensure the safety and effectiveness of the integrated system. Adaptive clinical trials offer flexible trial designs for precision medicine but require regulatory frameworks that can accommodate evolving study protocols while maintaining scientific rigor (European Medicines Agency, 2025b; FDA, 2025).

11.7.3.3 International harmonization

Global PM development requires coordinated regulatory approaches that facilitate innovation while ensuring safety and efficacy standards. ICH guidelines provide International Conference on Harmonization standards that help align regulatory expectations across different countries and regions. Data sharing agreements enable cross-border data exchange frameworks that support international research collaboration while protecting patient privacy and national interests. Regulatory convergence efforts aim to align approval processes across countries, reducing duplicative requirements and accelerating global access to precision medicine innovations. Quality standards ensure consistent product quality globally, providing confidence in PM products regardless of their country of origin. Intellectual property frameworks must balance protecting innovations with enabling access to life-saving treatments, particularly in resource-limited settings.

11.7.4 Healthcare equity and access

11.7.4.1 Diversity in genomic databases

Most genomic databases are derived from populations of European ancestry, significantly limiting PM benefits for other groups and creating health disparities. Ancestral bias in genomic databases leads to underrepresentation of diverse populations, resulting in reduced effectiveness of PM approaches for non-European populations. Variant interpretation becomes particularly challenging when classifying genetic variants in underrepresented groups, as reference databases may lack sufficient diversity to accurately assess variant significance. Drug response differences among populations reflect population-specific pharmacogenomic variants that may not be captured in predominantly European databases. Disease susceptibility patterns vary among populations due to population-specific risk factors that may not be adequately represented in current genomic resources. Research participation barriers prevent diverse population enrollment, perpetuating the cycle of underrepresentation and limiting the generalizability of PM findings.

11.7.4.2 Rural healthcare applications

Rural areas face unique challenges in PM implementation that require targeted solutions and innovative delivery models. Provider shortages limit access to genetic counselors and specialists who are essential for implementing PM approaches effectively. Technology infrastructure inadequacies, including limited broadband and IT systems, hinder the implementation of PM technologies that rely on sophisticated computational resources and connectivity. Transportation barriers create difficulties in accessing specialized care, particularly for genetic counseling and follow-up services required for PM implementations. Cost considerations become particularly acute in rural settings, where higher per-patient costs may make PM approaches economically challenging. Education needs among rural providers require targeted training programs to build PM knowledge and capabilities in areas with limited access to specialized medical education.

11.7.4.3 Global health implications

Precision medicine applications in low- and middle-income countries face specific challenges that require innovative approaches and international cooperation. Infrastructure limitations include inadequate laboratory and IT infrastructure necessary for implementing PM technologies effectively. Cost constraints reflect limited healthcare budgets and resources that make expensive PM approaches difficult to justify or implement. Regulatory capacity limitations result from insufficient regulatory oversight capabilities to evaluate and approve PM products safely and effectively. Training needs reflect limited PM expertise among healthcare providers, requiring comprehensive education and capacity-building programs. Disease priorities in these settings often focus on infectious diseases rather than chronic conditions, requiring adaptation of PM approaches to address local health needs and priorities.

11.7.5 Economic implications

11.7.5.1 Cost-effectiveness analysis

While PM holds immense promise for improving patient outcomes, its widespread adoption faces several critical challenges. These challenges span economic, ethical, and regulatory domains, impacting accessibility, data security, and clinical implementation. Addressing these barriers is essential for ensuring that PM becomes an equitable and effective healthcare solution.

11.7.5.2 Cost and accessibility of precision medicine

One of the most significant barriers to PM is its high cost. The expenses associated with genomic sequencing, biomarker identification, and targeted therapies often place these advancements out of reach for many patients, particularly those in low- and middle-income countries. The financial burden extends to healthcare systems as well, as precision treatments often require specialized diagnostic tools, trained personnel, and long-term patient monitoring.

Potential solutions to improve accessibility include subsidized programs, public-private partnerships, and government-led initiatives aimed at reducing the cost of genomic testing and precision treatments. Global health organizations, such as the World Health Organization (WHO), have emphasized the importance of equity in healthcare access. WHO health equity reports highlight strategies for integrating PM into national healthcare systems while ensuring affordability for all populations. Collaborative efforts between governments, pharmaceutical companies, and nonprofit organizations can help bridge the affordability gap and expand access to life-saving treatments.

Precision medicine interventions must demonstrate economic value to justify their implementation within healthcare systems facing resource constraints. Development costs for PM approaches are typically high due to the extensive research and development required to identify biomarkers, develop targeted therapies, and validate their effectiveness. Implementation costs include infrastructure requirements and training needs that healthcare systems must absorb to successfully deploy PM approaches. Diagnostic costs associated with molecular testing and analysis can be substantial, particularly for comprehensive genomic profiling required for many precision medicine applications. Treatment costs for targeted therapies are often high due to their specialized nature and limited market size, though they may offer improved outcomes compared to standard treatments. Long-term savings potential exists through reduced healthcare costs over time, as PM may prevent ineffective treatments and reduce adverse events, though these benefits may take years to realize.

11.7.5.3 Reimbursement challenges

Healthcare payers face complex decisions about covering precision medicine interventions, requiring new evaluation frameworks and payment models. Evidence requirements for reimbursement include demonstrating clinical utility and cost-effectiveness, which can be challenging for PM approaches that may benefit small patient populations. Coverage policies must develop appropriate reimbursement frameworks that account for the unique characteristics of PM, including companion diagnostics and personalized treatment approaches. Prior authorization processes require careful design to manage access to expensive treatments while ensuring appropriate utilization. Outcomes measurement becomes crucial for tracking the real-world effectiveness of precision medicine interventions to justify continued coverage and payment. Budget impact considerations require payers to manage short-term costs for long-term benefits, balancing immediate financial pressures with potential future savings and improved patient outcomes.

11.8 The future of precision medicine

The future of PM holds tremendous promise as emerging technologies, evolving regulatory frameworks, and changing healthcare delivery models converge to create new possibilities for personalized patient care. This transformation will fundamentally alter how we prevent, diagnose, and treat diseases, moving toward a more proactive, predictive, and personalized approach to healthcare.

11.8.1 Emerging technologies

11.8.1.1 Spatial transcriptomics and proteomics

Spatial omics technologies represent a revolutionary advancement in molecular analysis by preserving tissue architecture while providing detailed molecular information about cellular function and interaction. These technologies enable researchers to understand how cellular location affects function, revealing the critical importance of spatial context in biological processes. Disease mechanisms can now be studied by identifying spatial patterns in pathological processes, providing insights into how diseases develop and progress within specific tissue environments. Drug targeting approaches are being developed that take advantage of location-specific therapeutic opportunities, potentially improving treatment efficacy while reducing side effects. Biomarker discovery efforts are increasingly focused on finding spatially resolved disease signatures that can provide more precise diagnostic and prognostic information than traditional approaches.

Single-cell multiomics: The simultaneous analysis of multiple molecular layers in individual cells represents a paradigm shift in our understanding of biological systems and disease processes. This technology enables researchers to understand cellular heterogeneity by revealing the extensive cell-to-cell variation that exists within tissues and organ systems. Developmental biology applications allow scientists to track cell fate decisions in real-time, providing unprecedented insights into how cells differentiate and develop into specialized cell types. Disease progression can now be monitored at the cellular level, revealing how individual cells change over time during disease development and treatment. Treatment response studies can identify resistant cell populations that may contribute to therapeutic failure, enabling the development of more effective combination therapies.

Quantum computing applications: Quantum computers may revolutionize PM by solving complex computational problems that are currently intractable with classical computing approaches. Drug discovery applications could benefit from quantum computing's ability to simulate molecular interactions with unprecedented accuracy, potentially accelerating the identification of new therapeutic targets and compounds. Protein folding prediction represents a particularly promising application, as quantum computers may be able to predict three-dimensional protein structures more accurately than current methods. Optimization problems in treatment selection could be solved more efficiently using quantum algorithms, helping clinicians find optimal treatment combinations for individual patients. ML applications may be accelerated through quantum computing approaches, enabling faster pattern recognition algorithms that can process vast amounts of biomedical data.

11.8.1.2 Regulatory and policy evolution

Adaptive regulatory pathways: Regulatory agencies are developing flexible frameworks for PM that can accommodate the unique characteristics of personalized therapies while maintaining safety and efficacy standards. Breakthrough therapy designation provides expedited review processes for promising treatments that address unmet medical needs, accelerating patient access to innovative therapies. Regenerative medicine advanced therapy pathways offer streamlined approval processes for cell and gene therapies, recognizing their unique development and manufacturing requirements. Software precertification programs implement risk-based oversight for digital health tools, enabling faster approval of low-risk applications while maintaining rigorous review for high-risk devices. Real-world evidence utilization allows regulatory agencies to use post-market data for regulatory decisions, providing ongoing assessment of treatment safety and effectiveness in real-world clinical settings.

International collaboration: Global cooperation is essential for PM advancement, as the complexity and scale of personalized medicine research require coordinated international efforts. Data sharing initiatives are creating international genomic databases that pool resources and expertise from multiple countries, enabling larger-scale studies and more diverse population representation. Regulatory harmonization efforts aim to coordinate approval processes across different countries, reducing duplicative requirements and accelerating global access to precision medicine innovations. Research collaborations increasingly involve multinational clinical trials that can recruit diverse patient populations and generate more generalizable results. Capacity-building programs support PM development globally by providing training, infrastructure, and technical assistance to developing countries.

11.8.1.3 Healthcare system integration

Provider education and training: Healthcare professionals need specialized training in PM to effectively implement personalized treatment approaches in clinical practice. Genomic literacy programs help providers understand genetic test interpretation and its clinical implications, enabling them to make informed treatment decisions based on genetic information. Bioinformatics skills training provides healthcare professionals with the ability to analyze molecular data and interpret complex biomarker results. Ethical considerations training addresses privacy and discrimination issues that arise with genetic and molecular testing, ensuring that providers can navigate these complex issues appropriately. Communication skills development helps healthcare professionals explain complex genetic and molecular concepts to patients in understandable terms, facilitating informed decision-making.

Clinical decision support systems: AI-powered tools will assist healthcare providers in making more informed and personalized treatment decisions by integrating vast amounts of clinical and molecular data. Treatment recommendation systems provide evidence-based therapy selection based on patient characteristics, disease features, and predicted treatment responses. Risk assessment tools help predict patient outcomes by analyzing multiple risk factors and biomarkers simultaneously. Drug interaction identification systems can identify potential adverse effects by analyzing complex interactions between medications, patient genetics, and comorbidities. Workflow integration capabilities ensure seamless EHR integration, making precision medicine tools accessible within existing clinical workflows.

Patient engagement: Patients must be active participants in PM, as personalized treatment approaches require greater patient involvement in decision-making and care management. Health literacy initiatives help patients understand genetic and molecular information, enabling them to participate more effectively in treatment decisions. Shared decision-making approaches involve patients in collaborating with healthcare providers in treatment choices, ensuring that patient preferences and values are incorporated into care plans. Data ownership frameworks give patients control over their personal health information, including genetic data and biomarker results. Advocacy efforts encourage patients to support precision medicine research and access initiatives, helping to advance the field and improve care for all patients.

11.8.1.4 Research priorities

Biomarker validation: Robust biomarker validation is essential for clinical translation of PM discoveries, requiring comprehensive evaluation across multiple domains. Analytical validation ensures test accuracy and precision by demonstrating that biomarker assays produce consistent and reliable results across different laboratories and testing conditions. Clinical validation demonstrates clinical utility by showing that biomarker results actually improve patient outcomes when used to guide treatment decisions. Regulatory validation involves meeting approval requirements established by regulatory agencies, ensuring that biomarker tests meet safety and efficacy standards. Health economic validation proves cost-effectiveness by demonstrating that biomarker-guided care provides value relative to its cost.

Real-world evidence generation: Post-market studies should provide crucial evidence about the effectiveness and safety of PM interventions in real-world clinical settings. Effectiveness studies measure real-world treatment outcomes by comparing the performance of PM approaches to standard care in diverse patient populations. Safety surveillance systems monitor adverse events and long-term safety outcomes to ensure that PM interventions remain safe as they are used more widely. Healthcare utilization studies assess the economic impact of PM by measuring changes in healthcare costs, resource utilization, and care patterns. Patient outcome tracking focuses on measuring quality of life improvements and patient-reported outcomes to assess the broader impact of precision medicine on patient well-being.

Health services research: Understanding PM implementation requires a systematic study of how these innovations are adopted and integrated into healthcare systems. Implementation science research studies adoption barriers and facilitators, identifying factors that promote or hinder the successful implementation of precision medicine approaches. Workflow optimization studies focus on improving clinical processes to better accommodate PM testing and treatment approaches. Provider satisfaction assessments measure healthcare professionals' acceptance of PM tools and identify areas for improvement. Patient satisfaction studies assess patient experiences with PM approaches, ensuring that these innovations meet patient needs and expectations.

11.8.1.5 Long-term vision

Precision prevention: The future of PM extends beyond treatment to prevention, using personalized approaches to maintain health and prevent disease before it occurs. Risk prediction models will identify individuals at risk before disease onset by analyzing genetic, environmental, and lifestyle factors to provide personalized risk assessments. Lifestyle interventions will be tailored to individual risk profiles, providing personalized prevention strategies that address specific risk factors for each person. Environmental factor modification will address modifiable risk factors through personalized recommendations for diet, exercise, and lifestyle changes. Population health applications will apply PM principles to public health initiatives, enabling more targeted and effective prevention programs.

11.8.1.6 Precision health systems

The transformation of healthcare delivery through PM will create learning health systems that continuously improve through data analysis and real-world evidence generation. Learning health systems will use continuous data analysis to improve care quality and outcomes, creating feedback loops that enable ongoing optimization of treatment approaches. Predictive healthcare will anticipate health needs before problems arise, using advanced analytics to identify patients at risk and intervene proactively. Personalized care pathways will tailor entire care episodes to individual patient needs, from prevention through treatment and long-term management. Population segmentation approaches will customize interventions for specific groups based on shared characteristics, enabling more efficient and effective healthcare delivery.

11.8.1.7 Global health transformation

Extending PM benefits worldwide will require coordinated international efforts to ensure equitable access to these innovations across different healthcare systems and economic contexts. Technology transfer initiatives will share innovations with developing countries, providing access to PM tools and expertise. Capacity-building programs will train healthcare professionals globally, developing local expertise in PM implementation and management.

Sustainable implementation approaches will develop cost-effective methods for delivering PM in resource-limited settings. Health equity initiatives will ensure equitable access to PM benefits, addressing disparities in healthcare access and outcomes.

The future of PM promises to transform healthcare through the integration of advanced technologies, evolving regulatory frameworks, and patient-centered care approaches. This transformation will require continued innovation in technology development, regulatory adaptation, healthcare system integration, and global collaboration. As these elements converge, PM will evolve from a specialized approach used in select clinical situations to a fundamental component of healthcare delivery that improves outcomes for patients worldwide. The success of this transformation will depend on our ability to address current challenges while preparing for future opportunities, ensuring that the benefits of PM are accessible to all patients regardless of their geographic location, economic status, or cultural background.

The rapid advancements in our understanding of cancer development and evolution have led to the emergence of PM as a key approach in targeting specific disease characteristics. PM has revolutionized oncology by tailoring treatments to individual patients based on genetic, molecular, and environmental factors. However, despite these breakthroughs, many patients still lack access to precision therapies. The following review highlights the current technological trends and multidisciplinary efforts shaping the field. High cancer mortality rates necessitate innovative, safer therapeutic agents. Patient-derived organoids (PDOs) are promising preclinical models, with potential for translational research. When combined with CRISPR, PDOs can identify cancer driver genes and novel therapeutic targets. This review explores CRISPR-mediated functional screens and their potential in cancer immunotherapy (Zhu et al., 2025).

The success of next-generation precision oncology and its applications in other medical fields relies on multiple factors. These include discovering novel disease biomarkers, accurately diagnosing complex phenotypes, developing innovative clinical trial designs taking into account sex differences, and ensuring worldwide accessibility to targeted therapies. Addressing these challenges is crucial for expanding the benefits of precision medicine beyond select populations and making it a global standard in healthcare.

11.8.1.8 Emerging technologies in precision medicine

Cutting-edge technologies continue to drive the evolution of PM, enabling more effective and personalized treatments. Three of the most promising advancements include:

CRISPR and AlphaFold: Gene-editing tools like CRISPR (Das et al., 2022; Davies et al., 2024; Frangoul et al., 2021; McManus et al., 2024; Severi & Akbari, 2024) have revolutionized genetic research, offering precise modifications to DNA that may correct mutations responsible for various diseases. Meanwhile, AlphaFold (Abramson et al., 2024; Jumper et al., 2021), an AI-driven protein structure prediction tool, has transformed drug discovery and protein engineering, facilitating the design of novel therapeutics.

Digital twins: Virtual patient simulations, also known as "digital twins," (Corral-Acero et al., 2020; Mosquera-Lopez & Jacobs, 2024; Thangaraj et al., 2024) are being explored for their potential to model individual responses to treatments. By replicating a patient's physiology in a digital environment, researchers and clinicians can test treatment strategies before applying them in real-world scenarios, reducing risks and improving efficacy. Digital twin technology is emerging as a powerful tool for PM in chronic disease management, particularly for diabetes. This article explores digital twin models, including mechanistic, data-driven, and hybrid approaches, and highlights case studies demonstrating their potential to improve glucose outcomes in T1D and T2D. While digital twins offer promising clinical applications, challenges remain in translating research into practice (Mosquera-Lopez & Jacobs, 2024).

Continued research and development in these areas will play a pivotal role in expanding the applications of PM beyond its current scope.

11.8.1.9 Expanding precision medicine to noncommunicable diseases and mental health

While PM has primarily been associated with oncology, its applications are expanding to address noncommunicable diseases such as diabetes, hypertension, and cardiovascular diseases. Personalized treatment strategies, driven by genetic and lifestyle data, offer promising approaches to managing these conditions more effectively.

Additionally, PM is beginning to influence mental health care, particularly in the treatment of depression and other psychiatric disorders. Advances in pharmacogenomics allow clinicians to tailor antidepressant prescriptions based on a patient's genetic makeup, potentially reducing adverse effects and improving treatment outcomes. Further research is needed to establish standardized personalized approaches in these domains.

11.8.1.10 Global collaboration to improve accessibility

Despite technological advancements, access to PM remains a major challenge, particularly in low- and middle-income countries. Collaborative initiatives offer a pathway toward greater accessibility. Several organizations have demonstrated the power of global partnerships in ensuring equitable vaccine distribution. Similar frameworks could be adapted for PM, facilitating access to genetic testing, targeted therapies, and emerging biotechnologies in underserved regions.

Expanding international collaborations, strengthening healthcare infrastructure, and reducing the costs of precision treatments are essential steps toward making PM universally accessible.

Future policies should aim to bridge the gap between innovation and implementation, ensuring that all patients—regardless of geographic or economic status—can benefit from personalized healthcare solutions.

11.9 Conclusion

While PM holds immense promise for improving patient outcomes, its widespread adoption faces several critical challenges that span economic, ethical, and regulatory domains. These challenges impact accessibility, data security, and clinical implementation, requiring comprehensive solutions to ensure that PM becomes an equitable and effective healthcare solution.

One of the most significant barriers to PM is its high cost, with expenses associated with genomic sequencing, biomarker identification, and targeted therapies often placing these advancements out of reach for many patients, particularly those in low- and middle-income countries. The financial burden extends to healthcare systems as well, as precision treatments often require specialized diagnostic tools, trained personnel, and long-term patient monitoring. Potential solutions to improve accessibility include subsidized programs, public-private partnerships, and government-led initiatives aimed at reducing the cost of genomic testing and precision treatments. Global health organizations, such as the World Health Organization, have emphasized the importance of equity in healthcare access, with the WHO health equity reports highlighting strategies for integrating PM into national healthcare systems while ensuring affordability for all populations. Collaborative efforts between governments, pharmaceutical companies, and nonprofit organizations can help bridge the affordability gap and expand access to life-saving treatments.

The rise of PM has brought ethical dilemmas, particularly in the areas of genetic testing and data privacy. As genomic data becomes a crucial component of personalized treatments, concerns about how this sensitive information is collected, stored, and shared have intensified. Patients may be reluctant to undergo genetic testing due to fears of discrimination by insurers or employers, as well as potential misuse of their data. To address these concerns, regulatory frameworks such as the GDPR in Europe have established strict guidelines on genetic data protection, emphasizing informed consent, data anonymization, and security protocols. GDPR compliance reports highlight the importance of transparency in data handling and reinforce the need for patient-centric policies. Additionally, initiatives promoting secure data-sharing frameworks, such as blockchain-based health records, are being explored to enhance trust and security in PM.

The regulatory landscape for PM presents another significant challenge, with approval pathways for targeted therapies and companion diagnostics varying across regions, leading to inconsistencies in implementation. For example, the FDA and the EMA have different evaluation criteria and approval timelines for precision-based treatments. This divergence can delay the global availability of novel therapies and create barriers for pharmaceutical companies seeking international approval. Standardizing regulatory policies and establishing harmonized guidelines for clinical validation are essential for accelerating the adoption of precision medicine. FDA guidance documents outline the agency's approach to evaluating genomic-based therapies, including companion diagnostics and real-world evidence integration. Expanding such frameworks to align with international regulatory bodies would streamline approvals and enhance global access to precision treatments.

While PM has the potential to revolutionize healthcare, its implementation is filled with challenges related to cost, ethical considerations, and regulatory barriers. Overcoming these obstacles requires a multifaceted approach, including financial assistance programs, robust data protection policies, and streamlined regulatory frameworks like the European AI Act. By fostering global collaboration and adopting inclusive healthcare strategies, PM can transition from being an exclusive innovation to a widely accessible and transformative medical practice.

Despite the challenges, PM represents a fundamental shift toward more personalized, effective, and efficient healthcare. While significant challenges remain, the rapid pace of technological advancement and growing clinical evidence suggest that PM will become increasingly integrated into routine healthcare delivery.

Success in PM implementation will require:

1. **Continued technological innovation**: Advancing omics technologies, AI algorithms, and clinical tools
2. **Regulatory evolution**: Developing flexible frameworks that ensure safety while enabling innovation
3. **Healthcare system transformation**: Integrating PM into clinical workflows and decision-making
4. **Provider education**: Training healthcare professionals in genomic medicine and data interpretation
5. **Patient engagement**: Empowering patients to participate actively in their care
6. **Ethical frameworks**: Addressing privacy, equity, and discrimination concerns
7. **Economic sustainability**: Demonstrating cost-effectiveness and value
8. **Global collaboration**: Sharing knowledge and resources across countries and cultures

The future of PM holds tremendous promise for improving human health and reducing healthcare costs. By addressing current challenges and continuing to innovate, we can realize the full potential of personalized healthcare for all patients.

Precision medicine has the transformative potential to revolutionize healthcare by offering tailored treatments that enhance patient outcomes, improve disease management, and reduce adverse reactions. By leveraging genetic insights and advanced technologies, personalized and sex specific treatments can lead to more effective and targeted interventions across various medical fields.

To fully realize the promise of PM, strategic efforts must focus on expanding research, fostering global collaborations, and addressing cost barriers that limit accessibility. Increased investment in cutting-edge innovations, such as genomics and AI-driven diagnostics, will accelerate breakthroughs. Moreover, strengthening international partnerships and implementing equitable healthcare policies can ensure that PM benefits all patients, regardless of geographic or economic disparities. By prioritizing these pathways, the healthcare industry can transition from a one-size-fits-all approach to a future where treatments are tailored to individual needs, ultimately improving global health outcomes.

Editor's note

This chapter offers a comprehensive and authoritative examination of precision medicine as a defining paradigm in contemporary healthcare. By integrating advances in genomics, multiomics, artificial intelligence, and digital health technologies, the authors successfully demonstrate how precision approaches are reshaping prevention, diagnosis, and treatment across a wide range of medical specialties.

A particular strength of the chapter lies in its balanced treatment of scientific innovation and real-world complexity. Beyond showcasing technological breakthroughs—such as CRISPR-based therapies, AlphaFold-enabled drug discovery, and AI-driven decision support—the chapter critically addresses challenges related to data integration, regulatory heterogeneity, ethical governance, cost, and equity. This positioning is essential: precision medicine is not merely a technological shift, but a systemic transformation that requires alignment across clinical workflows, regulatory frameworks, health economics, and patient engagement.

The chapter is especially timely in its emphasis on global health implications. By highlighting issues of genomic diversity, access in low- and middle-income countries, and the need for international collaboration, it reinforces the importance of inclusive and responsible innovation. Readers are encouraged to interpret precision medicine not as an elite or niche intervention, but as a long-term strategy for building adaptive, learning health systems capable of delivering personalized care at scale.

Key takeaways

Precision medicine represents a systemic shift, moving healthcare from population averages to individualized prevention, diagnosis, and treatment based on genetic, molecular, environmental, and lifestyle data.

Multiomics integration is foundational, enabling a holistic understanding of disease mechanisms, treatment response, and patient heterogeneity across oncology, cardiology, endocrinology, RDs, and neurodegenerative conditions.

Artificial intelligence acts as a critical enabler, supporting data integration, predictive modeling, clinical decision support, and accelerated drug discovery—yet requires rigorous validation, transparency, and governance.

Clinical success depends on implementation readiness, including interoperable data infrastructures, trained healthcare professionals, ethical frameworks, and regulatory alignment.

Equity remains a central challenge, as underrepresentation in genomic datasets, high costs, and infrastructure gaps risk widening global health disparities.

The future of precision medicine extends beyond treatment, toward precision prevention, learning health systems, and global collaboration to ensure scalable, sustainable, and inclusive impact.

Learning activities

Learning activity 1: mapping precision medicine readiness

Format: Individual or pair work. **Time:** 30–40 minutes

Objective: Evaluate health system readiness for implementing precision medicine across clinical, technological, and ethical dimensions.

Instructions: Select a healthcare setting (e.g., academic hospital, regional health authority, LMIC health system).

Assess readiness across five dimensions:
Data infrastructure
Clinical workforce capability
Regulatory and ethical governance
Economic and reimbursement models
Patient engagement and trust
For each dimension, identify:
One key strength
One major gap
One feasible improvement within 12 months

Deliverable: A one-page readiness matrix with a short prioritization summary (150–200 words).

Learning activity 2: designing a precision medicine use case

Format: Team-based (3–5 students). **Time:** 45–60 minutes

Objective: Design a realistic precision medicine intervention that integrates technology, clinical practice, and governance.

Instructions: Each team designs a use case targeting one condition (e.g., breast cancer, diabetes, cardiovascular disease, and rare genetic disorder). The proposal must include:
Target population and unmet clinical need
Precision tools used (e.g., genomics, AI, digital twins, wearables)
Data sources and integration strategy
Ethical and regulatory safeguards
Success metrics (clinical + equity indicators)

Deliverable: A one-page concept note outlining the intervention, risks, and expected impact.

Glossary-abbreviations

Allele: One of two or more alternative forms of a gene that arise by mutation and are found at the same place on a chromosome.

Artificial intelligence (AI): Computer systems that can perform tasks that typically require human intelligence, such as learning, reasoning, and problem-solving.

Biomarker: A biological molecule found in blood, other body fluids, or tissues that is a sign of a normal or abnormal process, condition, or disease.

Bioinformatics: The science of collecting and analyzing complex biological data, such as genetic codes, using computational methods.

Chimeric antigen receptor (CAR T)-cell therapies: A type of treatment in which a patient's T cells are changed in the laboratory so they will attack cancer cells.

Circulating tumor DNA (ctDNA): Small fragments of DNA that are released from cancer cells into the bloodstream and can be detected through blood tests.

Companion diagnostic: A medical device that provides information essential for the safe and effective use of a corresponding therapeutic product.

CRISPR-Cas9: A revolutionary gene-editing technology that allows scientists to make precise changes to DNA sequences in living cells.

Deep learning: A subset of ML that uses neural networks with multiple layers to analyze and interpret complex data patterns.

Epigenetics: The study of heritable changes in gene expression that do not involve changes to the underlying DNA sequence.

Exome: The part of the genome formed by exons, which are the protein-coding sequences of genes.

Genotype: The genetic makeup of an individual organism, referring to the specific alleles present at particular gene loci.

Genome-Wide Association Study (GWAS): A research approach that involves scanning the entire genome to find genetic variations associated with diseases.

Liquid biopsy: A noninvasive diagnostic test that analyzes circulating tumor cells, DNA, or other biomarkers in blood or other body fluids.

Machine learning (ML): A type of artificial intelligence that enables computers to learn and improve from experience without being explicitly programmed.

Metabolomics: The comprehensive study of small molecules (metabolites) within cells, tissues, or organisms.

Multiomics: The integration of data from multiple "omics" fields including genomics, transcriptomics, proteomics, and metabolomics.

Mutation: A change in the DNA sequence that can affect gene function and potentially lead to disease.

Next-generation sequencing (NGS): Advanced DNA sequencing technologies that can rapidly sequence entire genomes or specific regions of interest.

Pharmacogenomics: The study of how genetic variations affect individual responses to medications.

Phenotype: The observable characteristics of an organism resulting from the interaction between its genotype and environment.

Polygenic risk score (PRS): A numerical score that estimates an individual's genetic predisposition to a disease based on multiple genetic variants.

Precision medicine/personalized medicine (PM): An approach to medical treatment that takes into account individual variability in genes, environment, and lifestyle.

Proteomics: The large-scale study of proteins, their structures, functions, and interactions within an organism.

Single nucleotide polymorphism (SNP): A variation in a single nucleotide (DNA building block) that occurs at the same position in the genome across different individuals.

Targeted therapy: A type of treatment that uses drugs or other substances to identify and attack specific cancer cells or disease mechanisms.

Transcriptomics: The study of all RNA molecules produced by cells, providing insights into gene expression and cellular activity.

Variant of uncertain significance (VUS): A genetic variant for which there is insufficient evidence to determine whether it is disease-causing or benign.

Whole exome sequencing (WES): A technique that sequences all protein-coding regions of the genome.

Whole genome sequencing (WGS): A comprehensive method that determines the complete DNA sequence of an organism's genome.

References

Abramson, J., Adler, J., Dunger, J., Evans, R., Green, T., Pritzel, A., Ronneberger, O., Willmore, L., Ballard, A. J., Bambrick, J., Bodenstein, S. W., Evans, D. A., Hung, C. C., O'Neill, M., Reiman, D., Tunyasuvunakool, K., Wu, Z., Žemgulytė, A., Arvaniti, E., ... Jumper, J. M. (2024). Accurate structure prediction of biomolecular interactions with AlphaFold 3. *Nature, 630*(8016), 493–500. https://doi.org/10.1038/s41586-024-07487-w, https://www.nature.com/nature/.

Abul-Husn, N. S., & Kenny, E. E. (2019). Personalized medicine and the power of electronic health records. *Cell, 177*(1), 58–69. https://doi.org/10.1016/j.cell.2019.02.039, https://www.sciencedirect.com/journal/cell.

Ada. (2025). https://ada.com/

Adashi, E. Y., & Stratakis, C. A. (2024). End of an era: The passing of pioneers of cloning. *Hormones (Athens, Greece), 23*(3), 361–362. https://doi.org/10.1007/s42000-024-00581-8.

Adler, R. A., Feingold, K. R., Anawalt, B., Blackman, M. R., Boyce, A., Chrousos, G., Corpas, E., De Herder, W. W., Dhatariya, K., Dungan, K., Hofland, J., Kalra, S., Kaltsas, G., Kapoor, N., & Koch, C. (2000). *Osteoporosis in Men*. Endotext. MDText.com, Inc.

Ahmed, Z. (2020). Practicing precision medicine with intelligently integrative clinical and multi-omics data analysis. *Human Genomics, 14*(1). https://doi.org/10.1186/s40246-020-00287-z.

Ahmed, Z. (2022). Precision medicine with multi-omics strategies, deep phenotyping, and predictive analysis. *Progress in Molecular Biology and Translational Science, 190*, 101–125. https://doi.org/10.1016/bs.pmbts.2022.02.002, http://www.elsevier.com/books/book-series/progress-in-molecular-biology-and-translational-science#.

AI ACT. (2025). https://eur-lex.europa.eu/legal-content/EN/TXT/?uri=CELEX%3A32024R1689

Akhoon, N. (2021). Precision medicine: A new paradigm in therapeutics. *International Journal of Preventive Medicine, 12*(1), 12. https://doi.org/10.4103/ijpvm.ijpvm_375_19.

Alfonso-Cristancho, R., Andia, T., Barbosa, T., & Watanabe, J. H. (2015). Definition and classification of generic drugs across the world. *Applied Health Economics and Health Policy, 13*, 5–11. https://doi.org/10.1007/s40258-014-0146-1, http://rd.springer.com/journal/40258.

Almotiri, A., Abogosh, A., Abdelfattah, A., Alowaisy, D., & Rodrigues, N. P. (2025). Treating genetic blood disorders in the era of CRISPR-mediated genome editing. *Molecular Therapy, 33*(6), 2645–2662. https://doi.org/10.1016/j.ymthe.2025.01.031, https://www.sciencedirect.com/science/journal/15250016.

AmeliMojarad, M. (2024). The neuroinflammatory role of microglia in Alzheimer's disease and their associated therapeutic targets. *CNS Neuroscience & Therapeutics, 30*(7). https://doi.org/10.1111/cns.14856.

Ananya, Panchariya, D. C., Karthic, A., Singh, S. P., Mani, A., Chawade, A., & Kushwaha, S. (2024). Vaccine design and development: Exploring the interface with computational biology and AI. *International Reviews of Immunology, 43*(6), 361–380. https://doi.org/10.1080/08830185.2024.2374546, http://www.tandfonline.com/loi/iiri20.

Andrews, Fullarton, & Holtzman, N. A. (1994). *Assessing Genetic Risks: Implications for Health and Social Policy*. National Academies Press.

Antonopoulos, A. S., Xintarakou, A., Protonotarios, A., Lazaros, G., Miliou, A., Tsioufis, K., & Vlachopoulos, C. (2024). Imagenetics for precision medicine in dilated cardiomyopathy. *Circulation: Genomic and Precision Medicine, 17*(2), E004301. https://doi.org/10.1161/CIRCGEN.123.004301, https://www.ahajournals.org/journal/circgen.

Aplakidou, E., Vergoulidis, N., Chasapi, M., Venetsianou, N. K., Kokoli, M., Panagiotopoulou, E., Iliopoulos, I., Karatzas, E., Pafilis, E., Georgakopoulos-Soares, I., Kyrpides, N. C., Pavlopoulos, G. A., & Baltoumas, F. A. (2024). Visualizing metagenomic and metatranscriptomic data: A comprehensive review. *Computational and Structural Biotechnology Journal, 23*, 2011–2033. https://doi.org/10.1016/j.csbj.2024.04.060, https://www.sciencedirect.com/science/journal/20010370.

Arga, K. Y., Attia, H., & Aziz, R. K. (2024). Pharmacomicrobiomics-guided precision oncology: A new frontier of P4 (predictive, personalized, preventive, and participatory) medicine and microbiome-based therapeutics. *OMICS A Journal of Integrative Biology, 28*(1), 5–7. https://doi.org/10.1089/omi.2023.0254, www.liebertonline.com/omi.

Aronson, S. J., & Rehm, H. L. (2015). Building the foundation for genomics in precision medicine. *Nature, 526*(7573), 336–342. https://doi.org/10.1038/nature15816, http://www.nature.com/nature/index.html.

Asgharzade, S., Sheikhshabani, S. H., Ghasempour, E., Heidari, R., Rahmati, S., Mohammadi, M., Jazaeri, A., & Amini-Farsani, Z. (2020). The effect of oleuropein on apoptotic pathway regulators in breast cancer cells. *European Journal of Pharmacology, 886*. https://doi.org/10.1016/j.ejphar.2020.173509, www.elsevier.com/locate/ejphar.

Baltagiannis, E. G., Kyrochristos, I. D., Ziogas, D. E., Goussia, A., Mitsis, M., & Roukos, D. H. (2020). From personalized to precision cancer medicine. *Personalized Medicine, 17*(4), 245–250. https://doi.org/10.2217/pme-2020-0056, http://www.futuremedicine.com/loi/pme;jsessionid=iDlhLxr7W4pgLWINGK.

Bando, H. (2021). Type 2 Diabetes mellitus (T2DM) may have four subtypes beneficial for adequate treatment. *Asploro Journal of Biomedical and Clinical Case Reports, 4*(1), 38–41.

Bargar, C., Wang, W., Gunzler, S. A., LeFevre, A., Wang, Z., Lerner, A. J., Singh, N., Tatsuoka, C., Appleby, B., Zhu, X., Xu, R., Haroutunian, V., Zou, W. Q., Ma, J., & Chen, S. G. (2021). Streamlined alpha-synuclein RT-QuIC assay for various biospecimens in Parkinson's disease and dementia with Lewy bodies. *Acta Neuropathologica Communications, 9*(1). https://doi.org/10.1186/s40478-021-01175-w, https://actaneurocomms.biomedcentral.com/.

Barrangou, R. (2020). Nobel dreams come true for doudna and charpentier. *The CRISPR Journal, 3*(5), 317–318. https://doi.org/10.1089/crispr.2020.29109.rba.

Bartha, Á., & Győrffy, B. (2019). Comprehensive outline of whole exome sequencing data analysis tools available in clinical oncology. *Cancers, 11*(11). https://doi.org/10.3390/cancers11111725.

Bastepe, M., Gensure, R. C., Blackman, M. R., Boyce, A., Chrousos, G., Corpas, E., De Herder, W. W., Dhatariya, K., Dungan, K., Hofland, J., Kalra, S., Kaltsas, G., Kapoor, N., & Koch, C. (2000). *Hypoparathyroidism and Pseudohypoparathyroidism*. Endotext. MDText.com, Inc.

Baynam, G., Bowman, F., Lister, K., Walker, C. E., Pachter, N., Goldblatt, J., Boycott, K. M., Gahl, W. A., Kosaki, K., Adachi, T., Ishii, K., Mahede, T., McKenzie, F., Townshend, S., Slee, J., Kiraly-Borri, C., Vasudevan, A., Hawkins, A., Broley, S., ... Dawkins, H. J. S. (2017). Improved diagnosis and care for rare diseases through implementation of precision public health framework. *Advances in Experimental Medicine and Biology, 1031*, 55–94. https://doi.org/10.1007/978-3-319–67144-4_4, http://www.springer.com/series/5584.

Behl, T., Kaur, I., Sehgal, A., Singh, S., Albarrati, A., Albratty, M., Najmi, A., Meraya, A. M., & Bungau, S. (2022). The road to precision medicine: Eliminating the "One Size Fits All" approach in Alzheimer's disease. *Biomedicine & Pharmacotherapy, 153*, 113337. https://doi.org/10.1016/j.biopha.2022.113337.

Benrubi, L., Sato, T., Westgard, L. K., Zollo-Venecek, K., Socrates, B., Sweigart, B., Ridgway, J. P., Suzuki, J., Morales, Y., Goodman-Meza, D., & Wurcel, A. G. (2025). Sensitivity and specificity of natural language processing systems for identification of hospitalized people who use drugs. *Open Forum Infectious Diseases*, 2328–8957. https://doi.org/10.1093/ofid/ofaf370.

Bera, K., Schalper, K. A., Rimm, D. L., Velcheti, V., & Madabhushi, A. (2019). Artificial intelligence in digital pathology — New tools for diagnosis and precision oncology. *Nature Reviews Clinical Oncology, 16*(11), 703–715. https://doi.org/10.1038/s41571-019-0252-y, http://www.nature.com/nrclinonc/archive/index.html.

Berry, D., Loy, A., Coburn, B., Guttman, D. S., Luca, F., Kupfer, S. S., Knights, D., Khoruts, A., Blekhman, R., Matsen, F. A., McBain, A. J., O'Neill, C. A., Amezquita, A., Price, L. J., Faust, K., Tett, A., Segata, N., Swann, J. R., Smith, A. M., & Kiers, E. T. (2018). Organ-on-a-chip in vitro models of the brain and the blood-brain barrier and their value to study the microbiota-gut-brain axis in neurodegeneration. *Current Opinion in Biotechnology, 13*(5).

betterhelp. (2025). https://www.betterhelp.com/

Bhinder, B., Gilvary, C., Madhukar, N. S., & Elemento, O. (2021). Artificial intelligence in cancer research and precision medicine. *Cancer Discovery, 11*(4), 900–915. https://doi.org/10.1158/2159–8290.CD-21–0090, https://cancerdiscovery.aacrjournals.org/content/11/4/900.full.pdf.

Big Health. (2025). https://www.bighealth.com/sleepio

Bonkhoff, A. K., & Grefkes, C. (2022). Precision medicine in stroke: Towards personalized outcome predictions using artificial intelligence. *Brain, 145*(2), 457–475. https://doi.org/10.1093/brain/awab439, http://brain.oxfordjournals.org/.

Bouris, V., & Avgerinos, E. (2024). AI applications in cardiovascular disease diagnosis and management. *IGI Global,* 169–184. https://doi.org/10.4018/979-8-3693–4422-4.ch009.

Boycott, K. M., Hartley, T., Biesecker, L. G., Gibbs, R. A., Innes, A. M., Riess, O., Belmont, J., Dunwoodie, S. L., Jojic, N., Lassmann, T., Mackay, D., Temple, I. K., Visel, A., & Baynam, G. (2019). A diagnosis for all rare genetic diseases: The horizon and the next frontiers. *Cell, 177*(1), 32–37. https://doi.org/10.1016/j.cell.2019.02.040, https://www.sciencedirect.com/journal/cell.

Brlek, P., Bulić, L., Bračić, M., Projić, P., Škaro, V., Shah, N., Shah, P., & Primorac, D. (2024). Implementing whole genome sequencing (WGS) in clinical practice: Advantages, challenges, and future perspectives. *Cells, 13*(6). https://doi.org/10.3390/cells13060504.

Brundin, P., Nath, A., & Beckham, J. D. (2020). Is COVID-19 a perfect storm for Parkinson's disease? *Trends in Neurosciences, 43*(12), 931–933. https://doi.org/10.1016/j.tins.2020.10.009, www.elsevier.com/locate/tins.

Bugiardini, R., Yoon, J., Mendieta, G., Kedev, S., Zdravkovic, M., Vasiljevic, Z., Miličić, D., Manfrini, O., van der Schaar, M., Gale, C. P., Bergami, M., Badimon, L., & Cenko, E. (2022). Reduced heart failure and mortality in patients receiving statin therapy before initial acute coronary syndrome. *Journal of the American College of Cardiology, 79*(20), 2021–2033. https://doi.org/10.1016/j.jacc.2022.03.354, www.elsevier.com/locate/jacc.

Bulotta, S., Corradino, R., Celano, M., D'Agostino, M., Maiuolo, J., Oliverio, M., Procopio, A., Iannone, M., Rotiroti, D., & Russo, D. (2011). Antiproliferative and antioxidant effects on breast cancer cells of oleuropein and its semisynthetic peracetylated derivatives. *Food Chemistry, 127*(4), 1609–1614. https://doi.org/10.1016/j.foodchem.2011.02.025.

Calabretta, M. M., Zangheri, M., Lopreside, A., Marchegiani, E., Montali, L., Simoni, P., & Roda, A. (2020). Precision medicine, bioanalytics and nanomaterials: Toward a new generation of personalized portable diagnostics. *Analyst, 145*(8), 2841–2853. https://doi.org/10.1039/c9an02041a, http://pubs.rsc.org/en/journals/journal/an.

Calinski, D. M., Hoefer, C., & Kisor, D. (2021). An interprofessional education experience to promote the role of the pharmacist in precision medicine. *Currents in Pharmacy Teaching and Learning, 13*(10), 1370–1375. https://doi.org/10.1016/j.cptl.2021.07.017, http://www.elsevier.com/wps/find/journaldescription.cws_home/718643/description#description.

Cappon, G., Vettoretti, M., Sparacino, G., & Facchinetti, A. (2019). Continuous glucose monitoring sensors for diabetes management: A review of technologies and applications. *Diabetes & Metabolism Journal, 43*(4), 383. https://doi.org/10.4093/dmj.2019.0121.

CardMedic. (2025). https://www.cardmedic.com/

Carreira, A. L., Korbonits, M., Blackman, M. R., Boyce, A., Chrousos, G., Corpas, E., De Herder, W. W., Dhatariya, K., Dungan, K., Hofland, J., Kalra, S., Kaltsas, G., Kapoor, N., Koch, C., Kopp, P., Korbonits, M., & Kovacs, C. S. (2000). ,. In *Familial Isolated Pituitary Adenoma*. Endotext. MDText.com, Inc.

Cecchin, E., & Stocco, G. (2020). Pharmacogenomics and personalized medicine. *Genes, 11*(6), 679. https://doi.org/10.3390/genes11060679.

Çelik, A., Öztürk, G. Z., Çavuşoğlu, Y., Ardıç, C., Nalbantgil, S., Arıca, S., Temizhan, A., Altay, H., Yılmaz, M. B., Özsarı, H., & Ural, D. (2025). Guideline for the use of natriuretic peptides in the early diagnosis and management of heart failure in primary care (Joint Consensus Report by the Eurasian Society of Heart Failure and the Turkish Association of Family Medicine). *Balkan Medical Journal, 42*(2), 94–107. https://doi.org/10.4274/balkanmedj.galenos.2025.2024-12-110, https://balkanmedicaljournal.org/pdf.php?&id=2692.

Chan, J. C. N., & Chan, A. T. C. (2017). Biologics and biosimilars: What, why and how? *ESMO Open, 2*(1). https://doi.org/10.1136/esmoopen-2017-000180, esmoopen.bmj.com/.

Chapleau, M., Iaccarino, L., Soleimani-Meigooni, D., & Rabinovici, G. D. (2022). The role of amyloid PET in imaging neurodegenerative disorders: A review. *Journal of Nuclear Medicine, 63*. https://doi.org/10.2967/jnumed.121.263195.

Chatterjee, M., Özdemir, S., Fritz, C., Möbius, W., Kleineidam, L., Mandelkow, E., Biernat, J., Doğdu, C., Peters, O., Cosma, N. C., Wang, X., Schneider, L. S., Priller, J., Spruth, E., Kühn, A. A., Krause, P., Klockgether, T., Vogt, I. R., Kimmich, O., ... Schneider, A. (2024). Plasma extracellular vesicle tau and TDP-43 as diagnostic biomarkers in FTD and ALS. *Nature Medicine, 30*(6), 1771–1783. https://doi.org/10.1038/s41591-024-02937-4, https://www.nature.com/nm/.

Chavanne, A., & Jacobi, D. (2024). Precision medicine in endocrinology: Unraveling metabolic health through time-restricted eating. *Annales d'Endocrinologie, 85*(1), 63–69. https://doi.org/10.1016/j.ando.2023.12.001.

Chen, Z.-H., Lin, L., Wu, C.-F., Li, C.-F., Xu, R.-H., & Sun, Y. (2021). Artificial intelligence for assisting cancer diagnosis and treatment in the era of precision medicine. *Cancer Communications, 41*(11), 1100–1115. https://doi.org/10.1002/cac2.12215.

Chen, X., Mangala, L. S., Rodriguez-Aguayo, C., Kong, X., Lopez-Berestein, G., & Sood, A. K. (2018). RNA interference-based therapy and its delivery systems. *Cancer and Metastasis Reviews, 37*(1), 107–124. https://doi.org/10.1007/s10555-017-9717-6.

Chiu, W., Lin, T. Y., Chang, Y. C., Lai, H. I. A. M., Lin, S. C., Ma, C., Yarmishyn, A. A., Lin, S. C., Chang, K. J., Chou, Y. B., Hsu, C. C., Lin, T. C., Chen, S. J., Chien, Y., Yang, Y. P., & Hwang, D. K. (2021). An update on gene therapy for inherited retinal dystrophy: Experience in leber congenital amaurosis clinical trials. *International Journal of Molecular Sciences, 22*(9). https://doi.org/10.3390/ijms22094534, https://www.mdpi.com/1422-0067/22/9/4534/pdf.

Cho, W. C., Wong, C. F., Li, K. P., Fong, A. H., Fung, K. Y., & Au, J. S. (2023). miR-145 as a potential biomarker and therapeutic target in patients with non-small cell lung cancer. *International Journal of Molecular Sciences, 24*(12). https://doi.org/10.3390/ijms241210022, http://www.mdpi.com/journal/ijms.

Chua, I. S., Gaziel-Yablowitz, M., Korach, Z. T., Kehl, K. L., Levitan, N. A., Arriaga, Y. E., Jackson, G. P., Bates, D. W., & Hassett, M. (2021). Artificial intelligence in oncology: Path to implementation. *Cancer Medicine, 10*(12), 4138–4149. https://doi.org/10.1002/cam4.3935, http://onlinelibrary.wiley.com/journal/10.1002/(ISSN)2045-7634.

clicktherapeutics. (2025). https://www.clicktherapeutics.com/

Colclough, K., Ellard, S., Hattersley, A., & Patel, K. (2022). Syndromic monogenic diabetes genes should be tested in patients with a clinical suspicion of maturity-onset diabetes of the young. *Diabetes, 71*(3), 530–537. https://doi.org/10.2337/db21-0517.

Coler, E. A., Chen, W., Melnik, A. V., Morton, J. T., & Aksenov, A. A. (2024). Metabolomics in the era of artificial intelligence. *Microbiota and Host, 2*(1). https://doi.org/10.1530/mah-23-0017.

Collins, F. S., & Varmus, H. (2015). A new initiative on precision medicine. *New England Journal of Medicine, 372*(9), 793–795. https://doi.org/10.1056/NEJMp1500523, http://www.nejm.org/doi/pdf/10.1056/NEJMp1500523.

Colombatti, R., & Sainati, L. (2016). Management of children with sickle cell disease in Europe: Current situation and future perspectives. *EMJ Hematology,* 129–135. https://doi.org/10.33590/emjhematol/10310534.

Corral-Acero, J., Margara, F., Marciniak, M., Rodero, C., Loncaric, F., Feng, Y., Gilbert, A., Fernandes, J. F., Bukhari, H. A., Wajdan, A., Martinez, M. V., Santos, M. S., Shamohammdi, M., Luo, H., Westphal, P., Leeson, P., DiAchille, P., Gurev, V., Mayr, M., ... Lamata, P. (2020). The 'Digital Twin' to enable the vision of precision cardiology. *European Heart Journal, 41*(48), 4556–4564. https://doi.org/10.1093/eurheartj/ehaa159, http://eurheartj.oxfordjournals.org/.

Coskun, A., Ertaylan, G., Pusparum, M., Van Hoof, R., Kaya, Z. Z., Khosravi, A., & Zarrabi, A. (2024). Advancing personalized medicine: Integrating statistical algorithms with omics and nano-omics for enhanced diagnostic accuracy and treatment efficacy. *Biochimica et Biophysica Acta (BBA) - Molecular Basis of Disease, 1870*(7), 167339. https://doi.org/10.1016/j.bbadis.2024.167339.

Dahl, A., & Kumar, S. (2020). Recent advances in neonatal diabetes. *Diabetes, Metabolic Syndrome and Obesity, 13*, 355–364. https://doi.org/10.2147/DMSO.S198932.

Das, S., Bano, S., Kapse, P., & Kundu, G. C. (2022). CRISPR based therapeutics: A new paradigm in cancer precision medicine. *Molecular Cancer, 21*(1). https://doi.org/10.1186/s12943-022-01552-6, http://www.molecular-cancer.com/start.asp.

Davies, K., Philippidis, A., & Barrangou, R. (2024). Five years of progress in CRISPR clinical trials (2019–2024). *The CRISPR Journal, 7*(5), 227–230. https://doi.org/10.1089/crispr.2024.0081.

Davis, H. A., Spanakis, E. K., Cryer, P. E., Siamashvili, M., Davis, S. N., Feingold, K. R., Anawalt, B., Blackman, M. R., Boyce, A., Chrousos, G., Corpas, E., Herder, W. W. D., Dhatariya, K., Dungan, K., Hofland, J., Kalra, S., Kaltsas, G., Kapoor, N., Koch, C., ... Kovacs, C. S. (2000). *Hypoglycemia During Therapy of Diabetes*. Endotext. MDText.com, Inc.

Dean, K. (2012). Mar Medical Genetics Summaries National Center for Biotechnology Information Clopidogrel Therapy and CYP2C19 Genotype

Declerck, P., Danesi, R., Petersel, D., & Jacobs, I. (2017). The language of biosimilars: Clarification, definitions, and regulatory aspects. *Drugs, 77*(6), 671–677. https://doi.org/10.1007/s40265-017-0717-1.

Delgado, A., Cholevas, C., & Theoharides, T. C. (2021). Neuroinflammation in Alzheimer's disease and beneficial action of luteolin. *BioFactors, 47*(2), 207–217. https://doi.org/10.1002/biof.1714, http://iubmb.onlinelibrary.wiley.com/hub/journal/10.1002/(ISSN)1872-8081/.

de Margerie-Mellon, C., & Chassagnon, G. (2023). Artificial intelligence: A critical review of applications for lung nodule and lung cancer. *Diagnostic and Interventional Imaging, 104*(1), 11–17. https://doi.org/10.1016/j.diii.2022.11.007.

Derry, W. B. (2021). CRISPR: Development of a technology and its applications. *FEBS Journal, 288*(2), 358–359. https://doi.org/10.1111/febs.15621, http://onlinelibrary.wiley.com/journal/10.1111/(ISSN)1742-4658.

Dewidar, B., Kahl, S., Pafili, K., & Roden, M. (2020). Metabolic liver disease in diabetes – From mechanisms to clinical trials. *Metabolism: Clinical and Experimental, 111*. https://doi.org/10.1016/j.metabol.2020.154299.

Dhatariya, K., Umpierrez, G. E., Anawalt, B., Blackman, M. R., Boyce, A., Chrousos, G., Corpas, E., Herder, W. W. D., Dhatariya, K., Dungan, K., Hofland, J., Kalra, S., Kaltsas, G., Kapoor, N., Koch, C., Kopp, P., Korbonits, M., & Kovacs, C. S. (2000). *Management of Diabetes and Hyperglycemia in Hospitalized Patients*. Endotext. MDText.com.

Domingo, F. R., Waddell, L. A., Cheung, A. M., Cooper, C. L., Belcourt, V. J., Zuckermann, A. M. E., Corrin, T., Ahmad, R., Boland, L., Laprise, C., Idzerda, L., Khan, A., Morissette, K., & Garcia, A. J. (2021). *Prevalence of Long-term Effects in Individuals Diagnosed with COVID-19: An Updated Living Systematic Review*. Canada: medRxiv. https://www.medrxiv.org/.

Doudna, J. A., & Charpentier, E. (2014). The new frontier of genome engineering with CRISPR-Cas9. *Science, 346*(6213). https://doi.org/10.1126/science.1258096, http://www.sciencemag.org/content/346/6213/1258096.full.pdf.

Duan, D., Goemans, N., Takeda, S.'ichi, Mercuri, E., & Aartsma-Rus, A. (2021). Duchenne muscular dystrophy. *Nature Reviews Disease Primers, 7*(1). https://doi.org/10.1038/s41572-021-00248-3.

Elamin, M. H., Daghestani, M. H., Omer, S. A., Elobeid, M. A., Virk, P., Al-Olayan, E. M., Hassan, Z. K., Mohammed, O. B., & Aboussekhra, A. (2013). Olive oil oleuropein has anti-breast cancer properties with higher efficiency on ER-negative cells. *Food and Chemical Toxicology, 53*, 310–316. https://doi.org/10.1016/j.fct.2012.12.009.

El Cheikh, J., Hamed, F., Rifi, H., Dakroub, A. H., & Eid, A. H. (2025). Genetic polymorphisms influencing antihypertensive drug responses. *British Journal of Pharmacology, 182*(4), 929–950. https://doi.org/10.1111/bph.17414.

European Commission. (2025). Rare diseases.

Equils, O., Bakaj, A., Wilson-Mifsud, B., & Chatterjee, A. (2023). Restoring trust: The need for precision medicine in infectious diseases, public health and vaccines. *Human Vaccines & Immunotherapeutics, 19*(2). https://doi.org/10.1080/21645515.2023.2234787.

European Medicines Agency. (2025a). https://www.ema.europa.eu/en/news/new-gene-therapy-rare-inherited-disorder-causing-vision-loss-recommended-approval.

European Medicines Agency. (2025b). https://www.ema.europa.eu/en/medicines/human/EPAR/zolgensma

European Medicines Agency. (2025c). https://www.ema.europa.eu/en/news/new-gene-therapy-treat-rare-inherited-blood-condition

European Medicines Agency. (2025d). https://www.ema.europa.eu/en/homepage

Eurordis, EURORDIS. (2025).

Evidation. (2025). https://evidation.com/

Farooqi, I. S., Feingold, K. R., Anawalt, B., Blackman, M. R., Boyce, A., Chrousos, G., Corpas, E., De Herder, W. W., Dhatariya, K., Dungan, K., Hofland, J., Kalra, S., Kaltsas, G., Kapoor, N., & Koch, C. (2000). *Genetic Obesity Syndromes*. Endotext. MDText.com, Inc.

FDA. (2025). https://www.fda.gov/news-events/press-announcements/fda-approves-first-gene-therapies-treat-patients-sickle-cell-disease

Feingold, K. R., Anawalt, B., Blackman, M. R., Boyce, A., Chrousos, G., Corpas, E., De Herder, W. W., Dhatariya, K., Dungan, K., Hofland, J., Kalra, S., Kaltsas, G., Kapoor, N., Koch, C., Kopp, P., Korbonits, M., & Kovacs, C. S. (2000). *The Effect of Diet on Cardiovascular Disease and Lipid and Lipoprotein Levels*. Endotext. MDText.com, Inc.

Feingold, K. R., Feingold, K. R., Anawalt, B., Blackman, M. R., Boyce, A., Chrousos, G., Corpas, E., De Herder, W. W., Dhatariya, K., Dungan, K., Hofland, J., Kalra, S., Kaltsas, G., Kapoor, N., & Koch, C. (2000a). *Cholesterol Lowering Drugs*. Endotext. MDText.com, Inc.

Feingold, K. R., Feingold, K. R., Anawalt, B., Blackman, M. R., Boyce, A., Chrousos, G., Corpas, E., De Herder, W. W., Dhatariya, K., Dungan, K., Hofland, J., Kalra, S., Kaltsas, G., Kapoor, N., & Koch, C. (2000b). *Introduction to Lipids and Lipoproteins*. Endotext. MDText.com, Inc.

Feingold, K. R., Feingold, K. R., Anawalt, B., Blackman, M. R., Boyce, A., Chrousos, G., Corpas, E., De Herder, W. W., Dhatariya, K., Dungan, K., Hofland, J., Kalra, S., Kaltsas, G., Kapoor, N., Koch, C., Kopp, P., Korbonits, M., & Kovacs, C. S. (2000c). *Oral and Injectable (Non-Insulin) Pharmacological Agents for the Treatment of Type 2 Diabetes*. Endotext. MDText.com, Inc.

Frangoul, H., Altshuler, D., Cappellini, M. D., Chen, Y. S., Domm, J., Eustace, B. K., Foell, J., De La Fuente, J., Grupp, S., Handgretinger, R., Ho, T. W., Kattamis, A., Kernytsky, A., Lekstrom-Himes, J., Li, A. M., Locatelli, F., Mapara, M. Y., De Montalembert, M., Rondelli, D., ... Corbacioglu, S. (2021). CRISPR-Cas9 gene editing for sickle cell disease and β-thalassemia. *New England Journal of Medicine, 384*(3), 252–260. https://doi.org/10.1056/NEJMoa2031054, http://www.nejm.org/medical-index.

FreeStyle Libre. (2025). https://www.freestyle.abbott/us-en/products/freestyle-libre-3.html?srsltid=AfmBOooT5I576e_g9u_kPNLIoXPuOjDRjZbP9nQq-sahe3xCUutvh7nx

Gabay, M. (2019). The orphan drug act: An appropriate approval pathway for treatments of rare diseases? *Hospital Pharmacy, 54*(5), 283–284. https://doi.org/10.1177/0018578719867665.

Genomics England. (2011). The 100,000 Genomes Project.

Galli, M., Ortega-Paz, L., Franchi, F., Rollini, F., & Angiolillo, D. J. (2022). Precision medicine in interventional cardiology: Implications for antiplatelet therapy in patients undergoing percutaneous coronary intervention. *Pharmacogenomics, 23*(13), 723–737. https://doi.org/10.2217/pgs-2022-0057, http://www.futuremedicine.com/loi/pgs?cookieSet=1.

Gallo Marin, B., Aghagoli, G., Lavine, K., Yang, L., Siff, E. J., Chiang, S. S., Salazar-Mather, T. P., Dumenco, L., Savaria, M. C., Aung, S. N., Flanigan, T., & Michelow, I. C. (2021). Predictors of COVID-19 severity: A literature review. *Reviews in Medical Virology, 31*(1), 1–10. https://doi.org/10.1002/rmv.2146, http://onlinelibrary.wiley.com/journal/10.1002/(ISSN)1099-1654.

Gao, T., Yang, L., Zhang, Y., Bajinka, O., & Yuan, X. (2024). Cancer metabolic reprogramming and precision medicine-current perspective. *Frontiers in Pharmacology, 15*. https://doi.org/10.3389/fphar.2024.1450441.

GDPR. (2025). https://eur-lex.europa.eu/eli/reg/2016/679/oj/eng

Gibson, J., Dhungana, A., Pokhrel, M., Arthur, B., Suresh, P., Adebayo, O., & Cottle, R. N. (2025). Validation of clinical-grade electroporation systems for CRISPR-Cas9-mediated gene therapy in primary hepatocytes for the correction of inherited metabolic liver disease. *Cells, 14*(10), 711. https://doi.org/10.3390/cells14100711.

Global Thalassaemia Review. (2023).

Gonçalves, M., Costa, M., Paiva-Martins, F., & Silva, P. (2024). Olive oil industry by-products as a novel source of biophenols with a promising role in Alzheimer disease prevention. *Molecules, 29*(20), 4841. https://doi.org/10.3390/molecules29204841.

Goričar, K., Dolžan, V., & Lenassi, M. (2021). Extracellular vesicles: A novel tool facilitating personalized medicine and pharmacogenomics in oncology. *Frontiers in Pharmacology, 12*. https://doi.org/10.3389/fphar.2021.671298.

Grétarsdóttir, H. M., Widman, E., Johansson, A., & Nyholm, D. (2021). Personalized medicine approach in treating parkinson's disease, using oral administration of levodopa/carbidopa microtablets in clinical practice. *Journal of Personalized Medicine, 11*(8). https://doi.org/10.3390/jpm11080720, https://www.mdpi.com/2075-4426/11/8/720/pdf.

Guideline on similar biological medicinal products. European Medicines Agency, (2025).

Hajj-Boutros, G., Landry-Duval, M. A., Comtois, A. S., Gouspillou, G., & Karelis, A. D. (2023). Wrist-worn devices for the measurement of heart rate and energy expenditure: A validation study for the Apple Watch 6, Polar Vantage V and Fitbit Sense. *European Journal of Sport Science, 23*(2), 165–177. https://doi.org/10.1080/17461391.2021.2023656, http://www.tandf.co.uk/journals/journal.asp?issn=1746-1391&linktype=1.

Ham, H., Jing, H., Lamborn, I. T., Kober, M. M., Koval, A., Berchiche, Y. A., Anderson, D. E., Druey, K. M., Mandl, J. N., Isidor, B., Ferreira, C. R., Freeman, A. F., Ganesan, S., Karsak, M., Mustillo, P. J., Teo, J., Zolkipli-Cunningham, Z., Chatron, N., Lecoquierre, F., ... Su, H. C. (2024). Germline mutations in a G protein identify signaling cross-talk in T cells. *Science (New York, N.Y.), 385*(6715), eadd8947. https://doi.org/10.1126/science.add8947.

Hampel, H., Caraci, F., Cuello, A. C., Caruso, G., Nisticò, R., Corbo, M., Baldacci, F., Toschi, N., Garaci, F., Chiesa, P. A., Verdooner, S. R., Akman-Anderson, L., Hernández, F., Ávila, J., Emanuele, E., Valenzuela, P. L., Lucía, A., Watling, M., Imbimbo, B. P., ... Lista, S. (2020). A path toward precision medicine for neuroinflammatory mechanisms in Alzheimer's disease. *Frontiers in Immunology, 11*. https://doi.org/10.3389/fimmu.2020.00456, https://www.frontiersin.org/journals/immunology#.

Han, Y. (2024). *Biomarker Analysis in Drug Development*. Boosting Precision Medicine - Crown Bioscience.

Hasenfuß, G., Schuster, A., Bergau, L., & Toischer, K. (2024). Precision medicine enhances personalized medicine in cardiology. *Innere Medizin (Germany), 65*(3), 239–247. https://doi.org/10.1007/s00108-024-01663-w, https://www.springer.com/journal/108.

Hassan, M., Awan, F. M., Naz, A., Deandrés-Galiana, E. J., Alvarez, O., Cernea, A., Fernández-Brillet, L., Fernández-Martínez, J. L., & Kloczkowski, A. (2022). Innovations in genomics and big data analytics for personalized medicine and health care: A review. *International Journal of Molecular Sciences, 23*(9). https://doi.org/10.3390/ijms23094645, https://www.mdpi.com/1422-0067/23/9/4645/pdf.

He, X., Liu, X., Zuo, F., Shi, H., & Jing, J. (2023). Artificial intelligence-based multi-omics analysis fuels cancer precision medicine. *Seminars in Cancer Biology, 88*, 187–200. https://doi.org/10.1016/j.semcancer.2022.12.009, http://www.elsevier.com/inca/publications/store/6/2/2/9/4/3/index.htt.

Heath, E., Dyson, G., Ribeiro, J. R., Xiu, J., Poorman, K., Mamdani, H., Al-Hallak, M. N., Shields, A. F., Elayoubi, J. A., Winer, I. S., Cackowski, F. C., Puckrein, G. A., Lopes, G.de L., Jones, N., Hauke, R. J., Kareff, S. A., Radovich, M., Sledge, G. W., Spetzler, D. B., ... Marshall, J. L. (2024). Health disparities among patients with cancer who received molecular testing for biomarker-directed therapy. *Cancer Research Communications, 4*(10), 2598–2609. https://doi.org/10.1158/2767-9764.CRC-24-0321, https://aacrjournals.org/cancerrescommun/issue/4/10.

Herder, C., & Roden, M. (2022). A novel diabetes typology: Towards precision diabetology from pathogenesis to treatment. *Diabetologia, 65*(11), 1770–1781. https://doi.org/10.1007/s00125-021-05625-x.

Hernández-García, S., García-Cano, B., Martínez-Rodríguez, P., Henarejos-Escudero, P., & Gandía-Herrero, F. (2024). Olive oil tyrosols reduce α-synuclein aggregation in vitro and in vivo after ingestion in a Caenorhabditis elegans Parkinson's model. *Food & Function, 15*(13), 7214–7223. https://doi.org/10.1039/d4fo01663g.

Hoffman, Fox, T. A., & Anastasopoulou (2023). *Maturity Onset Diabetes in the Young*. Treasure Island (FL): StatPearls Publishing.

Hollenbeck, D., Williams, C. L., Drazba, K., Descartes, M., Korf, B. R., Rutledge, S. L., Lose, E. J., Robin, N. H., Carroll, A. J., & Mikhail, F. M. (2017). Clinical relevance of small copy-number variants in chromosomal microarray clinical testing. *Genetics in Medicine. 19*(4), 377–385. https://doi.org/10.1038/gim.2016.132.

Hollunder, B., Rajamani, N., Siddiqi, S. H., Finke, C., Kühn, A. A., Mayberg, H. S., Fox, M. D., Neudorfer, C., & Horn, A. (2022). Toward personalized medicine in connectomic deep brain stimulation. *Progress in Neurobiology, 210*. https://doi.org/10.1016/j.pneurobio.2021.102211, www.elsevier.com/locate/pneurobio.

Hossain, F., Majumder, S., David, J., & Miele, L. (2021). Precision medicine and triple-negative breast cancer: Current landscape and future directions. *Cancers, 13*(15), 3739. https://doi.org/10.3390/cancers13153739.

Huang, H. H., Li, J., & Cho, W. C. (2023). Editorial: Integrative analysis for complex disease biomarker discovery. *Frontiers in Bioengineering and Biotechnology, 11*. https://doi.org/10.3389/fbioe.2023.1273084, http://journal.frontiersin.org/journal/bioengineering-and-biotechnology#archive.

Hutt, A. J. (2002). The development of single-isomer molecules: Why and how. *CNS Spectrums, 7*(4), 14–22. https://doi.org/10.1017/s1092852900028558, http://journals.cambridge.org/action/displayJournal?jid=CNS.

Hutt, A. J., & Tan, S. C. (1996). Drug chirality and its clinical significance. *Drugs, 52*(Supplement 5), 1–12. https://doi.org/10.2165/00003495-199600525-00003.

Imani, S., Roozitalab, G., Emadi, M., Moradi, A., Behzadi, P., & Jabbarzadeh Kaboli, P. (2024). The evolution of BRAF-targeted therapies in melanoma: overcoming hurdles and unleashing novel strategies. *Frontiers in Oncology, 14*. https://doi.org/10.3389/fonc.2024.1504142.

Ingle, R. G., M. Elossaily, G., Ansari, M. N., & Makhijani, S. (2025). Unlocking the potential: Advancements and applications of gene therapy in severe disorders. *Annals of Medicine, 57*(1). https://doi.org/10.1080/07853890.2025.2516697, http://www.tandfonline.com/loi/iann20.

Jack, C. R., Knopman, D. S., Jagust, W. J., Petersen, R. C., Weiner, M. W., Aisen, P. S., Shaw, L. M., Vemuri, P., Wiste, H. J., Weigand, S. D., Lesnick, T. G., Pankratz, V. S., Donohue, M. C., & Trojanowski, J. Q. (2013). Tracking pathophysiological processes in Alzheimer's disease: An updated hypothetical model of dynamic biomarkers. *The Lancet Neurology, 12*(2), 207–216. https://doi.org/10.1016/S1474-4422(12)70291-0.

Jia, F., Fellner, A., & Kumar, K. R. (2022). Monogenic Parkinson's disease: Genotype, phenotype, pathophysiology, and genetic testing. *Genes, 13*(3). https://doi.org/10.3390/genes13030471.

Jinek, M., Chylinski, K., Fonfara, I., Hauer, M., Doudna, J. A., & Charpentier, E. (2012). A programmable dual-RNA-guided DNA endonuclease in adaptive bacterial immunity. *Science, 337*(6096), 816–821. https://doi.org/10.1126/science.1225829, http://www.sciencemag.org/content/337/6096/816.full.pdf.

John, A., Qin, B., Kalari, K. R., Wang, L., & Yu, J. (2020). Patient-specific multi-omics models and the application in personalized combination therapy. *Future Oncology, 16*(23), 1737–1750. https://doi.org/10.2217/fon-2020-0119, http://www.futuremedicine.com/loi/fon.

Joshi, K., Taliou, A., & Stratakis, C. A. (2024). Diagnostic and management challenges in paediatric Cushing's syndrome. *Clinical Endocrinology, 101*(6), 631–639. https://doi.org/10.1111/cen.15096, http://onlinelibrary.wiley.com/journal/10.1111/(ISSN)1365-2265.

Jumper, J., Evans, R., Pritzel, A., Green, T., Figurnov, M., Ronneberger, O., Tunyasuvunakool, K., Bates, R., Žídek, A., Potapenko, A., Bridgland, A., Meyer, C., Kohl, S. A. A., Ballard, A. J., Cowie, A., Romera-Paredes, B., Nikolov, S., Jain, R., Adler, J., ... Hassabis, D. (2021). Highly accurate protein structure prediction with AlphaFold. *Nature, 596*(7873), 583–589. https://doi.org/10.1038/s41586-021-03819-2, http://www.nature.com/nature/index.html.

Juszczak, A., Morris, D., Grossman, A., Blackman, M. R., Boyce, A., Chrousos, G., Corpas, E., Herder, W. W. D., Dhatariya, K., Dungan, K., Hofland, J., Kalra, S., Kaltsas, G., Kapoor, N., Koch, C., Kopp, P., Korbonits, M., & Kovacs, C. S. (2000). *Cushing's Syndrome*. Endotext. MDText.com, Inc.

Kalra, S., Das, A. K., Bajaj, S., Priya, G., Ghosh, S., Mehrotra, R. N., Das, S., Shah, P., Deshmukh, V., Sanyal, D., Chandrasekaran, S., Khandelwal, D., Joshi, A., Nair, T., Eliana, F., Permana, H., Fariduddin, M. D., Shrestha, P. K., Shrestha, D., ... Shaikh, K. (2020). Utility of precision medicine in the management of diabetes: Expert opinion from an international panel. *Diabetes Therapy, 11*(2), 411–422. https://doi.org/10.1007/s13300-019-00753-5, http://www.springer.com/medicine/internal/journal/13300.

Kattamis, A., Kwiatkowski, J. L., & Aydinok, Y. (2022). Thalassaemia. *The Lancet, 399*(10343), 2310–2324. https://doi.org/10.1016/S0140-6736(22)00536-0, http://www.journals.elsevier.com/the-lancet/.

Kesik-Brodacka, M. (2018). Progress in biopharmaceutical development. *Biotechnology and Applied Biochemistry, 65*(3), 306–322. https://doi.org/10.1002/bab.1617.

Kikano, S., & Kannankeril, P. J. (2022). Precision medicine in pediatric cardiology. *Pediatric Annals, 51*(10), e390. https://doi.org/10.3928/19382359-20220803-05, http://www.pediatricsupersite.com/issue.aspx?pubid=PedAnn.

Kostopoulou, K., Lekka, D., Pnevmatikakis, A., Angelova, N., Stafylas, P., Tamouridis, S., Bargiota, A., & Kyriazakos, S. (2025). Multidomain behavioral change digital coaching for chronic disease management in patients with type 2 diabetes: Framework development and preliminary evaluation. *JMIR Formative Research, 9*, e73807. https://doi.org/10.2196/73807.

Krawczuk, P., Fox, Z. R., Petkov, V., Negoita, S., Doherty, J., Stroup, A., Schwartz, S., Penberthy, L., Hsu, E., Gounley, J., & Hanson, H. A. (2025). Large-scale deep learning for metastasis detection in pathology reports. *JAMIA Open, 8*(4). https://doi.org/10.1093/jamiaopen/ooaf070, https://academic.oup.com/jamiaopen.

Krittanawong, C., Khawaja, M., Rosenson, R. S., Amos, C. I., Nambi, V., Lavie, C. J., & Virani, S. S. (2022). Association of PCSK9 variants with the risk of atherosclerotic cardiovascular disease and variable responses to PCSK9 inhibitor therapy. *Current Problems in Cardiology, 47*(7). https://doi.org/10.1016/j.cpcardiol.2021.101043, http://www.elsevier.com/inca/publications/store/6/2/3/2/8/9/index.htt.

Larizza, L., & Cubellis, M. V. (2023). Rare diseases: Implementation of molecular diagnosis, pathogenesis insights and precision medicine treatment. *International Journal of Molecular Sciences, 24*(10), 9064. https://doi.org/10.3390/ijms24109064.

Lau, E., & Wu, J. C. (2018). Omics, big data, and precision medicine in cardiovascular sciences. *Circulation Research, 122*(9), 1165–1168. https://doi.org/10.1161/CIRCRESAHA.118.313161, http://circres.ahajournals.org.

Laurent, M., Geoffroy, M., Pavani, G., & Guiraud, S. (2024). CRISPR-based gene therapies: From preclinical to clinical treatments. *Cells, 13*(10). https://doi.org/10.3390/cells13100800, https://www.mdpi.com/journal/cells.

Le Ngoc, K., Pham, T. T. H., Nguyen, T. K., & Huong, P. T. (2024). Pharmacomicrobiomics in precision cancer therapy: Bench to bedside. *Frontiers in Immunology, 15*. https://doi.org/10.3389/fimmu.2024.1428420, https://www.frontiersin.org/journals/immunology#.

Leong, I. U. S., Cabrera, C. P., Cipriani, V., Ross, P. J., Turner, R. M., Stuckey, A., Sanghvi, S., Pasko, D., Moutsianas, L., Odhams, C. A., Elgar, G. S., Chan, G., Giess, A., Walker, S., Foulger, R. E., Williams, E. M., Daugherty, L. C., Rueda-Martin, A., Rhodes, D. J., ... McDonagh, E. M. (2024). Large-scale pharmacogenomics analysis of patients with cancer within the 100,000 genomes project combining whole-genome sequencing and medical records to inform clinical practice. *Journal of Clinical Oncology*((). https://doi.org/10.1200/JCO.23.02761, https://ascopubs.org/loi/jco.

Li, J., Li, L., You, P., Wei, Y., & Xu, B. (2023). Towards artificial intelligence to multi-omics characterization of tumor heterogeneity in esophageal cancer. *Seminars in Cancer Biology, 91*, 35–49. https://doi.org/10.1016/j.semcancer.2023.02.009, http://www.elsevier.com/inca/publications/store/6/2/2/9/4/3/index.htt.

Li, L., Sun, M., Wang, J., & Wan, S. (2024). Multi-omics based artificial intelligence for cancer research. *Advances in Cancer Research, 163*, 303–356. https://doi.org/10.1016/bs.acr.2024.06.005, https://www.sciencedirect.com/science/bookseries/0065230X.

Li, X., & Warner, J. L. (2020). A review of precision oncology knowledgebases for determining the clinical actionability of genetic variants. *Frontiers in Cell and Developmental Biology, 8*. https://doi.org/10.3389/fcell.2020.00048, https://www.frontiersin.org/journals/cell-and-developmental-biology#.

Lista, S., Imbimbo, B. P., Grasso, M., Fidilio, A., Emanuele, E., Minoretti, P., López-Ortiz, S., Martín-Hernández, J., Gabelle, A., Caruso, G., Malaguti, M., Melchiorri, D., Santos-Lozano, A., Imbimbo, C., Heneka, M. T., & Caraci, F. (2024). Tracking neuroinflammatory biomarkers in Alzheimer's disease: A strategy for individualized therapeutic approaches? *Journal of Neuroinflammation, 21*(1). https://doi.org/10.1186/s12974-024-03163-y, https://jneuroinflammation.biomedcentral.com.

Litman, A., Sauerwald, N., Green Snyder, L. A., Foss-Feig, J., Park, C. Y., Hao, Y., Dinstein, I., Theesfeld, C. L., & Troyanskaya, O. G. (2025). Decomposition of phenotypic heterogeneity in autism reveals underlying genetic programs. *Nature Genetics*. https://doi.org/10.1038/s41588-025-02224-z.

Ma, E., Chen, K., Shi, H., Wasko, K. M., Esain-Garcia, I., Trinidad, M. I., Zhou, K., Ye, J., & Doudna, J. A. (2025). *Directed Evolution Expands CRISPR-Cas12a Genome Editing Capacity*. United States: bioRxiv. https://www.biorxiv.org.

Martinez-Lopez, N., Mattar, P., Toledo, M., Bains, H., Kalyani, M., Aoun, M. L., Sharma, M., McIntire, L. B. J., Gunther-Cummins, L., Macaluso, F. P., Aguilan, J. T., Sidoli, S., Bourdenx, M., & Singh, R. (2023). mTORC2–NDRG1–CDC42 axis couples fasting to mitochondrial fission. *Nature Cell Biology, 25*(7), 989–1003. https://doi.org/10.1038/s41556-023-01163-3.

Mc.Conathy, J., & Owens, M. J. (2003). Stereochemistry in drug action. *The Primary Care Companion to The Journal of Clinical Psychiatry, 05*(02), 70–73. https://doi.org/10.4088/PCC.v05n0202.

McManus, M., Frangoul, H., & Steinberg, M. H. (2024). CRISPR-based gene therapy for the induction of fetal hemoglobin in sickle cell disease. *Expert Review of Hematology, 17*(12), 957–966. https://doi.org/10.1080/17474086.2024.2429605, http://www.tandfonline.com/loi/ierr20.

Montin, D., Santilli, V., Beni, A., Costagliola, G., Martire, B., Mastrototaro, M. F., Ottaviano, G., Rizzo, C., Sgrulletti, M., Miraglia Del Giudice, M., & Moschese, V. (2024). Towards personalized vaccines. *Frontiers in Immunology, 15*. https://doi.org/10.3389/fimmu.2024.1436108, https://www.frontiersin.org/journals/immunology#.

Morenas-Rodríguez, E., Li, Y., Nuscher, B., Franzmeier, N., Xiong, C., Suárez-Calvet, M., Fagan, A. M., Schultz, S., Gordon, B. A., Benzinger, T. L. S., Hassenstab, J., McDade, E., Feederle, R., Karch, C. M., Schlepckow, K., Morris, J. C., Kleinberger, G., Nellgard, B., Vöglein, J., ... Xu, X. (2022). Soluble TREM2 in CSF and its association with other biomarkers and cognition in autosomal-dominant Alzheimer's disease: A longitudinal observational study. *The Lancet Neurology, 21*(4), 329–341. https://doi.org/10.1016/S1474-4422(22)00027-8, http://www.journals.elsevier.com/the-lancet-neurology/.

Mosquera-Lopez, C., & Jacobs, P. G. (2024). Digital twins and artificial intelligence in metabolic disease research. *Trends in Endocrinology and Metabolism, 35*(6), 549–557. https://doi.org/10.1016/j.tem.2024.04.019, https://www.sciencedirect.com/science/journal/10432760.

Mukherjee, S., Stamatis, D., Li, C. T., Ovchinnikova, G., Kandimalla, M., Handke, V., Reddy, A., Ivanova, N., Woyke, T., Eloe-Fardosh, E. A., Chen, I. M. A., Kyrpides, N. C., & Reddy, T. B. K. (2025). Genomes OnLine Database (GOLD) v.10: New features and updates. *Nucleic Acids Research, 53*(1), D989. https://doi.org/10.1093/nar/gkae1000, https://academic.oup.com/nar/issue.

Mullard, A. (2017). FDA approves first CAR T therapy. *Nature Reviews Drug Discovery, 16*(10), 669. https://doi.org/10.1038/nrd.2017.196, http://www.nature.com/nrd/index.html.

Musallam, K. M., Cappellini, M. D., Coates, T. D., Kuo, K. H. M., Al-Samkari, H., Sheth, S., Viprakasit, V., & Taher, A. T. (2024). Alpha-thalassemia: A practical overview. *Blood Reviews, 64*. https://doi.org/10.1016/j.blre.2023.101165, https://www.sciencedirect.com/science/journal/0268960X.

MyChart. (2025). https://www.mychart.org/

Nabizadeh, F., Weiner, M. W., Aisen, P., Petersen, R., Jack, C. R., Jagust, W., Trojanowski, J. Q., Toga, A. W., Beckett, L., Green, R. C., Saykin, A. J., Morris, J., Shaw, L. M., Khachaturian, Z., Sorensen, G., Kuller, L., Raichle, M., Paul, S., Davies, P., ... Furst, A. J. (2025). Local molecular and connectomic contributions of tau-related neurodegeneration. *GeroScience, 47*(1), 227–246. https://doi.org/10.1007/s11357-024-01339-1.

Naithani, N., Atal, A. T., Tilak, T. V. S. V. G. K., Vasudevan, B., Misra, P., & Sinha, S. (2021). Precision medicine: Uses and challenges. *Medical Journal Armed Forces India, 77*(3), 258–265. https://doi.org/10.1016/j.mjafi.2021.06.020, http://www.journals.elsevier.com/Medical-Journal-Armed-Forces-India.

Naithani, N., Sinha, S., Misra, P., Vasudevan, B., & Sahu, R. (2021). Precision medicine: Concept and tools. *Medical Journal Armed Forces India, 77*(3), 249–257. https://doi.org/10.1016/j.mjafi.2021.06.021.

Natarajan, S., Ponde, C. K., Rajani, R. M., Jijina, F., Gursahani, R., Dhairyawan, P. P., & Ashavaid, T. F. (2013). Effect of CYP2C9 and VKORC1 genetic variations on warfarin dose requirements in Indian patients. *Pharmacological Reports, 65*(5), 1375–1382. https://doi.org/10.1016/s1734-1140(13)71496-8.

Naveed Ahmad, J., He, B., Schroeder, B., & Rosales, J. (2022). Two distinct primary EGFR-mutated lung adenocarcinoma within the same patient: A case report. *International Journal of Cancer Care and Delivery, 2*(2). https://doi.org/10.53876/001c.37213.

Ndjonko, L. C. M., Chakraborty, A., Petri, F., Alavi, S. M. A., Matsuo, T., Borgonovo, F., Comba, I. Y., Murad, M. H., Nassr, A., El-Zein, S., & Berbari, E. F. (2025). Evaluating predictive performance and generalizability of traditional and artificial intelligence models in predicting surgical site infections post-spinal surgery: A systematic review. *The Spine Journal*. https://doi.org/10.1016/j.spinee.2025.07.032.

Neagu, A. N., Bruno, P., Johnson, K. R., Ballestas, G., & Darie, C. C. (2024). Biological basis of breast cancer-related disparities in precision oncology era. *International Journal of Molecular Sciences, 25*(7). https://doi.org/10.3390/ijms25074113, http://www.mdpi.com/journal/ijms.

Neagu, A. N., Whitham, D., Bruno, P., Morrissiey, H., Darie, C. A., & Darie, C. C. (2023). Omics-based investigations of breast cancer. *Molecules, 28*(12). https://doi.org/10.3390/molecules28124768, http://www.mdpi.com/journal/molecules.

Nguyen, M., Maria, A. G., Faucz, F. R., Trivellin, G., Stratakis, C. A., & Tatsi, C. (2024). FAF1 gene involvement in pituitary corticotroph. *Tumors. Hormone and Metabolic Research, 56*(08), 604–610. https://doi.org/10.1055/a-2192-1761.

Novotni, G., Jakimovska, M., Plaseska-Karanfilska, D., Tanovska, N., Kuzmanovski, I., Aleksovski, V., Karanfilovik, K., Baneva-Dolnenec, N., Stankovic, M., Milutinovik, M., Iloski, S., Isjanovska, R., Blazevska-Stoilkovska, B., Duma, A., & Novotni, A. (2019). Evaluation of APOE genotype and vascular risk factors as prognostic and risk factors for alzheimer's disease and their influence on age of symptoms onset. *Open Access Macedonian Journal of Medical Sciences, 7*(4), 516–520. https://doi.org/10.3889/oamjms.2019.166.

Olawade, D. B., Teke, J., Fapohunda, O., Weerasinghe, K., Usman, S. O., Ige, A. O., & Clement David-Olawade, A. (2024). Leveraging artificial intelligence in vaccine development: A narrative review. *Journal of Microbiological Methods, 224*. https://doi.org/10.1016/j.mimet.2024.106998, https://www.sciencedirect.com/science/journal/01677012.

Olivier, M., Asmis, R., Hawkins, G. A., Howard, T. D., & Cox, L. A. (2019). The need for multi-omics biomarker signatures in precision medicine. *International Journal of Molecular Sciences, 20*(19). https://doi.org/10.3390/ijms20194781, https://www.mdpi.com/1422-0067/20/19/4781/pdf.

Onoue, T., Nishida, K., Nakata, Y., Hayashi, F., Marutani, M., Sakane, J., Moriguchi, S., Muto, K., Kato, Masuda, T., Okamura, K., Matsuzaki, T., Kawamura, K., & Tsushita, K. (2025). Effectiveness of recommendations in promoting the use of Mobile health applications in health guidance: a randomized controlled trial. *Journal of occupational health*. https://doi.org/10.1093/joccuh/uiaf036.

Orphanou, N., Papatheodorou, E., & Anastasakis, A. (2022). Dilated cardiomyopathy in the era of precision medicine: Latest concepts and developments. *Heart Failure Reviews, 27*(4), 1173–1191. https://doi.org/10.1007/s10741-021-10139-0.

Ortega-Batista, A., Jaén-Alvarado, Y., Moreno-Labrador, D., Gómez, N., García, G., & Guerrero, E. N. (2025). Single-cell sequencing: Genomic and transcriptomic approaches in cancer cell biology. *International Journal of Molecular Sciences, 26*(5). https://doi.org/10.3390/ijms26052074.

Ossenkoppele, R., van der Kant, R., & Hansson, O. (2022). Tau biomarkers in Alzheimer's disease: Towards implementation in clinical practice and trials. *The Lancet Neurology, 21*(8), 726–734. https://doi.org/10.1016/S1474-4422(22)00168-5.

Papadopoulou, P., & Lytras, M. (2023). Advancing precision medicine in medical education: Integrated, precise and data-driven smart solutions. *Applied Research, 2*(6). https://doi.org/10.1002/appl.202200131.

Papadopoulou, P., Polissidis, A., Kythreoti, G., Sagnou, M., Stefanatou, A., & Theoharides, T. C. (2024). Anti-inflammatory and neuroprotective polyphenols derived from the european olive tree, Olea europaea L., in long COVID and other conditions involving cognitive impairment. *International Journal of Molecular Sciences, 25*(20), 11040. https://doi.org/10.3390/ijms252011040.

Parhi, R., Jena, G. K., Patra, C. N., & Jammula, S. (2025). Biomarkers as diagnostic and prognostic tools in cardiac disorders: A comprehensive review. *Journal of Bio-X Research, 8*. https://doi.org/10.34133/jbioxresearch.0030.

Parums, D. V. (2024). Editorial: First regulatory approvals for CRISPRCas9 therapeutic gene editing for sickle cell disease and transfusion-dependent b-thalassemia. *Medical Science Monitor, 30*. https://doi.org/10.12659/MSM.944204, https://medscimonit.com/abstract/full/idArt/944204.

Personalized Medicine Coalition (PMC) The Personalized Medicine Report-Opportunity, Challenges and the Future. (2017).

Picher-Martel, V., Valdmanis, P. N., Gould, P. V., Julien, J. P., & Dupré, N. (2016). From animal models to human disease: A genetic approach for personalized medicine in ALS. *Acta Neuropathologica Communications, 4*(1). https://doi.org/10.1186/s40478-016-0340-5, https://actaneurocomms.biomedcentral.com/.

Popescu, C., Munteanu, C., Anghelescu, A., Ciobanu, V., Spînu, A., Andone, I., Mandu, M., Bistriceanu, R., Băilă, M., Postoiu, R. L., Vlădulescu-Trandafir, A. I., Giuvara, S., Malaelea, A. D., & Onose, G. (2024). Novelties on neuroinflammation in Alzheimer's disease–Focus on gut and oral microbiota involvement. *International Journal of Molecular Sciences, 25*(20). https://doi.org/10.3390/ijms252011272, http://www.mdpi.com/journal/ijms.

Purnell, J. Q., Feingold, K. R., Anawalt, B., Blackman, M. R., Boyce, A., Chrousos, G., Corpas, E., Herder, W. W. D., Dhatariya, K., Dungan, K., Hofland, J., Kalra, S., Kaltsas, G., Kapoor, N., Koch, C., & Kopp, P. (2000). *Definitions, Classification, and Epidemiology of Obesity*. Endotext. MDText.com, Inc.

QuestPrehab. (2025). https://questprehab.com/

Rasmussen, J., & Langerman, H. (2019). Alzheimer's disease – Why we need early diagnosis. *Degenerative Neurological and Neuromuscular Disease, 9*, 123–130. https://doi.org/10.2147/dnnd.s228939.

Raverdy, V., Cohen, R. V., Caiazzo, R., Verkindt, H., Petry, T. B. Z., Marciniak, C., Legendre, B., Bauvin, P., Chatelain, E., Duhamel, A., Drumez, E., Oukhouya-Daoud, N., Chetboun, M., Baud, G., Ahlqvist, E., Wierup, N., Asplund, O., Laferrère, B., Groop, L., & Pattou, F.Ç. (2022). Data-driven subgroups of type 2 diabetes, metabolic response, and renal risk profile after bariatric surgery: A retrospective cohort study. *The Lancet Diabetes and Endocrinology, 10*(3), 167–176. https://doi.org/10.1016/S2213-8587(22)00005-5.

Rodriguez-Vieitez, E., Kumar, A., Malarte, M. L., Ioannou, K., Rocha, F. M., & Chiotis, K. (2024). Imaging neuroinflammation: Quantification of astrocytosis in a multitracer PET approach. *Methods in molecular biology (Clifton, N.J.), 2785*, 195–218. https://doi.org/10.1007/978-1-0716-3774-6_13.

Roshani, A., Mohammadi, M., Bahadori, T., Ahmadi Zare, H., Judaki, M. A., Mobini, M., Golsaz-Shirazi, F., Jeddi-Tehrani, M., Amiri, M. M., & Shokri, F. (2023). Comparison of different transient gene expression systems for the production of a new humanized anti-HER2 monoclonal antibody (Hersintuzumab). *DARU, Journal of Pharmaceutical Sciences, 31*(2), 221–231. https://doi.org/10.1007/s40199-023-00477-9, https://www.springer.com/journal/40199.

Sadee, W. (2017). Personalized therapeutics and pharmacogenomics: Integral to personalized health care. *Pharmaceutical Research, 34*(8), 1535–1538. https://doi.org/10.1007/s11095-017-2170-y.

Sadee, W., Wang, D., Hartmann, K., & Toland, A. E. (2023). Pharmacogenomics: Driving personalized medicine. *Pharmacological Reviews, 75*(4), 789–814. https://doi.org/10.1124/pharmrev.122.000810, http://pharmrev.aspetjournals.org/.

Samanthula, K. S., Alli, R., & Gorre, T. (2021). Preliminary studies on optimization of anti-parkinson drug loaded lipid nanoparticles enriched hydrogel formulations for management of parkinson's disease. *Current Nanomedicine, 11*(2), 112–126. https://doi.org/10.2174/2468187311666210311114908, https://www.eurekaselect.com/192219/article.

Schyvens, A. M., Van Oost, N. C., Aerts, J. M., Masci, F., Peters, B., Neven, A., Dirix, H., Wets, G., Ross, V., & Verbraecken, J. (2024). Accuracy of fitbit charge 4, garmin vivosmart 4, and WHOOP versus polysomnography: Systematic review. *JMIR mHealth and uHealth, 12*, e52192. https://doi.org/10.2196/52192.

Severi, A. A., & Akbari, B. (2024). CRISPR-Cas9 delivery strategies and applications: Review and update. *genesis, 62*(3). https://doi.org/10.1002/dvg.23598.

Shen, Y., Liu, F., & Zhang, M. (2024). Therapeutic potential of plant-derived natural compounds in Alzheimer's disease: Targeting microglia-mediated neuroinflammation. *Biomedicine & Pharmacotherapy, 178*, 117235. https://doi.org/10.1016/j.biopha.2024.117235.

Shippy, D. C., Oliai, S. F., & Ulland, T. K. (2024). Zinc utilization by microglia in Alzheimer's disease. *Journal of Biological Chemistry, 300*(5). https://doi.org/10.1016/j.jbc.2024.107306, https://www.sciencedirect.com/science/journal/00219258.

Singh, R., Kaushik, S., Wang, Y., Xiang, Y., Novak, I., Komatsu, M., Tanaka, K., Cuervo, A. M., & Czaja, M. J. (2009). Autophagy regulates lipid metabolism. *Nature, 458*(7242), 1131–1135. https://doi.org/10.1038/nature07976.

Singh, S., Sarma, D. K., Verma, V., Nagpal, R., & Kumar, M. (2023). Unveiling the future of metabolic medicine: Omics technologies driving personalized solutions for precision treatment of metabolic disorders. *Biochemical and Biophysical Research Communications, 682*, 1–20. https://doi.org/10.1016/j.bbrc.2023.09.064, http://www.sciencedirect.com/science/journal/0006291X.

Song, Y., Wang, Y., Man, J., Xu, Y., Zhou, G., Shen, W., Chao, Y., Yang, K., Pei, P., & Hu, L. (2025). Chimeric antigen receptor cells solid tumor immunotherapy assisted by biomaterials tools. *ACS Applied Materials and Interfaces, 17*(7), 10246–10264. https://doi.org/10.1021/acsami.4c20275, http://pubs.acs.org/journal/aamick.

Stewart, A. (2013). SLCO1B1 polymorphisms and statin-induced myopathy. *PLoS Currents*. https://doi.org/10.1371/currents.eogt.d21e7f0c58463571bb0d9d3a19b82203 (DEC).

Stratakis, C. A. (2024a). Apropos thyroid endocrinology and EndoBridge, as well as more on reproductive medicine. *Hormones, 23*(2), 179–181. https://doi.org/10.1007/s42000-024-00577-4, https://www.springer.com/journal/42000.

Stratakis, C. A. (2024b). The passing of the creator of dolly and other pioneers, endocrine disruptors, metabolic syndrome, and more. *Hormones, 23*(3), 359–360. https://doi.org/10.1007/s42000-024-00601-7, https://www.springer.com/journal/42000.

Su, M., Pan, T., Chen, Q.-Z., Zhou, W.-W., Gong, Y., Xu, G., Yan, H.-Y., Li, S., Shi, Q.-Z., Zhang, Y., He, X., Jiang, C.-J., Fan, S.-C., Li, X., Cairns, M. J., Wang, X., & Li, Y.-S. (2022). Data analysis guidelines for single-cell RNA-seq in biomedical studies and clinical applications. *Military Medical Research, 9*(1). https://doi.org/10.1186/s40779-022-00434-8.

Sultova, E., Westphalen, C. B., Jung, A., Kumbrink, J., Kirchner, T., Mayr, D., Rudelius, M., Ormanns, S., Heinemann, V., Metzeler, K. H., Greif, P. A., Burges, A., Trillsch, F., Mahner, S., Harbeck, N., & Wuerstlein, R. (2021). NGS-guided precision oncology in metastatic breast and gynecological cancer: First experiences at the CCC Munich LMU. *Archives of Gynecology and Obstetrics, 303*(5), 1331–1345. https://doi.org/10.1007/s00404-020-05881-z, https://www.springer.com/medicine/gynecology/journal/404.

Swain, S. M., Shastry, M., & Hamilton, E. (2023). Targeting HER2-positive breast cancer: Advances and future directions. *Nature Reviews Drug Discovery, 22*(2), 101–126. https://doi.org/10.1038/s41573-022-00579-0.

Takeda, S., Clemens, P. R., & Hoffman, E. P. (2021). Exon-skipping in duchenne muscular dystrophy. *Journal of neuromuscular diseases, 8*(2), S343. https://doi.org/10.3233/JND-210682.

Tang, Q., Chen, Y., Li, X., Long, S., Shi, Y., Yu, Y., Wu, W., Han, L., & Wang, S. (2022). The role of PD-1/PD-L1 and application of immune-checkpoint inhibitors in human cancers. *Frontiers in Immunology. 13*. https://doi.org/10.3389/fimmu.2022.964442.

Tchang, B. G., Aras, M., Kumar, R. B., Aronne, L. J., Feingold, K. R., Anawalt, B., Blackman, M. R., Boyce, A., Chrousos, G., Corpas, E., Herder, W. W. D., Dhatariya, K., Dungan, K., Hofland, J., Kalra, S., Kaltsas, G., Kapoor, N., Koch, C., Kopp, P., ... Kovacs, C. S. (2000). *Pharmacologic Treatment of Overweight and Obesity in Adults*. Endotext. MDText.com, Inc.

Testa, D., Salma, I., Iborra, V., Roussel, V., Dutech, M., Minvielle, E., & Cabanes, E. (2025). Remote patient monitoring system for polypathological older adults at high risk for hospitalization: Retrospective cohort study. *Journal of Medical Internet Research, 27*, e71527. https://doi.org/10.2196/71527.

Thakur, V., & Kutty, R. V. (2019). Recent advances in nanotheranostics for triple negative breast cancer treatment. *Journal of Experimental and Clinical Cancer Research, 38*(1). https://doi.org/10.1186/s13046-019-1443-1, http://www.jeccr.com/.

Thangaraj, P. M., Benson, S. H., Oikonomou, E. K., Asselbergs, F. W., & Khera, R. (2024). Cardiovascular care with digital twin technology in the era of generative artificial intelligence. *European Heart Journal, 45*(45), 4808–4821. https://doi.org/10.1093/eurheartj/ehae619.

The Lancet Global Health. (2024). The landscape for rare diseases in 2024. *The Lancet Global Health. 12*(3), e341. https://doi.org/10.1016/S2214-109X(24)00056-1, https://www.sciencedirect.com/science/journal/2214109X.

The National Institutes of Health:The Promise of Precision Medicine. (2025). https://www.nih.gov/about-nih/nih-turning-discovery-into-health/promise-precision-medicine

Theoharides, T. C. (2017). Neuroendocrinology of mast cells: Challenges and controversies. *Experimental Dermatology, 26*(9), 751–759. https://doi.org/10.1111/exd.13288, http://onlinelibrary.wiley.com/journal/10.1111/(ISSN)1600-0625.

Theoharides, T. C. (2020). Stress, inflammation, and autoimmunity: The 3 modern erinyes. *Clinical Therapeutics, 42*(5), 742–744. https://doi.org/10.1016/j.clinthera.2020.04.002, www.elsevier.com/locate/clinthera.

Theoharides, T. C. (2021). Luteolin: The wonder flavonoid. *BioFactors, 47*(2), 139–140. https://doi.org/10.1002/biof.1729, http://iubmb.onlinelibrary.wiley.com/hub/journal/10.1002/(ISSN)1872-8081/.

Theoharides, T. C., & Leeman, S. E. (2019). Effect of IL-33 on de novo synthesized mediators from human mast cells. *Journal of Allergy and Clinical Immunology, 143*(1), 451. https://doi.org/10.1016/j.jaci.2018.09.014, http://www.elsevier.com/inca/publications/store/6/2/3/3/6/8/index.htt.

Tsigos, C., Kyrou, I., Kassi, E., Chrousos, G. P., Anawalt, B., Blackman, M. R., Boyce, A., Chrousos, G., Corpas, E., Herder, W. W. D., Dhatariya, K., Dungan, K., Hofland, J., Kalra, S., Kaltsas, G., Kapoor, N., & Koch, C. (2000). *Stress: Endocrine Physiology and Pathophysiology*. Endotext. MDText.com, Inc.

Two Distinct Primary EGFR-Mutated Lung Adenocarcinoma Within the Same Patient: A Case Report. (n.d.)

Tzeplaeff, L., Wilfling, S., Requardt, M. V., & Herdick, M. (2023). Current state and future directions in the therapy of ALS. *Cells, 12*(11), 1523. https://doi.org/10.3390/cells12111523.

Vanhooydonck, M., De Neef, E., De Saffel, H., Boel, A., Willaert, A., Callewaert, B., & Claes, K. B. M. (2025). Prime editing outperforms homology-directed repair as a tool for CRISPR-mediated variant knock-in in zebrafish. *Lab Animal, 54*(6), 165–172. https://doi.org/10.1038/s41684-025-01560-1, https://www.springer.com/journal/41684.

Varricchi, G., & Poto, R. (2024). Towards precision medicine in COPD: Targeting type 2 cytokines and alarmins. *European Journal of Internal Medicine, 125*, 28–31. https://doi.org/10.1016/j.ejim.2024.05.011.

Vogiatzi, G., Lazaros, G., Oikonomou, E., Lazarou, E., Vavuranakis, E., & Tousoulis, D. (2022). Role of genetic testing in cardiomyopathies: A primer for cardiologists. *World Journal of Cardiology, 14*(1), 29–39. https://doi.org/10.4330/wjc.v14.i1.29.

Walton, N. A., & Christensen, G. B. (2023). Paving a pathway for large-scale utilization of genomics in precision medicine and population health. *Frontiers in Sociology, 8*. https://doi.org/10.3389/fsoc.2023.1122488, www.frontiersin.org/journals/sociology.

Wang, J., Yu, Y., Lin, Q., Zhang, J., & Song, C. (2024). Efficacy and safety of first-line therapy in patients with HER2-positive advanced breast cancer: A network meta-analysis of randomized controlled trials. *Journal of Cancer Research and Clinical Oncology, 150*(1). https://doi.org/10.1007/s00432-023-05530-3.

Wang, R. S., Maron, B. A., & Loscalzo, J. (2023). Multiomics network medicine approaches to precision medicine and therapeutics in cardiovascular diseases. *Arteriosclerosis, Thrombosis, and Vascular Biology, 43*(4), 493–503. https://doi.org/10.1161/ATVBAHA.122.318731, https://www.ahajournals.org/journal/atvb.

Warden, B. A., Fazio, S., Shapiro, M. D., Feingold, K. R., Anawalt, B., Blackman, M. R., Boyce, A., Chrousos, G., Corpas, E., Herder, W. W. D., Dhatariya, K., Dungan, K., Hofland, J., Kalra, S., Kaltsas, G., Kapoor, N., Koch, C., Kopp, P., Korbonits, M., & Kovacs, C. S. (2000). *Familial Hypercholesterolemia: Genes and Beyond*. Endotext. MDText.com, Inc.

Weerarathna, I. N., Doelakeh, E. S., Kiwanuka, L., Kumar, P., & Arora, S. (2024). Prophylactic and therapeutic vaccine development: Advancements and challenges. *Molecular Biomedicine, 5*(1). https://doi.org/10.1186/s43556-024-00222-x, https://www.springer.com/journal/43556.

What is the Health Information Portal?. European Health Information Portal. (2025).

Wilton-Clark, H., & Yokota, T. (2023). Recent trends in antisense therapies for duchenne muscular dystrophy. *Pharmaceutics. 15*(3). https://doi.org/10.3390/pharmaceutics15030778.

Woodward, E. A., Wang, E., Wallis, C., Sharma, R., Tie, A. W. J., Murthy, N., & Blancafort, P. (2024). Protocol for delivery of CRISPR/dCas9 systems for epigenetic editing into solid tumors using lipid nanoparticles encapsulating RNA. *Methods in Molecular Biology, 2842*, 267–287. https://doi.org/10.1007/978-1-0716-4051-7_14, https://www.springer.com/series/7651.

Wu, Y., Battalapalli, D., Hakeem, M. J., Selamneni, V., Zhang, P., Draz, M. S., & Ruan, Z. (2021). Engineered CRISPR-Cas systems for the detection and control of antibiotic-resistant infections. *Journal of Nanobiotechnology, 19*(1). https://doi.org/10.1186/s12951-021-01132-8, http://www.jnanobiotechnology.com/start.asp.

Xiao, Y., Ma, D., Yang, Y. S., Yang, F., Ding, J. H., Gong, Y., Jiang, L., Ge, L. P., Wu, S. Y., Yu, Q., Zhang, Q., Bertucci, F., Sun, Q., Hu, X., Li, D. Q., Shao, Z. M., & Jiang, Y. Z. (2022). Comprehensive metabolomics expands precision medicine for triple-negative breast cancer. *Cell Research, 32*(5), 477–490. https://doi.org/10.1038/s41422-022-00614-0, http://www.nature.com/cr/index.html.

Xie, F., Chan, J. C. N., & Ma, R. C. W. (2018). Precision medicine in diabetes prevention, classification and management. *Journal of Diabetes Investigation, 9*(5), 998–1015. https://doi.org/10.1111/jdi.12830.

Yang, J., Liang, J., Hu, N., He, N., Liu, B., Liu, G., & Qin, Y. (2024). The gut microbiota modulates neuroinflammation in alzheimer's disease: elucidating crucial factors and mechanistic underpinnings. *CNS Neuroscience & Therapeutics, 30*(10). https://doi.org/10.1111/cns.70091.

Yildiz, B. O., Boguszewski, C. L., da Silva Boguszewski, M. C., Busetto, L., Celik, O., Fuleihan, G. E. H., Goulis, D. G., Hammer, G. D., Haymart, M. R., Kaltsas, G., Law, J. R., Lim, A. Y. L., Luger, A., Macut, D., McGowan, B., McClung, M., Miras, A. D., Patti, M. E., Peeters, R. P., ... Yazici, D. (2024). EndoBridge 2023: Highlights and pearls. *Hormones, 23*(2), 183–204. https://doi.org/10.1007/s42000-024-00549-8, https://www.springer.com/journal/42000.

Yin, Q., Ni, J.-jiao, & Ying, J.-er (2024). Potential mechanisms and targeting strategies of the gut microbiota in antitumor immunity and immunotherapy. *Immunity, Inflammation and Disease, 12*(7). https://doi.org/10.1002/iid3.1263.

Yousef, R., Gupta, G., Yousef, N., & Khari, M. (2022). A holistic overview of deep learning approach in medical imaging. *Multimedia Systems, 28*(3), 881–914. https://doi.org/10.1007/s00530-021-00884-5.

Zang, S. S., Zhang, R., Zhang, J. R., Zhang, X., & Li, J. (2025). Progress, applications and prospects of CRISPR-based genome editing technology in gene therapy for cancer and sickle cell disease. *Human Gene Therapy, 36*(11-12), 858–869. https://doi.org/10.1089/hum.2024.262, www.liebertonline.com/hum.

Zhang, P., & Xu, Z. (2025). The advancements in precision medicine for Leber congenital amaurosis: Breakthroughs from genetic diagnosis to therapy. *Survey of Ophthalmology*. https://doi.org/10.1016/j.survophthal.2025.04.005.

Zhang, R., Wang, Y., Peng, Y., Zhao, J., & Zhang, Z. (2023). Advanced progress of the relationship between PCSK9 monoclonal antibodies and hyperglycemic adverse events. *Frontiers in Cardiovascular Medicine, 10*. https://doi.org/10.3389/fcvm.2023.1117143.

Zhao, L., & Cao, Y. J. (2019). Engineered T cell therapy for cancer in the clinic. *Frontiers in Immunology, 10*. https://doi.org/10.3389/fimmu.2019.02250, https://www.frontiersin.org/journals/immunology#.

Zhao, Q., Chen, Y., Huang, W., Zhou, H., & Zhang, W. (2023). Drug-microbiota interactions: An emerging priority for precision medicine. *Signal Transduction and Targeted Therapy, 8*(1). https://doi.org/10.1038/s41392-023-01619-w.

Zhou, K., Lansang, M. C., Blackman, M. R., Boyce, A., Chrousos, G., Corpas, E., Herder, W. W. D., Dhatariya, K., Dungan, K., Hofland, J., Kalra, S., Kaltsas, G., Kapoor, N., Koch, C., Kopp, P., Korbonits, M., & Kovacs, C. S. (2000). *Diabetes Mellitus and Infection*. Endotext. MDText.com, Inc.

Zhu, Q., Wang, J., Yu, H., Hu, Q., Bateman, N. W., Long, M., Rosario, S., Schultz, E., Dalgard, C. L., Wilkerson, M. D., Sukumar, G., Huang, R. Y., Kaur, J., Lele, S. B., Zsiros, E., Villella, J., Lugade, A., Moysich, K., Conrads, T. P., ... Odunsi, K. (2022). Whole-genome sequencing identifies PPARGC1A as a putative modifier of cancer risk in BRCA1/2 mutation carriers. *Cancers, 14*(10). https://doi.org/10.3390/cancers14102350, https://www.mdpi.com/2072-6694/14/10/2350/pdf?version=1652170913.

Zhu, Z., Shen, J., Ho, P. C.-L., Hu, Y., Ma, Z., & Wang, L. (2025). Transforming cancer treatment: Integrating patient-derived organoids and CRISPR screening for precision medicine. *Frontiers in Pharmacology, 16*. https://doi.org/10.3389/fphar.2025.1563198.

CHAPTER 12

Future outlook: Anticipating trends and opportunities in the AI-driven pharmaceutical industry

Miltiadis Lytras[1] and Patricia Ordonez de Pablos[2]

[1]*Computer Science Department, College of Engineering, Effat University, Jeddah, Saudi Arabia,* [2]*Department of Business Administration, The University of Oviedo, Oviedo, Spain*

12.1 Introducing Pharma 2040: vision and strategic imperatives

By the year 2040, the pharmaceutical industry will have undergone a radical transformation shaped by artificial intelligence (AI), data-driven innovation, and a relentless focus on personalized, preventive, and precision healthcare. This evolution, while built on decades of innovation, will represent a structural break from traditional pharma models. Rather than functioning in isolated, linear pipelines, future-proof pharmaceutical organizations will operate as agile, integrated, and intelligent ecosystems (Argiyantari et al., 2020; Della Corte et al., 2022; Harrer et al., 2023; Hull & Coutts, 2021; Tantray et al., 2025).

The Pharma 2040 vision is shaped by five strategic shifts that redefine how value is created across the lifecycle:

- **AI as an operating capability (not a tool):** AI is embedded in discovery, development, manufacturing, safety, regulatory intelligence, and commercial decision-making—shifting pharma from episodic analysis to continuous learning and optimization.
- **Personalization becomes the default standard of care:** Genomics, biomarkers, real-world evidence, and longitudinal patient data enable precision stratification, adaptive dosing, and therapy pathways designed for individuals and micro-populations.
- **Platforms replace pipelines:** Competitive advantage moves from linear stage-gate execution to ecosystem orchestration—integrating diagnostics, therapeutics, patient services, and outcome tracking through interoperable platforms.
- **Compliance becomes predictive and continuous:** Pharmacovigilance, quality, and regulatory submissions evolve into real-time systems powered by AI, automation, and validated real-world evidence—reducing lag while strengthening transparency and safety.

The Future of Pharma Across All Sectors in the Artificial Intelligence Era. DOI: https://doi.org/10.1016/B978-0-443-40572-3.00010-1

- **Responsible innovation becomes the license to scale:** Trust, equity, sustainability, and explainability shift from "nice-to-have" principles to operational requirements—shaping adoption, partnerships, reimbursement, and societal legitimacy.

Taken together, these shifts signal a structural break from traditional pharma models: Future leaders will compete on learning speed, governance maturity, and measurable patient outcomes—not volume alone.

12.1.1 Strategic imperatives for Pharma 2040

The road to Pharma 2040 is paved with complexity, requiring forward-looking organizations to develop and adopt a new set of strategic imperatives:

- **Reinvent business models:** Shift from volume to outcomes and value-based contracting.
- **Build data-centric operating models:** Invest in interoperable data foundations, federated learning, and AI governance.
- **Develop digital-ready talent:** Scale AI literacy, ethics, clinical informatics, and cross-functional teams.
- **Institutionalize collaboration:** Embed startup, academia, regulator, and patient partnerships into the innovation ecosystem to accelerate responsible AI adoption and sustainable value creation.

Table 12.1 outlines the five foundational pillars that define the Pharma 2040 transformation. These are not abstract aspirations, but actionable goals driving innovation strategies in forward-thinking organizations. AI integration, for example, is already visible in the accelerating timelines for drug discovery, with platforms like AlphaFold and IBM Watson Health paving the way. Precision medicine is making its mark in oncology and in rare diseases therapeuticst through deep phenotyping and genomic analytics. Ethical innovation—long considered aspirational—has become operational through access-oriented licensing models and environmental stewardship in pharmaceutical production.

Table 12.1 Pillars of the Pharma 2040 vision.

Pillar	Description
AI integration	Use of AI in R&D, clinical trials, and manufacturing
Precision medicine	Patient-specific treatment pathways using genomics and biomarkers
Digital platforms	Ecosystems for data, collaboration and remote clinical engagement
Predictive compliance	Real-time pharmacovigilance and adaptive regulatory strategies
Ethical and sustainable impact	Inclusion, equity, access and ecological sustainability

Source: AI, Artificial intelligence; *R&D*, research and development.

As we set the scene for Pharma 2040, it becomes evident that technological innovation alone will not suffice. True transformation will require a holistic reimagining of the entire pharmaceutical value chain. In the following section, we explore the detailed structure and the key phases of this value chain, including research, development, manufacturing, and post-marketing surveillance. Understanding the internal mechanisms of pharmaceutical processes is critical for evaluating how AI and digital transformation can generate tangible improvements in efficiency, transparency, and outcomes.

12.2 Strategic foresight: ten core scenarios across the pharma industry

The future of the pharmaceutical industry will be defined by how effectively it adapts to a convergence of transformative forces—Artificial intelligence (AI), digitization, regulatory evolution, patient empowerment, and sustainability imperatives. In preparing for Pharma 2040, it is critical to project strategic foresight into plausible, actionable scenarios which shape investment priorities and innovation pipelines (Artico et al., 2022; Ghodke et al., 2023; Harrer et al., 2023).

The Pharma 2040 North Star: Seven Non-Negotiables for AI-Driven Pharma

Core insight: Pharma 2040 leaders will not win by "using AI." They will win by building **AI-governed, outcome-driven learning systems** that scale trust, equity, and resilience.

Seven non-negotiables (executive test)

Outcome first: AI investments must be tied to clinical outcomes and patient value—not efficiency alone.

Data as a regulated asset: Treat data pipelines, models, and real-world evidence as controlled, auditable assets (good practice-grade).

Human accountability by design: Clarify decision rights; what AI recommends, what humans approve, how exceptions may escalate.

Interoperability as strategy: Platforms must connect research and development (R&D), trials, manufacturing, safety, and access—without any silos.

Bias, drift, and misuse readiness: Continuous monitoring for bias and model drift; safeguards against misuse are built-in, rather than- added to later.

Resilience built into the architecture: Distributed operations, stress-tested supply chains, and digital twins ensure continuity under shocks.

Ethics and equity as competitive advantage: Trust, inclusion, and access are not constraints; they are prerequisites for scalability and legitimacy.

Executive takeaway: If an initiative fails two or more of these nonnegotiables, it is not "Pharma 2040-ready"—it is a tech pilot.

Below, we present **ten core scenarios** that represent high-impact areas across the pharmaceutical value chain. These scenarios are not merely trends—they are directional blueprints for organizational readiness and opportunity assessment. Each scenario addresses a specific frontier where digital transformation and AI are projected to create disruptive and strategic shifts in capabilities, services, and outcomes.

12.2.1 Callout

Table 12.2 summarizes the ten strategic scenarios for Pharma 2040, structured across their key drivers, expected outcomes, and required enablers. This table can serve as a foresight map for executives, researchers, and regulators planning for long-term sustainability and innovation in the industry.

From scenarios to strategic action

While the ten scenarios outlined above describe plausible futures for Pharma 2040, their real value lies in how they guide **strategic prioritization and execution today**. These scenarios are not predictions; they are decision lenses. Organizations that treat them merely as trend narratives, risk fragmentation and slower adaptation. In contrast, future-ready pharma firms are those who translate scenarios into **tangible investments, governance choices, and portfolio bets**.

Three principles help convert foresight into action:

First, not all scenarios require equal investment. Leading organizations select 3–4 scenarios that best align with their core assets, therapeutic focus, regulatory exposure, and market sizet. For example, a firm with strong real-world evidence infrastructure may prioritize digital-first clinical trials and predictive pharmacovigilance, while a manufacturing-centric organization may emphasize autonomous production and sustainable supply chains.

Second, scenarios should be sequenced, not pursued in parallel. Attempting to address all futures simultaneously creates dilution. Effective strategies establish a clear sequencing logic—building foundational data and governance capabilities first, followed by advanced AI applications and ecosystem orchestration. This sequencing reduces execution risk while preserving options.

Third, scenarios must be owned by leadership, not functions. Strategic foresight fails when scenarios are delegated to innovation units without executive sponsorship. Each prioritized scenario should have accountable leadership, measurable milestones, and explicit links to investment planning, talent acquisition, and regulatory engagement.

In this sense, scenarios act as **alignment mechanisms**—connecting vision, capability development, and operational execution across the enterprise.

This foresight framework provides both strategic clarity and operational depth. For example, scenario 2 (Digital-First Clinical Trials) leverages AI and RWD (real-world data) to not only decentralize trials, but they also make them more inclusive and globally scalable. Similarly,

Table 12.2 Strategic scenarios for Pharma 2040.

#	Scenario	Key drivers	Expected outcomes	Core enablers
1	AI-enabled precision medicine	Genomic AI, wearables, patient data	Hyper-personalized therapies and dosage optimization	Interoperable data, regulatory frameworks
2	Digital-first clinical trials	Decentralized trials, RWD, e-consent	Faster, inclusive, and cost-effective clinical research	Remote tools, patient engagement platforms
3	Autonomous pharma manufacturing	Robotics, IoT, predictive AI	Smart factories, minimal wasteand reduced time-to-market	Digital twins, edge computing
4	Real-time pharmacovigilance	AI NLP, social listening, EHR mining	Early safety signal detection and regulatory transparency	AI dashboards, integrated data pipelines
5	AI-augmented drug repurposing	Machine learning, literature mining	Discovery of new indications for existing molecules	High-throughput screening, AI inference engines
6	Dynamic value-based pricing	Predictive modeling, outcome tracking	Pricing tied to patient outcomes and pay-for-performance models	Blockchain, payor-provider integration
7	Sustainable pharma supply chains	ESG frameworks, lifecycle analytics	Carbon-neutral operations and ethical sourcing	Circular economy principles, green chemistry
8	Regulatory co-innovation hubs	Digital sandboxing, agile compliance	Continuous approval models and reduced regulatory lag	Regulatory partnerships, AI simulation tools
9	AI-enabled patient support systems	AI chatbots, digital health coaches	Improved adherence, real-time feedbackand patient outcomes	Conversational AI, wearable integrations
10	Workforce of the future in pharma	Hybrid roles, digital talent	Agile, AI-literate, cross-functional pharma teams	Lifelong learning, microcredential programs

Source: AI, Artificial intelligence; *EHR*, electronic health records, *IOT*, Internet of Things, *NLP*, natural language processing.

scenario 6 reflects the growing momentum toward **value-based pricing**, where AI can track treatment outcomes and dynamically adjust prices based on clinical merit.

In scenario 7, the industry aligns with the global push for sustainability, where **green chemistry** and supply chain optimization will no longer be optional but critical to investor confidence and global regulatory compliance. Finally, scenario 10 addresses the **transformation of the pharmaceutical workforce**, where job roles will increasingly require fluency in data science, AI ethics, and interdisciplinary collaboration.

Table 12.3 translates these scenarios into a strategic matrix connecting each scenario with specific capabilities and innovation areas. This allows organizations to prioritize investments, develop roadmaps, and ensure internal alignment across R&D, marketing, regulatory, and operations.

Table 12.3 acts as a **capability roadmap** that pharma executives can use for strategic planning and workforce development. It reinforces the importance of not only recognizing what changes are coming but also how to prepare and operationalize those changes through investment in people, platforms, and governance.

Table 12.3 Mapping future scenarios to core capabilities and innovation domains.

Scenario	Strategic capabilities	Innovation focus areas
AI-enabled precision medicine	Data governance, algorithm validation	Digital biomarkers, N-of-1 trials
Digital-first clinical trials	Virtual trial design, remote monitoring	Patient stratification, eSource data
Autonomous pharma manufacturing	Robotics integration, process AI	Smart batch processing, quality-by-design (QbD)
Real-time pharmacovigilance	NLP models, adverse event tracking	Automated signal detection, real-world safety dashboards
AI-augmented drug repurposing	Knowledge graphs, ML models	Computational drug discovery, repurposing pipelines
Dynamic value-based pricing	Economic modeling, payer alignment	Outcome-based contracts, digital ledgers
Sustainable pharma supply chains	ESG analytics, lifecycle assessment	Clean production technologies, smart packaging
Regulatory co-innovation hubs	Digital twins for trials, risk modeling	Simulation-based regulation, adaptive licensing
AI-enabled patient support systems	Conversational interfaces, mobile health	Personalized education, feedback loops
Workforce of the future in pharma	Talent analytics, digital literacy programs	Interdisciplinary teams, virtual learning academies

Source: AI, Artificial intelligence; *ML*, machine learning.

Executive Lens: How to Use Pharma 2040 Scenarios

Do not ask: "Which scenario will happen?"

Ask instead:

Which scenarios expose our greatest strategic vulnerability?

Which scenarios amplify our existing strengths?

Which capabilities appear across multiple scenarios and therefore justify early investment?

Where does inaction create irreversible disadvantage?

Executive takeaway: In Pharma 2040, advantage belongs to organizations that prepare for *multiple futures* while committing decisively to a *small number of strategic paths*.

The scenarios and capabilities described above signal the critical need for cohesive transformation. They paint a compelling vision of the future pharma enterprise: one that is intelligent, adaptive, sustainable, and purpose-driven. To realize this future, companies must implement a deliberate, structured roadmap that connects aspirations with systems and execution. This roadmap and its enabling pillars are the focus of the next section.

12.3 A strategic roadmap for AI-driven pharma

12.3.1 Reframing the roadmap: from artificial intelligence adoption to governed transformation

The strategic roadmap for AI-driven pharma should not be interpreted as a technology deployment plan. Rather, it represents a governance-led transformation of how decisions are made, risks are managed, and value is created across the pharmaceutical enterprise. In highly regulated, high-stakes environments such as pharma, artificial intelligence does not create advantage by speed alone—but by **trustworthy integration into operating models, accountability structures, and regulatory-grade processes**.

Consequently, the roadmap presented in this section is best understood as an **enterprise transformation framework**, where technology enablement follows governance clarity, human accountability, and organizational readiness. Firms that reverse this logic—deploying AI before establishing decision rights, ethical safeguards, and cross-functional ownership—are likely to encounter resistance, regulatory friction, and erosion of trust.

The transformation of the pharmaceutical industry through artificial intelligence is not a one-time initiative—it requires a **structured roadmap** that encompasses systems innovation, workforce readiness, ethical governance, and product development. For future-proofing pharma operations, AI must be adopted through a **phased, strategic approach** that aligns with regulatory expectations, market needs, and organizational capabilities.

This roadmap unfolds in three dimensions:

- **Technology systems and infrastructure**
- **Talent and organizational culture**
- **Products, services, and process innovation**

Each phase builds on foundational elements and advances toward a comprehensive AI-integrated business model. The following narrative explains these dimensions and culminates in a detailed roadmap table.

12.3.2 Technology systems and infrastructure

To begin with, organizations must **digitally mature** their infrastructure before they can scale AI deployment. This means transitioning from siloed databases to **interoperable platforms** that integrate clinical, operational, and commercial data streams. Cloud computing, data lakes, blockchain for traceability, and advanced cybersecurity protocols are essential prerequisites.

Moreover, AI applications—such as **natural language processing (NLP)**, machine learning (ML), and computer vision—must be embedded within systems that support end-to-end value chain integration, from R&D and production to supply chain and pharmacovigilance.

Importantly, infrastructure decisions in Pharma 2040 are governance decisions: they determine traceability, auditability, explainability, and ultimately regulatory confidence in AI-supported outcomes.

12.3.3 Talent and organizational culture

The second pillar is developing a digitally literate, AI-ready workforce. Pharma companies must cultivate roles such as **clinical data scientists**, **AI ethics officers**, and **digital transformation leads**. Additionally, reskilling existing teams in areas like data analytics, automation tools, and agile management is nonnegotiable.

In this context, talent readiness is not defined by technical proficiency alone, but by the organization's ability to assign responsibility, interpret AI outputs critically, and uphold ethical judgment in decision-making.

Organizations must move toward a culture of **continuous learning**, foster experimentation, and embrace failure as a form of iterative progress. Knowledge-sharing platforms, mentorship programs, and cross-functional innovation labs are foundational enablers.

12.3.4 Product, services, and process innovation

AI is not simply a back-office function—it is a **value driver** for novel products, services, and patient-centered delivery models. AI can dramatically shorten drug discovery cycles, enable adaptive clinical trials, and automate adverse event reporting. Meanwhile, **new digital products** like virtual coaches, adherence apps, and personalized dosing algorithms are redefining patient engagement and loyalty.

To navigate this future, the strategic roadmap must also prioritize **interoperability**, **scalability**, and **regulatory agility** to handle evolving compliance requirements.

12.3.4.1 Callout

Table 12.4 outlines a **strategic roadmap** for AI integration in the pharmaceutical industry. It breaks down stages of maturity and identifies key actions, focus areas, and investment priorities for each phase.

Read vertically rather than horizontally, Table 17.4 reveals a critical insight: as organizations move toward transformation, **governance intensity increases alongside technological autonomy**. The more decisions AI systems influence, the greater the need for ethical oversight, explainability, and institutional accountability. This progression underscores why AI maturity in pharma must be evaluated not only by capability depth, but by governance readiness.

This roadmap shows a **realistic progression** that organizations can follow, recognizing that digital maturity and cultural transformation do not happen overnight. In the foundation phase, organizations must invest in **baseline digital readiness** and attract AI-savvy talent. As we move toward the optimization and transformation phases, pharma firms are expected to deliver not just efficiency gains but **entirely new patient value propositions**. Moreover, the

Table 12.4 Strategic roadmap for AI-driven pharma (2025–40).

Phase	Focus areas	Key actions	Investment priorities
Foundation (2025–27)	Data governance, digitization, pilot AI projects	Develop unified data architecture, launch pilot projects	Cloud platforms, cybersecurity, talent acquisition
Integration (2027–30)	End-to-end AI integration, RPA, decision support	Deploy AI in R&D, supply chain, pharmacovigilance	NLP tools, ML algorithms, system interoperability
Optimization (2030–35)	AI-driven innovation, predictive analytics	Launch AI-designed products, value-based contracts, adaptive trials	Predictive AI, AI-enabled CRM, digital twin applications
Transformation (2035–40)	Autonomous operations, AI strategy at core	Establish AI ethics boards, continuous feedback loops	Ethical AI governance, generative AI, lifelong learning

Source: AI, Artificial intelligence; *R&D,* research and development.

transformation phase incorporates **autonomous decision-making systems**, enabling companies to manage supply chain interruptions, predict adverse events, and recommend treatment adjustments in real-time. Strategic investments in this final phase should focus on AI safety, **explainable AI (XAI)**, and social impact alignment.

The outlined roadmap underscores that success in Pharma 2040 will not stem from incremental progress alone. It will require **bold leadership**, long-term vision, and an unwavering commitment to ethical, human-centric innovation. In the next section, we explore how the pharma industry can translate this roadmap into real-world opportunities by aligning technological capabilities with new business models and patient-centric strategies.

Product and service innovation in Pharma 2040, therefore, becomes inseparable from governance design, as every AI-enabled offering embeds assumptions about accountability, consent, risk tolerance, and societal impact.

12.4 Unlocking opportunities: innovation, capabilities, and value-driven pharma

As the pharmaceutical industry advances into the AI-driven era, a paradigm shift is underway—one that redefines how value is created, how care is delivered, and how organizations evolve. No longer can pharmaceutical firms rely solely on legacy pipelines and traditional operating models (Basit, 2020; Dupuy et al., 2024; Gelis et al., 2023; Hong et al., 2024; Ladner et al., 2025; Malheiro et al., 2023; Mirzaei & Rijcken, 2023; Pörtner et al., 2025; Seewald et al., 2020). The future belongs to those who can proactively identify opportunities, align them with core capabilities, and implement AI-powered solutions to address both patient needs and business goals.

This section maps out the **strategic opportunity landscape** of the pharmaceutical sector and presents how organizations can leverage **artificial intelligence**, **advanced analytics**, and **digital transformation** to create **scalable, high-impact innovations**. The aim is to enable a **future-proof pharmaceutical ecosystem**—resilient, adaptive, and deeply aligned with the principles of personalized, efficient, and ethical care (Steinwandter et al., 2019; Taifa & Nzowa, 2025; Tantray et al., 2025; Wang et al., 2024; Williams et al., 2022; Wölfle et al., 2025; Xu et al., 2022; Yoshiura, Kawata and Sengoku, 2025).

12.4.1 Strategic opportunity domains in the AI-driven pharma

Below are key opportunity domains where AI integration can transform processes, elevate outcomes, and foster long-term sustainability:

12.4.1.1 Precision medicine and individualized therapies

- Enable tailored drug development based on patient genotypes and phenotypes
- Accelerate treatment matching through predictive diagnostics and biomarker discovery
- Enhance efficacy while minimizing adverse effects via adaptive dosing algorithms

12.4.1.2 Smart clinical development

- Use AI to design optimized protocols and simulate trial outcomes
- Automate patient screening and recruitment with electronic health data integration
- Monitor trial adherence and safety in real-time using wearable and Internet of Things technologies

12.4.1.3 AI-augmented drug discovery and preclinical testing

- Reduce R&D cycle times with deep learning algorithms for molecule screening
- Predict pharmacokinetics and toxicity profiles computationally before lab testing
- Identify repurposing candidates using large-scale knowledge graphs and AI reasoning

12.4.1.4 Intelligent manufacturing and supply chain operations

- Forecast demand and detect bottlenecks using AI-powered supply chain analytics
- Implement predictive maintenance in manufacturing to reduce downtime
- Apply real-time quality control systems based on computer vision and pattern recognition

12.4.1.5 Next-generation pharmacovigilance and regulatory intelligence

- Automate adverse event detection from unstructured data sources (e.g., social media, EMRs)
- Use NLP tools to analyze regulatory updates and support compliance documentation
- Identify safety signals early and suggest remedial actions with AI-based models

12.4.1.6 Digital therapeutics and patient engagement platforms

- Deliver behavioral therapies and disease management solutions through AI-powered apps
- Personalize content delivery and reminders to improve adherence and satisfaction
- Collect patient-reported outcomes and integrate them into continuous care loops

12.4.1.7 Health economics and market access (HEOR)

- Model cost-effectiveness using real-world evidence and predictive modeling
- Support pricing decisions with simulations of treatment uptake and population impact
- Identify market gaps and optimize portfolio strategies through AI-driven insights

12.4.1.8 Workforce transformation and digital talent development

- Reskill employees to embrace AI workflows, agile methodologies, and interdisciplinary roles

- Foster a culture of innovation and collaboration across silos
- Promote leadership in data science, regulatory innovation, and translational medicine

12.4.2 Building AI-enabled capabilities

To capitalize on the aforementioned opportunity domains, organizations must develop **capabilities in four key dimensions**:

12.4.2.1 Technological capabilities

- Invest in cloud infrastructure, AI platforms, and high-performance computing
- Build data lakes with structured and unstructured data for multi-modal analytics
- Ensure robust cybersecurity, data interoperability, and regulatory-grade auditability

12.4.2.2 Human capabilities

- Attract and retain AI-savvy talent, including data scientists, bioinformaticians, and digital strategists
- Foster interdisciplinary collaboration among clinicians, engineers, and commercial teams
- Upskill traditional functions (e.g., regulatory, R&D, manufacturing) with digital literacy

12.4.2.3 Organizational capabilities

- Create agile governance frameworks for responsible AI innovation
- Integrate AI into decision-making across the enterprise
- Adopt open innovation ecosystems with startups, academia, and regulators

12.4.2.4 Strategic vision and alignment

- Link AI and digital health investments to long-term value creation
- Anticipate disruptions and adapt business models accordingly
- Embed ethical, inclusive, and patient-centered principles at the core of every strategy

12.4.3 Concluding thoughts for the road ahead

The real promise of AI in pharma is not simply automation or cost savings—it lies in **unlocking previously inaccessible forms of value**, accelerating scientific breakthroughs, and transforming the relationship between industry and society. Pharma companies that embrace this vision will not only improve health outcomes but also redefine the boundaries of what is possible in life sciences.

As we now move into the strategic roadmap of transition (Section 5), we will examine how these innovations and capabilities must be embedded in a comprehensive framework that balances investment, risk, and impact to shape the **Pharma 2040** vision.

12.5 Embracing patient-centric pharma and the social impact of artificial intelligence

12.5.1 From technological progress to leadership responsibility

By 2040, patient-centricity will no longer be a differentiating aspiration—it will be a leadership obligation. As artificial intelligence reshapes discovery, development, and delivery, pharmaceutical organizations will be judged not only by innovation outcomes but by how responsibly, equitably, and transparently those outcomes are achieved. This section, therefore, reframes patient-centric pharma not as a design preference, but as a **governance mandate**, requiring deliberate leadership choices across strategy, ethics, and organizational culture.

The pharmaceutical industry is undergoing a historic transition—one that pivots from being primarily **product-centered** to becoming **deeply patient-centric**. In this evolution, **AI** is not only a driver of operational excellence and R&D acceleration but also a **powerful enabler of human-centered care**. Section 5 brings the chapter to a thoughtful conclusion by exploring how future pharmaceutical systems can be reshaped to prioritize **health equity**, **accessibility**, **inclusivity**, and **long-term societal wellbeing**.

12.5.2 The rise of the empowered patient

In the emerging healthcare ecosystem, patients are no longer passive recipients of care—they are **informed, proactive stakeholders** with access to data, digital tools, and personalized health solutions. The convergence of AI and pharma has opened up new avenues for:

- **Personalized care pathways**: AI algorithms synthesize genetic, lifestyle, and behavioral data to design treatment plans optimized for individual needs.
- **Real-time monitoring**: Wearables and remote diagnostic tools enable ongoing health tracking and early intervention strategies.
- **Patient education and communication**: Chatbots and AI-powered interfaces support multilingual, accessible engagement with patients and caregivers.
- **Shared decision-making**: Digital tools empower patients to participate actively in treatment decisions, improving adherence and satisfaction.

This shift demands a redesign of business models and value propositions to **focus on long-term outcomes** rather than short-term profit. In Pharma 2040, empowering patients is not an optional engagement strategy—it is a prerequisite for legitimacy, trust, and sustained value creation.

12.5.3 Artificial intelligence for social good and global health equity

While digital transformation brings efficiency and innovation, it must also serve as a vehicle for **bridging systemic inequities** in global healthcare access. Pharma companies, especially those with AI capabilities, can play a critical role by:

- Developing **affordable AI-enabled diagnostics** for underserved communities.
- Using **predictive analytics** to anticipate health crises in vulnerable regions.
- Partnering with governments to improve supply chain resilience and medication availability.
- Participating in **global data-sharing initiatives** for emerging diseases and epidemiological monitoring.

Failure to apply AI capabilities toward equity and access will increasingly be interpreted not as oversight, but as strategic neglect. Pharma's responsibility goes beyond delivering medications—it includes supporting **inclusive healthcare systems** and **public health preparedness** worldwide.

12.5.4 Safeguarding ethics, trust, and transparency

As AI becomes further embedded in the decision-making frameworks of pharma companies, **ethical safeguards** must keep pace. A patient-centric, AI-driven pharma industry requires:

- **Transparent algorithms** and explainable decision-making.
- **Bias mitigation protocols** in training data and model development.
- **Informed consent** procedures adapted to AI-assisted care.
- **Compliance with evolving international regulations** (e.g., EU AI Act, Health Insurance Portability and Accountability Act, General Data Protection Regulation).

The success of AI in pharma hinges not only on its technical performance but also on **societal trust**. Pharma leaders must prioritize **governance frameworks** and **AI ethics boards** which align innovation with humanity. Trust, once lost through opaque or biased AI systems, will be nearly impossible to restore in data-driven healthcare ecosystems.

12.5.5 Human-AI collaboration and the role of knowledge officers

AI does not replace people—it enhances their capabilities. Pharma organizations must empower:

- **Knowledge officers and clinical data stewards** to curate and contextualize AI-driven insights.
- **Patient advocates and community health specialists** to mediate between digital tools and real-world needs.
- **Ethics committees and AI governance experts** to shape responsible innovation pathways.

The human touch remains essential—particularly in **complex diagnoses, empathy-driven care, and health communication**. Pharma 2040 must be built on the **partnership between advanced technology and compassionate expertise**. The most advanced Pharma 2040 organizations will be those that formalize human judgment as a governance asset—rather than treating it as a residual control.

12.5.5.1 Leadership mandate for Pharma 2040

The future of the pharmaceutical industry will not be determined by algorithms, platforms, or automation alone. It will be determined by leadership choices—about where intelligence is applied, how responsibility is assigned, and whose interests are prioritized when trade-offs arise. Pharma 2040 demands leaders who can govern complexity, align innovation with societal trust, and ensure that technological power translates into human benefit. In this context, neutrality is not possible: organizations will either actively shape a responsible AI-driven future—or passively inherit its risks.

This chapter has outlined the **scenarios, strategies, and systems** that will define pharma in the AI era. But it is ultimately the **alignment of vision, ethics, and execution** that will determine whether the future of pharma becomes an **engine of equity and empowerment**—or a missed opportunity. The choice is ours to make, and the time is now.

12.5.5.2 Key takeaways for executives, policymakers, and innovation leaders

This chapter advances a clear message: **Pharma 2040 will reward organizations that govern intelligence—not merely deploy it**. Based on the foresight scenarios, strategic roadmaps, and ethical considerations explored, the following takeaways summarize the non-negotiable priorities for leadership:

AI is now a core strategic actor in pharma, not a support tool. Artificial intelligence will increasingly influence discovery, clinical decisions, manufacturing, pricing, and patient engagement. Leaders must therefore treat AI as part of the enterprise decision architecture, with explicit accountability, auditability, and escalation mechanisms.

Patient-centricity has evolved into a governance mandate. By 2040, organizations that fail to embed patient empowerment, transparency, and shared decision-making into digital systems will lose trust, legitimacy, and long-term relevance.

Resilience and adaptability outweigh efficiency as sources of advantage. Pharma firms optimized only for speed or cost will struggle in an era defined by uncertainty, shocks, and regulatory scrutiny. Resilient operating models—supported by AI, digital twins, and platform ecosystems—will define sustainable leadership.

Ethical AI is a strategic differentiator, not a compliance burden. Explainability, bias mitigation, and responsible data stewardship will directly influence regulatory approval, public trust, and ecosystem partnerships. Ethics-by-design enables scale; ethics-by-exception erodes it.

Talent, culture, and governance determine AI value realization. Technology investments alone are insufficient. Organizations must develop AI-literate leadership, interdisciplinary teams, and new roles (e.g., Knowledge Officers, AI Stewards) that translate intelligence into responsible action.

The future of pharma is platform-based and ecosystem-driven. Competitive advantage will increasingly come from orchestrating ecosystems—connecting data, partners, regulators, and patients—rather than owning isolated assets or linear pipelines.

Executive Brief: What Leaders Must Do Now to Be Ready for Pharma 2040

Core message

Pharma 2040 readiness is not about predicting technologies—it is about **designing organizations capable of governing continuous change**.

Six essential leadership actions:

1. **Adopt AI governance at the board level:** AI strategy, risk, and ethics must be overseen at the highest level. Boards should treat AI systems as regulated assets with defined ownership, performance thresholds, and accountability structures.
2. **Redesign decision rights for human–AI collaboration:** Clarify which decisions AI can recommend, which require human approval, and how responsibility is assigned when outcomes diverge. Any ambiguity riskssystemic errors.
3. **Invest in data as a public-interest capability:** Operationalize FAIR principles, ensure interoperability, and treat patient data as a stewardship responsibility—not a proprietary weapon.
4. **Align innovation incentives with outcomes, not volume:** Shift key performance indicators from speed and throughput toward patient outcomes, equity, trust, and long-term societal impact.
5. **Prepare the workforce for cognitive partnership:** Develop leaders and teams capable of working *with* intelligent systems—interpreting uncertainty, challenging recommendations, and embedding ethical judgment into workflows.
6. **Engage regulatory bodies and members of society as partners:** Regulatory bodies, patients, healthcare professionals and public institutions must be partners in innovation. Continuous dialogue reduces friction and accelerates trustworthy adoption, while minimizing downstream obstacles.

Executive warning

Organizations that delay these actions will not fail due to lack of technological advancements k-—but rather due to -**lack of governance, accountability, and trust**.

Executive opportunity

Those who act early will shape standards, influence regulation, attract ecosystem partners, and define what "responsible pharma leadership" means in the AI era.

Learning activities: Exploring the future of AI-driven pharma

These learning activities are designed to engage students and professionals in a deeper understanding of the trends, technologies, and strategies shaping the pharmaceutical industry in the age of AI. They promote critical thinking, digital literacy, and strategic foresight.

1. **Short essay prompts**
   Choose one of the following topics and write a short essay (500–700 words) with a clear structure, referencing scholarly and industry sources:
   - **Topic A:** "The Role of Artificial Intelligence in Driving Personalized Medicine in Pharma by 2040"
   - **Topic B**: "How Can Pharma Companies Balance Innovation and Ethics in an AI-Driven Environment?"
   - **Topic C:** "Building AI-Enabled Drug Discovery Pipelines: Challenges and Opportunities"
2. **Use case studies**
   Case study: Decentralized clinical trials and AI
   PharmaCo, a mid-sized pharmaceutical company, is investing in AI tools to manage decentralized clinical trials. These tools include wearable monitoring devices, virtual patient dashboards, and predictive modeling to identify patient dropout risks.
   Discussion questions:
   - What advantages and risks come with using AI in decentralized trials?
   - How can PharmaCo ensure ethical data usage and compliance?
   - What strategies would improve patient adherence and trust?
3. **Digital research and navigation**
   Objective: Conduct guided internet research using the following resources and answer the questions below:
   Resources:
   - https://www.pharmavoice.com
   - https://aiin.healthcare
   - https://www.ema.europa.eu
   - https://www.fda.gov/drugs
   Tasks:
   - Find and summarize a recent AI innovation in pharmaceutical R&D.
   - Identify two regulatory policies affecting AI usage in clinical trials.
   - Explore one pharma startup using AI and describe its value proposition.
4. **Bloom's taxonomy-based activities**
   See Table 12.5

Table 12.5 Bloom's taxonomy-based activities.

Cognitive level	Activity
Remember	List 5 use cases of AI in pharma supply chains
Understand	Describe how AI improves predictive analytics for drug demand
Apply	Draft a patient engagement model using AI chatbots
Analyze	Compare AI applications in preclinical vs. post-market drug surveillance
Evaluate	Critique the current limitations of AI in regulatory compliance
Create	Design an AI-driven pharma service that targets underrepresented populations

5. Team activity: roadmap to Pharma 2040

Form teams and design a strategic roadmap for transforming a traditional pharmaceutical company into a digitally enabled, AI-driven, patient-centric enterprise by 2040. Include:

- Key technologies and capabilities
- Organizational structure
- Talent development and leadership
- Ethical and regulatory safeguards

Present the roadmap in class with a brief pitch (5–7 minutes).

References

Argiyantari, B., Simatupang, T. M., & Basri, M. H. (2020). Pharmaceutical supply chain transformation through application of the lean principle: A literature review. *Journal of Industrial Engineering and Management, 13*(3), 475–494. Available from: https://doi.org/10.3926/jiem.3100, http://jiem.org/index.php/jiem/article/download/3100/941.

Artico, F., Edge, A. L., & Langham, K. (2022). The future of artificial intelligence for the biotech big data landscape. *Current Opinion in Biotechnology, 76*. https://doi.org/10.1016/j.copbio.2022.102714 Available from: http://www.elsevier.com/locate/copbio.

Basit, A. (2020). Recent innovations in 3D-printed personalized medicines: An interview with Abdul Basit. *Journal of 3D Printing in Medicine, 4*(1), 5–7. https://doi.org/10.2217/3dp-2020-0010.

Della Corte, D., Young, N., & Della Corte, K. A. (2022). Delivering digital transformation with self-reporting data assets. *Lecture Notes in Networks and Systems, 358*, 975–985. springer.com/series/15179, 10.1007/978-3-030-89906-6_62.

Dupuy, S., Opincar, L., Pandya, K., Wnorowski, S., Cuellar, M., Riggins, J., & Hermes-DeSantis, E. R. (2024). An update from the benchmark survey of phactMI™ member companies on providing medical information in the digital space. *Therapeutic Innovation and Regulatory Science, 58*(1), 200–213. https://doi.org/10.1007/s43441-023-00587-1 Available from: https://www.springer.com/journal/43441.

Gelis, L., Stoeckert, I., & Podhaisky, H. P. (2023). Digital tools—Regulatory considerations for application in clinical trials. *Therapeutic Innovation and Regulatory Science, 57*(4), 769–782. https://doi.org/10.1007/s43441-023-00535-z Available from: https://www.springer.com/journal/43441.

Ghodke, P. K., Reddy, P. S., Akiti, N., & Kilari, H. (2023). Artificial intelligence in the digital chemical industry, its application and sustainability. In *Recent Trends and Best Practices in Industry 4.0*. India: River Publishers, 1–29 Available from: https://www.riverpublishers.com/book_details.php?book_id=1059.

Harrer, S., Menard, J., Rivers, M., Green, D. V. S., Karpiak, J., Jeliazkov, J. R., Shapovalov, M. V., del Alamo, D., & Sternke, M. C. (2023). Artificial intelligence drives the digital transformation of pharma. In *Artificial Intelligence in Clinical Practice: How AI Technologies Impact Medical Research and Clinics*. Australia: Elsevier, 345–372. Available from: https://www.sciencedirect.com/book/9780443156885 10.1016/B978-0-443-15688-5.00049-8.

Hong, J., Bae, E. Y., Lee, H. J., Lee, T. J., & Clarke, P. (2024). Values, challenges, and responses associated with high-priced potential cures: perspectives of diverse stakeholders in South Korea. *Cost Effectiveness and Resource Allocation, 22*(1). https://doi.org/10.1186/s12962-024-00527-2 Available from: https://resource-allocation.biomedcentral.com.

Hull, W., & Coutts, R. (2021). Pci pharma's digital transformation: Reaching new levels of customer experience. *Drug Development and Delivery, 21*(6), 66–69. Available from: www.drug-dev.com.

Ladner, T., Weh, C., Dhillon, A., Giffard, M., & Iacovelli, D. (2025). Data computation platform (DCP): Empowering pharma 4.0 innovation through GxP-compliant and scalable software platform enabling advanced data analytics and real-time process monitoring in regulated environments. *Journal of Intelligent Manufacturing*. https://doi.org/10.1007/s10845-025-02574-9.

Malheiro, V., Duarte, J., Veiga, F., & Mascarenhas-Melo, F. (2023). Exploiting pharma 4.0 technologies in the non-biological complex drugs manufacturing: Innovations and implications. *Pharmaceutics, 15*(11), 2545. https://doi.org/10.3390/pharmaceutics15112545.

Mirzaei, A., & Rijcken, C. (2023). *Pharmaceutical Care in Digital Revolution: Blending Digital with Human Innovation* (Second Edition). Australia: Elsevier, 1–383. Available from: https://www.sciencedirect.com/book/9780443133602 10.1016/C2020-0-03995-2.

Pörtner, L., Riel, A., Schmidt, B., Leclaire, M., & Möske, R. (2025). Data management maturity model—Process dimensions and capabilities to leverage data-driven organizations towards industry 5.0. *Applied System Innovation, 8*(2), 41. https://doi.org/10.3390/asi8020041.

Seewald, M. J., Plumb, J. M., Gutierrez, B., Liwing, J., Tepie, M. F., Hammer, M., LoCasale, R., Khosla, S., Yin, D., Pashos, C. L., & Nagy, M. (2020). Strengthening pharma's contract with society: The value of trusted partnerships between pharma and healthcare facilitated by real-world data. *Journal of Comparative Effectiveness Research, 9*(3), 155–159. https://doi.org/10.2217/cer-2019-0183 Available from: https://becarispublishing.com/loi/cer.

Steinwandter, V., Borchert, D., & Herwig, C. (2019). Data science tools and applications on the way to Pharma 4.0. *Drug Discovery Today, 24*(9), 1795–1805. https://doi.org/10.1016/j.drudis.2019.06.005.

Taifa, I. W. R., & Nzowa, J. S. (2025). Implementing supply chain management 4.0: Potential driving forces and strategies from an empirical study of pharmaceutical industries. *Engineering Reports, 7*(6). https://doi.org/10.1002/eng2.70190 Available from: https://onlinelibrary.wiley.com/journal/25778196.

Tantray, J., Mohseen, S., Nazir Wani, S., Yusuf, J. B., Prajapati, R., & Pandey (2025). *Pharma Products Transformation Through Computer Vision (CV) and Internet of Everything (IoE) Computer Vision and Internet of Everything (IoE) for Societal Needs*. India: IGI Global, 241–265. Available from https://www.igi-global.com/book/computer-vision-internet-everything-ioe/350190, 10.4018/979-8-3693-8272-1.ch012.

Wang, Z., Tang, S., Guo, G., Yang, Y., He, D., Yang, L., Han, M., & Hou, Y. (2024). Adaptive quality control with uncertainty for a pharmaceutical cyber-physical system based on data and knowledge integration. *IEEE Transactions on Industrial Informatics, 20*(3), 3339–3350. https://doi.org/10.1109/tii.2023.3306355.

Williams, C., Kobashi, N., & Weber, N. (2022). Meeting an unmet pharma need: Pioneering the way to a connected future. *ONdrugDelivery, 2022*(134), 55–59 Available from: https://www.ondrugdelivery.com/wp-content/uploads/2022/06/134_2022_Jun_Connectivity_SHL_Medical.pdf.

Wölfle, R., Saur-Amaral, I., & Teixeira, L. (2025). Information model for pharmaceutical smart factory equipment design. *Information (Switzerland), 16*(5). https://doi.org/10.3390/info16050412 Available from: http://www.mdpi.com/journal/information/.

Xu, Q., Ahmadi, E., Amini, A., Rus, D., & Lo, A. W. (2022). Identifying and mitigating potential biases in predicting drug approvals. *Drug Safety, 45*(5), 521–533. https://doi.org/10.1007/s40264-022-01160-9 Available from: https://www.springer.com/journal/40264.

Yoshiura, H., Kawata, Y., & Sengoku, S. (2025). Open innovation and regulatory challenges in new modality development: The pivotal role of contract development and manufacturing organisations in advancing antibody drugs. *Therapeutic Innovation & Regulatory Science, 59*(1), 63–70. https://doi.org/10.1007/s43441-024-00701-x.

CHAPTER 13

The role of artificial intelligence in transforming clinical research and evidence generation

Miltiadis Lytras[1] and Chaido-Charalampia Lytra[2]

[1]*Computer Science Department, College of Engineering, Effat University, Jeddah, Saudi Arabia,*
[2]*Medical School, University of Patras, Patras, Greece*

13.1 Introduction: why AI is reshaping clinical research and evidence

Clinical research and evidence generation are undergoing a structural transformation driven by artificial intelligence (AI). This change is not simply the adoption of new software tools; it reflects a deeper shift in how evidence is designed, produced, interpreted, and translated into clinical and regulatory decisions. Traditionally, clinical research relied on a relatively linear pipeline: define a protocol, recruit participants, collect data, analyze results, and publish findings—often over several years. While this model has produced foundational medical advances, it also suffers from persistent limitations: high costs, long cycle times, operational inefficiencies, limited generalizability, and challenges in recruiting diverse populations. In parallel, healthcare systems now generate unprecedented volumes of data through electronic health records (EHRs), imaging, genomics, connected devices, and patient-reported outcomes. AI's capacity to synthesize high-dimensional information and learn predictive patterns from complex datasets positions it as a central enabler of modern clinical research.

The core contribution of AI is that it expands what is feasible in both scale and speed. In a conventional trial environment, many decisions are constrained by human bandwidth: manual chart review, protocol feasibility checks, patient matching, monitoring, and data cleaning. AI-enabled analytics can automate and augment these activities, reducing latency and improving consistency. For example, natural language processing (NLP) can interpret eligibility criteria and map them to structured and unstructured EHR information, accelerating the identification of eligible participants. Machine learning (ML) can forecast recruitment rates, screen failure risk, and site performance. Predictive models can detect missingness or anomalies in trial data streams early, supporting faster corrective action. These capabilities collectively improve operational resilience and reduce the high frequency of delays, amendments, and costly trial inefficiencies.

The Future of Pharma Across All Sectors in the Artificial Intelligence Era. DOI: https://doi.org/10.1016/B978-0-443-40572-3.00006-X

Beyond operational acceleration, AI changes the epistemology of evidence generation—how we build and justify conclusions. Evidence has historically been dominated by randomized controlled trials (RCTs), which remain the gold standard for causal inference. Yet RCTs face increasing pressure in a world of rare diseases, precision medicine, and rapidly evolving interventions where traditional trial designs may be impractical, slow, or ethically complex. AI facilitates alternative evidence strategies, including the use of real-world evidence (RWE) derived from clinical practice data, as well as the construction of external or synthetic control arms where suitable. AI also supports adaptive and platform trials, enabling trial designs that learn and evolve during execution. These approaches do not replace randomization as a principle; rather, they extend the evidence toolkit and allow research programs to answer more nuanced questions in shorter timeframes under controlled governance.

AI's impact is particularly visible at the intersection of clinical research and evidence translation. Evidence is not created for publication alone; it must inform regulators, clinicians, payers, and ultimately patient care. AI can enhance this translation by supporting more granular subgroup analyses, improving risk stratification, and identifying biomarkers that predict response or adverse outcomes. In oncology, cardiology, and immunology, for instance, multimodal modeling integrating imaging, molecular signatures, and longitudinal clinical trajectories is increasingly essential to understand heterogeneity in treatment response. AI methods help uncover latent patterns that can be overlooked by conventional statistical approaches, particularly when interactions are complex and non-linear. When governed appropriately, such insights can strengthen precision medicine and improve the alignment between research findings and real-world patient outcomes.

At the same time, AI introduces a set of challenges that are not optional to address. The most visible challenge is transparency and accountability. Many advanced AI models—especially deep learning systems—are perceived as "black boxes," producing outputs without clear explanations. In high-stakes clinical research, decisions must be traceable: why a patient was flagged as eligible, why a site was classified as high risk, why a safety signal was predicted, or why a subgroup effect was inferred. Explainable AI (XAI) offers tools to interpret model behavior, but explanation quality varies and can be misused if treated as a superficial add-on rather than a governance requirement. Closely linked is the issue of algorithmic bias: models trained on historical datasets may reproduce or amplify disparities, leading to inequitable recruitment, inaccurate risk prediction for underrepresented groups, or distorted evidence conclusions. Ethical evidence generation requires not only technical validation but fairness-aware evaluation across demographic and clinical subgroups.

Data governance is another strategic constraint. Clinical research increasingly depends on accessing sensitive health data across institutions, countries, and regulatory environments. This introduces requirements for privacy, consent, security, and auditability. Federated and privacy-preserving learning methods aim to enable collaborative model training without centralizing raw data, but they require strong interoperability and standardized data representations. Without robust data quality and harmonization, AI tools can perform well in controlled settings yet degrade under real-world heterogeneity, threatening the reliability of evidence claims.

Finally, the transformation of clinical research through AI is a socio-technical change. Tools do not deliver value in isolation; value emerges when AI is integrated into workflows, roles, training, and institutional governance. Researchers, data scientists, clinical teams, and regulators need shared language and shared expectations. This means establishing lifecycle processes for model development, validation, monitoring, updating, and retirement—especially when AI systems are used continuously rather than as one-off analyses. It also means building organizational readiness: AI literacy for clinical teams, defining accountability for decisions, and clear thresholds for when AI outputs can be acted upon or must be overridden.

This chapter examines the role of AI in transforming clinical research and evidence generation across the full lifecycle—from study design and trial operations to RWE strategies and trustworthy governance. It frames AI not as a replacement for clinical science, but as a capability layer that can accelerate discovery and strengthen evidence—provided it is implemented responsibly. The next sections map AI's contributions to the clinical research lifecycle, show how AI enables new evidence generation paradigms, and present the governance and operating models needed to scale AI safely in a patient-centric and regulation-aligned way.

13.2 AI across the clinical research lifecycle: from protocol to reporting

AI reshapes clinical research most tangibly when examined across the full study lifecycle. Rather than acting as a single intervention point, AI-enabled analytics now influence decisions from early protocol conceptualization to final reporting and post-study learning. This end-to-end integration is critical: isolated AI applications may yield local efficiencies, but lifecycle-wide adoption enables structural improvements in speed, quality, and evidentiary robustness.

13.2.1 Protocol design and feasibility assessment

Clinical trials often fail or require costly amendments because protocol assumptions do not align with real-world clinical practice. Eligibility criteria may be overly restrictive, endpoints impractical to measure, or site capacity underestimated. AI addresses these challenges by enabling data-driven protocol design. Using historical trial data and real-world clinical datasets, ML models can simulate eligibility criteria against actual patient populations, estimating recruitment feasibility before a protocol is finalized.

NLP plays a central role at this stage by parsing free-text eligibility criteria and mapping them to structured clinical variables found in EHRs. This allows sponsors and investigators to quantify how small protocol changes—such as modifying age ranges, laboratory thresholds, or comorbidity exclusions—affect the size and diversity of eligible populations. Predictive models can further forecast recruitment timelines, screen failure rates, and geographic variability in patient availability. As a result, protocol design shifts from expert intuition to evidence-informed optimization.

Importantly, AI-supported feasibility assessment contributes to equity goals. By identifying criteria that disproportionately exclude underrepresented populations, sponsors can proactively redesign protocols to improve inclusivity while maintaining scientific rigor. This capability is particularly relevant in precision medicine trials, where narrow inclusion criteria may unintentionally limit generalizability.

13.2.2 Site selection and study startup

Site selection has traditionally relied on historical performance metrics, investigator reputation, and feasibility questionnaires—methods that are often subjective and slow. AI introduces a more systematic approach by integrating multidimensional data sources, including prior enrollment performance, patient population characteristics, operational capacity indicators, and real-time healthcare utilization patterns.

ML models can rank sites based on predicted enrollment velocity, data quality risk, protocol adherence likelihood, and patient retention probability. These predictions allow sponsors to prioritize high-performing sites and allocate resources more effectively. In parallel, AI-supported startup tools can automate document review, identify missing regulatory elements, and flag inconsistencies in ethics submissions or contracts, reducing startup delays.

This stage illustrates a broader theme: AI shifts clinical research management from reactive problem-solving to proactive risk mitigation. Rather than responding to slow enrollment or protocol deviations after they occur, sponsors can anticipate challenges and intervene early.

13.2.3 Patient identification, recruitment, and retention

Recruitment remains one of the most persistent bottlenecks in clinical research. AI-enabled analytics transform recruitment by leveraging real-world data to identify eligible participants at scale. NLP systems can scan unstructured clinical notes to detect relevant diagnoses, disease severity markers, or prior treatment histories that may not be captured in structured fields. When combined with predictive scoring, AI can prioritize patients who are not only eligible but also likely to consent and remain engaged.

AI also enhances patient-centricity. Personalized outreach strategies, informed by behavioral analytics, can tailor communication to patient preferences, improving trust and participation rates. During the trial, predictive models can identify participants at risk of dropout based on visit adherence, symptom trajectories, or engagement patterns, enabling targeted retention interventions.

From an ethical perspective, recruitment algorithms must be carefully governed. Transparency in how patients are identified and contacted, safeguards against discriminatory targeting, and clear consent processes are essential to ensure that AI-supported recruitment aligns with regulatory and ethical standards.

13.2.4 Data collection, monitoring, and quality assurance

Once a trial is underway, AI contributes most strongly to data integrity and monitoring. Traditional monitoring relies heavily on manual source data verification and periodic site visits, which are resource-intensive and limited in scope. AI enables a shift toward risk-based and continuous monitoring.

ML models can detect anomalies, outliers, and inconsistent patterns in incoming data streams, flagging potential errors, protocol deviations, or even fraudulent behavior. These systems learn normal patterns of data generation across sites and participants, allowing them to surface subtle signals that might escape human review. In decentralized or hybrid trials, where data originates from wearable devices, mobile apps, and remote assessments, AI becomes essential for managing volume and variability.

Predictive safety analytics represent another critical application. By continuously analyzing adverse event reports, laboratory trends, and physiological data, AI systems can support early detection of safety signals. While such systems do not replace clinical judgment or regulatory reporting obligations, they enhance situational awareness and support timely escalation.

13.2.5 Analysis, interpretation, and reporting

AI's role extends beyond data collection into analysis and interpretation. In complex trials involving high-dimensional data—such as imaging, genomics, or digital biomarkers—traditional statistical methods may struggle to capture non-linear relationships and interactions. AI techniques can complement classical analyses by uncovering latent structures, subgroup effects, and response patterns that inform deeper scientific understanding.

However, this phase also highlights the importance of explainability. Regulators, clinicians, and scientific audiences require clear justification for analytical conclusions. AI-supported analyses must therefore be accompanied by interpretable outputs, sensitivity analyses, and transparent documentation of model assumptions. XAI methods can help translate complex model behavior into clinically meaningful insights, supporting both regulatory review and scientific communication.

Finally, AI can streamline reporting by automating parts of clinical study reports, generating structured summaries, and supporting consistency checks across tables, figures, and narratives. While human oversight remains indispensable, these tools reduce administrative burden and allow researchers to focus on interpretation and decision-making.

13.2.6 Lifecycle integration as a strategic capability

Taken together, AI-enabled analytics redefine the clinical research lifecycle as a connected system rather than a sequence of isolated tasks. Value emerges not from individual tools, but from integration: feasibility insights inform protocol design, which influences recruitment strategies, which shape monitoring priorities, which ultimately affect analysis and evidence quality. Organizations that treat AI as a lifecycle capability—supported by governance, training, and infrastructure—are better positioned to deliver faster, more reliable, and more equitable clinical evidence.

The next section builds on this foundation by examining how AI enables new paradigms of evidence generation beyond traditional trials, including RWE, synthetic controls, and digitally enabled study designs.

AI as an End-to-End Clinical Research Capability (Not a Point Solution)

Clinical research transformation through AI does not occur through isolated tools or single use cases. Its value emerges when AI-enabled analytics are integrated coherently across the full research lifecycle.

AI-enabled clinical research operates across five interdependent layers:

Design intelligence: AI informs protocol feasibility, eligibility criteria, endpoint selection, and recruitment projections using historical and real-world data.

Operational intelligence: Predictive analytics optimize site selection, enrollment velocity, monitoring intensity, and resource allocation.

Analytical intelligence: ML supports high-dimensional data analysis, subgroup discovery, and adaptive inference beyond traditional statistical methods.

Evidence intelligence: AI enables RWE integration, synthetic controls, and continuous outcome assessment.

Governance intelligence: Explainability, traceability, bias monitoring, and lifecycle oversight ensure regulatory acceptability and trust.

Executive insight: Organizations that deploy AI only at isolated stages (e.g., recruitment or monitoring) achieve incremental gains. Those that integrate AI as a **lifecycle capability** achieve structural transformation in speed, quality, and evidentiary credibility.

13.3 State of the art: AI and machine learning in clinical research and evidence generation

The application of AI and ML in clinical research has evolved from experimental pilot studies into a central driver of transformation in evidence generation. A growing body of interdisciplinary research demonstrates that AI is reshaping how clinical evidence is produced, synthesized, validated, and translated into practice. Rather than replacing established research paradigms, AI augments traditional clinical trials and evidence-based medicine by enabling scalability, adaptivity, and continuous learning across the full research lifecycle.

Early comprehensive assessments emphasize that ML techniques contribute across multiple stages of clinical research, including pre-trial planning, cohort identification, participant management, and data analysis (Weissler et al., 2021). These contributions are particularly significant in RCTs, where AI-enhanced design and monitoring can improve efficiency without undermining methodological rigor. ML is increasingly viewed as a mechanism for *augmenting*—not replacing—the gold standard of randomized evidence, improving trial feasibility and success rates while preserving scientific validity.

13.3.1 Artificial intelligence and the evolution of evidence-based medicine

Recent scholarship highlights a broader paradigm shift from traditional evidence-based medicine toward what has been described as "deep" or next-generation evidence generation. This transformation is driven by the convergence of AI, data science, wearable technologies, and large-scale digital health data (Subbiah, 2023). Clinical research is no longer confined to episodic trials but is increasingly embedded in continuous data streams that allow adaptive learning over time.

AI enables this shift by supporting advanced predictive modeling, real-time analytics, and longitudinal outcome tracking. Predictive models based on ML techniques—such as NLP and deep learning—have demonstrated the ability to outperform traditional risk scores in several clinical domains, enabling dynamic decision support and adaptive care strategies (Eloranta & Boman, 2022). Importantly, these models differ from classical statistical inference approaches by prioritizing prediction accuracy and real-world applicability, which is essential for personalized medicine and precision health.

13.3.2 Machine learning across the clinical trial lifecycle

A substantial body of evidence confirms that AI and ML are positioned to revolutionize the conduct of clinical trials. Technology-enabled trials leverage predictive analytics, digital biomarkers, and automated endpoint adjudication to improve efficiency and reduce operational burden (Marquis-Gravel et al., 2019). AI-driven recruitment strategies, for example, utilize behavioral and clinical data from digital sources to enhance patient matching and enrollment while supporting decentralized and hybrid trial models.

Multiple systematic reviews demonstrate that ML algorithms—such as random forests, gradient boosting methods, support vector machines, and logistic regression—have shown high potential for clinical applications, particularly for outcome prediction across oncology, inflammatory diseases, neuropsychiatric disorders, and infectious diseases (Nwanosike et al., 2022). These capabilities directly address longstanding challenges related to sample size, recruitment delays, and late-stage trial failure.

At the same time, scholars consistently emphasize that robust evidence generation for AI models faces hurdles similar to those encountered by pharmaceuticals and medical devices, including the need for external validation, prospective trials, and reproducibility across settings (Kolasa et al., 2024). The lack of replication studies and inconsistent reporting of harms remain critical translational barriers (Coiera & Liu, 2022).

13.3.3 Automated evidence synthesis and living reviews

Beyond trial execution, AI is transforming evidence synthesis itself. Automated and semiautomated approaches using NLP and ML are increasingly applied to systematic reviews, metaanalyses, and guideline development. AI-driven tools support evidence retrieval, screening, data extraction, bias assessment, and summarization at an unprecedented scale (Ofori-Boateng & Aceves-Martins, 2024).

Recent work proposes a future of *living* and interactive systematic reviews, where AI continuously updates evidence bases as new studies emerge (Riaz et al., 2024). Large language models are explored as enablers of real-time synthesis, although researchers consistently stress the necessity of human–AI collaboration to preserve methodological integrity. These developments align with broader ambitions to publish clinical trial data in computable formats, enabling immediate synthesis and translation into practice (Coiera & Liu, 2022).

13.3.4 Natural language processing and clinical knowledge extraction

NLP represents a foundational technology for AI-enabled evidence generation. Scoping reviews demonstrate that NLP supports all five steps of evidence-based medicine—Ask, Acquire, Appraise, Apply, and Assess—by enabling large-scale extraction and synthesis of clinical knowledge from unstructured text (Xu et al., 2025). NLP is increasingly used in trial design, eligibility identification, endpoint detection, and evidence summarization, thereby reducing manual workload and accelerating research cycles.

13.3.5 AI in drug development and translational research

In pharmaceutical research, AI-driven analytics accelerate drug discovery, development, and clinical evaluation by integrating chemical, biological, clinical, and real-world data. Reviews consistently report that AI improves trial design, patient stratification, toxicity prediction, and safety monitoring while reducing cost and development timelines (Tiwari et al., 2023; Bhatt et al., 2024). AI-enabled patient matching and adaptive protocols improve inclusivity and precision, supporting both conventional and decentralized trial formats (Mirakhori & Niazi, 2025).

Regulatory and translational perspectives emphasize that AI's impact extends across the entire drug lifecycle, from discovery through postauthorization surveillance (Shah et al., 2019; Oualikene-Gonin et al., 2024). However, the adoption of AI-generated evidence requires structured evaluation frameworks aligned with clinical trial principles. Recent proposals advocate for trial-informed frameworks that assess safety, efficacy, effectiveness, and ongoing monitoring of AI systems in real-world deployment (You et al., 2025).

13.3.6 Challenges, governance, and responsible integration

Despite strong evidence of potential, the literature converges on several unresolved challenges. Ethical concerns related to data quality, bias, interpretability, and regulatory uncertainty remain the primary obstacles to large-scale adoption (Askin et al., 2023; Thamson & Panahi, 2025). Scholars consistently stress that AI must augment—not replace—human expertise and that explainability, transparency, and accountability are prerequisites for trust and regulatory acceptance (Subbiah, 2023).

Overall, the state of the art indicates that AI and ML are no longer peripheral innovations in clinical research. They are foundational technologies reshaping evidence generation, synthesis, and translation. However, their sustainable impact depends on rigorous validation, transparent reporting, regulatory alignment, and continuous human oversight.

13.4 AI-enabled evidence generation beyond traditional clinical trials

While RCTs remain the gold standard for evaluating safety and efficacy, they are increasingly recognized as insufficient on their own to meet modern evidence demands. High costs, long timelines, limited generalizability, and ethical constraints—particularly in rare diseases and oncology—have created pressure to complement traditional trial paradigms. AI plays a pivotal role in this transition by enabling new models of evidence generation that extend beyond conventional trial boundaries.

AI-driven analytics allow clinical research to evolve from episodic, tightly controlled experimentation toward continuous, RWE generation. This shift is not a rejection of RCTs but an expansion of the evidentiary ecosystem, where multiple data sources and analytical strategies converge to support regulatory, clinical, and policy decisions.

13.4.1 Real-world evidence and learning health systems

RWE refers to clinical insights derived from routinely collected healthcare data, including EHRs, registries, claims databases, and patient-generated data from digital devices. Historically, the analytical complexity and heterogeneity of such data have limited its regulatory utility. AI fundamentally changes this equation.

ML models can integrate longitudinal, high-dimensional real-world datasets to identify treatment effects, safety signals, and patient subgroups that may not be observable in controlled trials. NLP enables the extraction of clinically meaningful information from unstructured sources such as physician notes, pathology reports, and discharge summaries. These capabilities support the emergence of learning health systems, where evidence generation is embedded within routine care and continuously updated.

AI-enhanced RWE is particularly valuable for post-marketing surveillance, comparative effectiveness research, and long-term safety monitoring. It enables regulators and healthcare systems to move from static evidence snapshots to dynamic, continuously evolving knowledge bases. However, the credibility of AI-generated RWE depends on rigorous validation, transparency in model design, and careful handling of bias and confounding—issues that require both technical and governance solutions.

13.4.2 Synthetic control arms and external comparators

One of the most impactful applications of AI in evidence generation is the creation of synthetic control arms. In trials where randomization is impractical or unethical—such as rare diseases or life-threatening conditions—AI can construct external comparators using historical trial data and real-world patient cohorts.

By applying causal inference techniques and advanced matching algorithms, AI systems can identify patients who closely resemble trial participants across demographic, clinical, and molecular characteristics. These synthetic cohorts serve as reference groups against which treatment effects can be evaluated, reducing reliance on placebo arms and minimizing patient exposure to ineffective interventions.

Regulatory interest in synthetic controls has grown rapidly, particularly when traditional trial designs are infeasible. However, their acceptance hinges on methodological rigor. AI-generated controls must demonstrate transparency in cohort construction, sensitivity to hidden confounders, and reproducibility across datasets. Explainability is again central: regulators must understand how patients were selected and how comparability was established.

13.4.3 Digital biomarkers and continuous outcome measurement

Traditional clinical endpoints often rely on episodic assessments conducted during scheduled study visits. These snapshots may miss important fluctuations in disease progression, treatment response, or adverse effects. AI-enabled digital biomarkers address this limitation by transforming continuous data streams into clinically meaningful endpoints.

Wearable devices, mobile applications, and connected sensors generate vast volumes of physiological and behavioral data, including activity patterns, sleep quality, heart rate variability, speech characteristics, and movement dynamics. AI algorithms analyze these signals to detect subtle changes that may precede clinical deterioration or improvement.

Digital biomarkers are particularly valuable in neurological, cardiovascular, and mental health research, where disease manifestations are dynamic and context-dependent. By enabling remote, continuous measurement, AI supports decentralized and hybrid trial designs, reduces patient burden, and improves data richness. At the same time, it raises new questions about validation, standardization, and regulatory qualification of novel endpoints.

13.4.4 Adaptive and pragmatic trial designs

AI also enables more flexible and responsive study designs. Adaptive trials adjust key parameters—such as dosing, randomization ratios, or enrollment criteria—based on interim data. While adaptive designs predate modern AI, ML enhances their sophistication by enabling more precise, data-driven adaptations.

Pragmatic trials, which evaluate interventions under real-world conditions, benefit from AI's ability to manage variability and complexity. AI systems can stratify patients, adjust analyses for confounding factors, and support real-time decision-making without compromising methodological integrity.

These designs align closely with patient-centric research priorities. They allow studies to evolve in response to emerging evidence, reducing waste and improving relevance. However, they also increase the importance of governance, documentation, and regulatory alignment, as adaptive decisions must be pre-specified, traceable, and auditable.

13.4.5 Regulatory perspectives on AI-generated evidence

Regulatory agencies increasingly recognize the potential of AI-enabled evidence generation, but acceptance is cautious and conditional. Regulators emphasize that AI should augment—not replace—scientific rigor. Evidence derived from AI-supported methods must meet standards of validity, reliability, and transparency comparable to traditional approaches.

Key regulatory concerns include data provenance, algorithmic bias, reproducibility, and explainability. AI systems used in evidence generation must be subject to validation across diverse populations and settings. Documentation of model development, training data, and performance monitoring is essential to establish trust.

Importantly, regulators are moving toward lifecycle-based oversight, recognizing that AI models evolve over time. This perspective aligns with the broader shift toward continuous evidence generation and adaptive governance frameworks.

13.4.6 Implications for the future of clinical research

AI-enabled evidence generation represents a structural evolution in how medical knowledge is produced. By integrating trials, real-world data, digital technologies, and advanced analytics, clinical research becomes more responsive, inclusive, and efficient. Yet this transformation is not purely technical. It requires new competencies, interdisciplinary collaboration, and robust governance models.

The next section addresses these challenges directly by examining the ethical, regulatory, and organizational frameworks needed to ensure that AI-driven clinical research remains trustworthy, accountable, and aligned with patient-centered values.

13.5 Governance, ethics, and regulatory readiness in AI-driven clinical research

The integration of AI into clinical research and evidence generation introduces transformative capabilities, but it also exposes fundamental challenges related to governance, ethics, and regulation. Unlike traditional statistical tools, AI systems are adaptive, data-hungry, and often opaque. In high-risk environments such as clinical research—where decisions directly affect patient safety, regulatory approval, and public trust—these characteristics necessitate a shift from ad hoc oversight to structured, lifecycle-based governance.

This section examines the governance architectures required to responsibly deploy AI in clinical research, with particular emphasis on explainability, accountability, regulatory alignment, and human oversight.

13.5.1 The governance gap in AI-enabled clinical research

Clinical research has long relied on well-established governance mechanisms, including ethics committees, protocol review boards, good clinical practice guidelines, and regulatory inspections. However, these mechanisms were designed for static study designs and deterministic analytical methods. AI disrupts this paradigm by introducing models that evolve over time, learn from new data, and generate probabilistic outputs rather than fixed conclusions.

This creates a governance gap. Without clear frameworks, AI systems may be deployed without adequate clarity regarding responsibility for decisions, mechanisms for performance monitoring, or procedures for intervention when models drift or fail. In clinical research, such gaps are unacceptable, as they undermine both scientific integrity and ethical accountability.

Effective governance must therefore treat AI not as a standalone tool but as a regulated clinical asset embedded within the research lifecycle. This requires explicit policies governing model development, validation, deployment, monitoring, updating, and retirement.

13.5.2 Explainability and accountability as ethical imperatives

Among the ethical challenges posed by AI, model opacity—the so-called "black box" problem—is the most consequential. Deep learning models may achieve high predictive accuracy, yet fail to provide intelligible explanations for their outputs. In clinical research, this opacity creates ethical and legal dilemmas.

First, clinicians cannot responsibly act on recommendations they do not understand. Second, patients cannot provide truly informed consent if the role of AI in decision-making is unclear. Third, regulators cannot approve evidence generated by systems whose reasoning cannot be audited.

XAI addresses these concerns by enabling insight into how models arrive at specific conclusions. Techniques such as feature attribution, counterfactual explanations, and uncertainty estimation allow stakeholders to interrogate model behavior and identify potential errors or biases. Importantly, explainability is not merely a technical enhancement—it is a prerequisite for accountability.

In AI-driven clinical research, accountability must be traceable. It must be possible to reconstruct how a model contributed to a decision, what data were used, which assumptions were embedded, and where human judgment intervened. XAI transforms AI systems from opaque decision engines into auditable, governable components of the research infrastructure.

When Is AI-Generated Evidence "Trustworthy" in Clinical Research?

For AI-generated evidence to be acceptable to regulators, clinicians, and patients, **predictive accuracy alone is insufficient**. Trustworthiness in clinical research requires satisfaction of five conditions:

Explainability: It must be possible to understand *why* an AI system contributed to a decision or inference.

Traceability: Data sources, preprocessing steps, model versions, and outputs must be auditable across the research lifecycle.

Reproducibility: Evidence must be stable across populations, sites, and settings—not confined to a single dataset.

Human oversight: AI outputs must inform—not replace—scientific judgment, with clear escalation and override pathways.

Lifecycle accountability: AI systems must be monitored, recalibrated, or retired as data, practice, and populations evolve.

Regulatory takeaway: In AI-enabled clinical research, *trust is an operational property*, not a philosophical one. It is engineered through governance, not assumed through performance metrics.

13.5.3 Regulatory alignment and evidence acceptability

Regulatory agencies increasingly recognize the potential of AI to enhance clinical research efficiency and evidence generation. However, acceptance is conditional on rigorous standards. Regulators emphasize that AI-derived evidence must meet the same—or higher—thresholds of validity, reliability, and transparency as traditional methods.

A central regulatory concern is reproducibility. AI models trained on proprietary or institution-specific datasets may perform well locally but fail to generalize across populations. This raises questions about bias, equity, and fairness, particularly when models are applied to underrepresented groups.

Another concern is lifecycle management. Unlike static statistical models, AI systems evolve. Regulators are therefore moving toward lifecycle-based oversight models, where approval is not a one-time event but an ongoing process involving continuous monitoring, performance evaluation, and revalidation.

For sponsors and research organizations, this means that regulatory readiness must be built into AI systems from the outset. Documentation, version control, data provenance tracking, and performance monitoring are not optional add-ons—they are foundational requirements for regulatory acceptability.

13.5.4 Human oversight and responsibility allocation

Despite advances in automation, AI does not eliminate the need for human judgment in clinical research. On the contrary, it heightens the importance of clearly defined human oversight. AI systems may generate insights, predictions, or recommendations, but responsibility for decisions must remain human-centered.

Effective governance frameworks explicitly define who is accountable at each decision point. This includes clarifying when AI outputs may inform decisions, when escalation is required, and when human judgment must override algorithmic recommendations. These rules should be embedded into protocols, standard operating procedures, and training programs.

Human oversight also extends to interdisciplinary collaboration. Data scientists, clinicians, ethicists, and regulatory experts must work together to ensure that AI systems align with clinical realities and ethical expectations. Governance is therefore as much an organizational challenge as a technical one.

13.5.5 Data governance, privacy, and trust

AI-driven clinical research depends on access to large volumes of sensitive health data. This reliance intensifies concerns about privacy, data security, and patient trust. Traditional consent models, which assume limited and predefined data use, are strained by AI systems that derive value from secondary analysis and data reuse.

Robust data governance frameworks are essential. These include clear policies on data access, anonymization, consent management, and secondary use. Privacy-preserving technologies such as federated learning and secure multiparty computation offer promising pathways by enabling model training without centralized data aggregation.

Trust is ultimately the currency of clinical research. Patients must trust that their data are used responsibly, clinicians must trust AI-generated insights, and regulators must trust the evidence presented for approval. Governance frameworks that prioritize transparency, accountability, and ethical integrity are critical to sustaining this trust.

13.5.6 From compliance to responsible innovation

A narrow focus on regulatory compliance risks reduces governance to a box-ticking exercise. Instead, AI-enabled clinical research requires a shift toward responsible innovation—a mindset that integrates ethical reflection, stakeholder engagement, and continuous learning.

Responsible innovation recognizes that not all risks can be eliminated in advance. Instead, it emphasizes adaptive governance, where systems are continuously evaluated, improved, and aligned with societal values. In this model, governance is not a barrier to innovation but a prerequisite for sustainable impact.

The final section of this chapter synthesizes these insights by outlining future directions for AI in clinical research and evidence generation, emphasizing strategic priorities for researchers, regulators, and healthcare leaders.

13.6 Future directions: AI as the foundation of next-generation clinical evidence

AI is no longer an experimental enhancement to clinical research—it is becoming the foundational infrastructure upon which next-generation evidence generation is built. As healthcare systems confront rising complexity, accelerating innovation cycles, and increasing regulatory scrutiny, AI-enabled clinical research offers a pathway to generate faster, more adaptive, and more representative evidence. However, realizing this potential requires a strategic shift in how evidence is conceived, produced, and evaluated.

This section outlines the emerging future of AI-driven clinical research, highlighting structural transformations in evidence generation, methodological innovation, and the evolving roles of institutions, regulators, and clinical professionals.

13.6.1 From episodic trials to continuous evidence generation

Traditional clinical research is organized around episodic studies—discrete trials with fixed protocols, predefined endpoints, and limited temporal scope. While effective for many purposes, this model struggles to keep pace with rapidly evolving therapies, personalized medicine, and real-world complexity.

AI enables a transition toward continuous evidence generation. By integrating real-world data, adaptive trial designs, and post-market surveillance, AI systems support evidence generation across the full lifecycle of a therapy—from early discovery to long-term safety monitoring. This continuity allows research questions to evolve dynamically, reflecting emerging signals rather than static assumptions.

In this future paradigm, evidence is not generated once and archived; it is continuously updated, contextualized, and refined. AI acts as the connective tissue linking clinical trials, observational studies, and real-world outcomes into an integrated evidence ecosystem.

13.6.2 Personalized and context-aware evidence

One of the most profound implications of AI in clinical research is the shift from population averages to personalized evidence. Traditional trials often aim to demonstrate average treatment effects, which may obscure meaningful variation across subgroups. AI-enabled analytics, particularly those leveraging multiomics data and longitudinal patient histories, enable context-aware evidence generation.

This approach allows researchers to identify which patients benefit most from specific interventions, under what conditions, and at what stages of disease progression. Evidence becomes stratified rather than aggregated, supporting precision medicine at scale.

However, personalized evidence raises methodological and ethical questions. How should regulators evaluate evidence that varies across subpopulations? How can bias be avoided when models learn from historically imbalanced datasets? Addressing these questions requires new regulatory thinking and methodological rigor—areas where AI must be complemented by strong governance frameworks.

13.6.3 Synthetic evidence and virtual trial augmentation

AI is also transforming the structure of trials themselves through the use of synthetic data and virtual controls. Synthetic control arms, generated using historical trial data and RWE, can reduce the need for placebo groups, particularly in rare diseases or ethically sensitive contexts.

These approaches promise faster recruitment, reduced costs, and improved patient experience. However, they also challenge traditional evidentiary standards. Regulators and sponsors must ensure that synthetic data are scientifically valid, transparent, and appropriately validated against real-world outcomes.

The future of clinical research will likely involve hybrid models that combine physical trials with AI-generated synthetic evidence. Success will depend on rigorous validation, transparent assumptions, and clear communication with regulatory authorities.

13.6.4 Institutional transformation and skills evolution

The widespread adoption of AI in clinical research necessitates institutional transformation. Research organizations must develop new capabilities in data science, AI governance, and interdisciplinary collaboration. Clinical researchers will increasingly work alongside data engineers, AI ethicists, and regulatory specialists.

This transformation extends to education and training. Future clinical researchers must be literate in AI concepts—not to become programmers, but to critically evaluate AI outputs, understand model limitations, and engage meaningfully in governance discussions. Without this institutional readiness, AI risks becoming a black box that undermines trust rather than enhancing insight.

Leadership also plays a critical role. Organizational leaders must foster cultures that value responsible innovation, transparency, and continuous learning. AI adoption is as much a change management challenge as a technological one.

13.6.5 Regulatory evolution and global harmonization

As AI reshapes evidence generation, regulatory frameworks must evolve accordingly. Regulators are increasingly exploring adaptive approval pathways, RWE integration, and lifecycle-based oversight models. AI can support these efforts by enabling continuous monitoring, automated signal detection, and dynamic risk assessment.

However, regulatory fragmentation remains a challenge. Divergent standards across jurisdictions can slow innovation and complicate global trials. International harmonization of AI governance principles—particularly around transparency, validation, and accountability—will be essential to fully realize the benefits of AI-driven clinical research.

In this evolving landscape, proactive engagement between researchers, sponsors, and regulators is critical. AI should be developed with regulatory expectations in mind from the outset, rather than retrofitted for compliance.

13.6.6 A human-centered vision for AI-driven evidence

Despite its transformative power, AI does not replace the human core of clinical research. Instead, it redefines roles and responsibilities. Human judgment remains essential for interpreting evidence, weighing risks and benefits, and making ethically grounded decisions.

The future of AI in clinical research is therefore human-centered. AI systems augment human capabilities by handling complexity, scale, and uncertainty—but humans retain responsibility for values, accountability, and trust. This balance is the cornerstone of sustainable innovation.

13.6.7 Strategic implications for the next decade

Looking ahead, several strategic priorities emerge:

Evidence ecosystems will replace isolated studies, integrating trials, real-world data, and post-market surveillance.

Explainability and governance will become central determinants of adoption and regulatory acceptance.

Personalized evidence will challenge traditional evaluation models and require new methodological standards.

Institutional readiness will determine which organizations successfully scale AI-enabled research.

Trust and transparency will remain the ultimate success factors, outweighing raw technical performance.

In conclusion, AI is redefining what clinical evidence means, how it is generated, and how it is trusted. Organizations that embrace AI responsibly—integrating technical innovation with ethical governance and human oversight—will lead the next era of clinical research. Those that fail to adapt risk obsolescence in an increasingly data-driven healthcare landscape.

Clinical Evidence in 2035: From Trials to Evidence Ecosystems

It is accelerating a transition from *study-centric* evidence generation to *ecosystem-based* evidence production.
By the next decade, leading clinical research systems will exhibit the following characteristics:
Continuous evidence streams: Evidence will evolve dynamically through integration of trials, real-world data, and post-market monitoring.
Hybrid experimental models: Physical trials will be augmented by synthetic controls, digital biomarkers, and virtual cohorts.
Personalized evidence frameworks: Evidence will be stratified by patient context rather than averaged across populations.
Regulatory coevolution: Approval processes will increasingly rely on lifecycle oversight rather than static submissions.
Human-centered AI governance: AI will operate as a decision-support layer embedded in accountable institutional structures.
Strategic insight: The future of clinical research is not "AI-driven" but **AI-governed**.
Competitive advantage will belong to organizations that master evidence integration, not algorithm complexity.

Editor's note

This chapter provides a comprehensive and forward-looking examination of the role of AI in transforming clinical research and evidence generation. It successfully situates AI not merely as a technological enhancement but as a structural enabler of a new research paradigm—one that is adaptive, data-intensive, and patient-centered.

A defining strength of the chapter lies in its balanced treatment of innovation and governance. While it clearly demonstrates how AI accelerates trial design, patient recruitment, monitoring, and RWE generation, it equally emphasizes the ethical, regulatory, and accountability challenges that accompany these advances. By foregrounding explainability, transparency, and human oversight, the chapter avoids techno-determinism and instead presents AI as a sociotechnical system embedded within clinical, institutional, and regulatory contexts.

The chapter is particularly timely in its articulation of continuous evidence generation and personalized analytics as the next frontier of clinical research. These themes reflect emerging regulatory directions and respond directly to the limitations of traditional episodic trial models. Importantly, the chapter recognizes that trust—not accuracy alone—will determine the long-term success of AI-enabled clinical research.

Overall, this contribution offers both conceptual depth and practical relevance. It is well-suited for researchers, healthcare leaders, regulators, and policymakers seeking to understand not only what AI can do for clinical research but also how it must be governed to ensure safety, legitimacy, and societal value.

Key takeaways

Artificial Intelligence is transforming clinical research from a static, trial-centric activity into a continuous, adaptive evidence generation process spanning the full therapeutic lifecycle.

AI-enabled analytics improve efficiency and feasibility across clinical research stages, including protocol design, patient recruitment, monitoring, and outcome prediction.

The integration of real-world data with traditional trials enables more representative and timely evidence, supporting regulatory decision-making beyond controlled experimental settings.

Personalized and context-aware evidence generation challenges population-average models and enables precision medicine, but requires new evaluation and governance frameworks.

Synthetic data and virtual control arms offer powerful opportunities to accelerate trials, particularly in rare or high-risk conditions, while demanding rigorous validation standards.

XAI is essential for clinical accountability, regulatory compliance, and trust, transforming opaque models into transparent, auditable decision-support tools.

Effective AI adoption depends on institutional readiness, interdisciplinary collaboration, and clinician education—not technology alone.

Regulatory evolution toward lifecycle-based oversight and adaptive approval models will be critical to enabling responsible AI-driven research.

Human oversight remains indispensable; AI augments clinical judgment but does not replace ethical responsibility or professional accountability.

The future of AI in clinical research is human-centered, governance-driven, and evidence-focused rather than technology-driven.

Mini case study vignette (anonymized)

Transforming evidence generation through AI-enabled adaptive research

A multinational research consortium launched an AI-enabled platform to support oncology clinical trials across multiple academic hospitals and regional care centers. The platform integrated EHRs, imaging data, genomic profiles, and real-world outcomes to support patient eligibility screening, adaptive trial monitoring, and post-market evidence collection.

During the initial deployment, the system demonstrated strong performance in identifying eligible patients and predicting treatment response trajectories. Recruitment timelines were shortened significantly, and early safety signals were detected sooner than in comparable historical trials.

Despite these successes, clinicians and regulators raised concerns regarding model transparency and accountability. While predictions were accurate, the system initially offered limited insight into why certain patients were flagged as high-risk or highly responsive. This lack of explainability slowed regulatory review and reduced clinician confidence in acting on recommendations.

In response, the consortium integrated XAI components, including feature attribution dashboards and confidence scoring. Clinicians were able to trace recommendations back to specific clinical variables and biomarkers, enabling informed validation and override where appropriate.

Following these changes, regulatory engagement improved, clinician adoption increased, and patient communication became more effective. The platform transitioned from a decision automation tool to a trusted decision-support system.

Key insight: The success of AI-enabled clinical research depends less on predictive accuracy alone and more on explainability, governance, and alignment with clinical accountability structures.

Learning activities

Learning activity 1: mapping artificial intelligence across the clinical research lifecycle

Format: Individual or small group. **Time:** 30–40 minutes

Objective: To understand how AI contributes to evidence generation across different stages of clinical research.

Instructions: Map AI applications across the following phases:
Study design and protocol development
Patient recruitment and eligibility screening
Trial monitoring and safety surveillance
Outcome analysis and reporting
Post-market evidence generation
For each phase, identify:
One AI-enabled capability
One key benefit
One governance or ethical challenge

Deliverable: A one-page lifecycle map with concise explanatory notes.

Learning activity 2: designing a responsible artificial intelligence evidence framework

Format: Team-based (3–5 participants). **Time:** 45–60 minutes

Objective: To develop a governance-aware framework for AI-enabled clinical research.

Instructions: Design a conceptual framework for deploying AI in a clinical research setting. Your framework should address:
Research objectives and evidence goals
Data sources and analytics methods
Explainability and validation mechanisms
Human oversight and accountability
Regulatory alignment and lifecycle monitoring

Deliverable: A structured framework summary (1–2 pages).

Learning activity 3: executive reflection exercise

Format: Individual. **Time:** 15–20 minutes

Objective: To encourage strategic reflection on trust and accountability in AI-enabled research.

Reflection prompt: Should regulatory approval prioritize explainability and governance even if it limits the use of highly complex AI models? Why or why not?

Deliverable: A reflective essay of 200–250 words.

References

Askin, S., Burkhalter, D., Calado, G., & El Dakrouni, S. (2023). Artificial intelligence applied to clinical trials: Opportunities and challenges. In *Health and Technology*. Springer.

Bhatt, P., Singh, S., Kumar, V., & Nagarajan, K. (2024). Artificial intelligence in pharmaceutical industry: Revolutionizing drug development and delivery. *Current Artificial Intelligence*.

Coiera, E., & Liu, S. (2022). Evidence synthesis, digital scribes, and translational challenges for artificial intelligence in healthcare. *Cell Reports Medicine, 3*(7).

Eloranta, S., & Boman, M. (2022). Predictive models for clinical decision making: Deep dives in practical machine learning. *Journal of Internal Medicine, 292*(3), 369–381.

Kolasa, K., Admassu, B., et al. (2024). Systematic reviews of machine learning in healthcare: A literature review. *Expert Review of Pharmacoeconomics & Outcomes Research.*

Marquis-Gravel, G., Roe, M. T., Turakhia, M. P., & Boden, W. (2019). Technology-enabled clinical trials: Transforming medical evidence generation. *Circulation, 140*(17), 1426–1436.

Mirakhori, F., & Niazi, S. K. (2025). Harnessing the AI/ML in drug and biological products discovery and development: The regulatory perspective. *Pharmaceuticals, 18*(2).

Nwanosike, E. M., Conway, B. R., Merchant, H. A., et al. (2022). Potential applications and performance of machine learning techniques and algorithms in clinical practice: A systematic review. *International Journal of Medical Informatics, 159.*

Ofori-Boateng, R., & Aceves-Martins, M. (2024). Towards the automation of systematic reviews using natural language processing, machine learning, and deep learning: A comprehensive review. *Artificial Intelligence Review.*

Riaz, I. B., Naqvi, S. A. A., Hasan, B., & Murad, M. H. (2024). Future of evidence synthesis: Automated, living, and interactive systematic reviews and meta-analyses. *Mayo Clinic Proceedings: Digital Health, 2*(1).

Shah, P., Kendall, F., Khozin, S., Goosen, R., & Hu, J. (2019). Artificial intelligence and machine learning in clinical development: A translational perspective. *NPJ Digital Medicine, 2*(1).

Subbiah, V. (2023). The next generation of evidence-based medicine. *Nature Medicine, 29*, 49–58.

Thamson, K., & Panahi, O. (2025). Challenges and opportunities for implementing AI in clinical trials. *Journal of Bio Advanced Science Research.*

Tiwari, P. C., Pal, R., & Chaudhary, M. J. (2023). Artificial intelligence revolutionizing drug development: Exploring opportunities and challenges. *Drug Development Research, 84*(5).

Weissler, E. H., Naumann, T., Andersson, T., Ranganath, R., et al. (2021). The role of machine learning in clinical research: Transforming the future of evidence generation. *Trials, 22*(537).

Xu, Z., Ma, H., Ding, Y., Zhang, G., & Weng, C. (2025). Natural language processing in support of evidence-based medicine: A scoping review. *Findings of the Association for Computational Linguistics.*

You, J. G., Hernandez-Boussard, T., & Pfeffer, M. A. (2025). Clinical trials informed framework for real world clinical implementation and deployment of artificial intelligence applications. *NPJ Digital Medicine, 8.*

CHAPTER 14

Artificial intelligence in clinical trials: a transformative force

Khizra Sultana[1,2,3]

[1]King Saud Bin Abdulaziz University for Health Sciences (KSAU-HS), Riyadh, Saudi Arabia, [2]Ministry of National Guard Health Affairs, Riyadh, Saudi Arabia, [3]King Abdullah International Medical Research Center (KAIMRC), Clinical Trial Management, Riyadh, Saudi Arabia

14.1 Artificial intelligence in modern healthcare

Artificial intelligence (AI) is fundamentally transforming the practice of medicine by performing tasks traditionally associated with human cognition, such as learning, reasoning, and problem-solving (Barhate et al., 2024; Rani et al., 2025). This transformation is driven by two major factors: the exponential growth of healthcare data and rapid advancements in computational techniques, including machine learning (ML) and deep learning (DL) (Kulkarni & Singh, 2023; Tasneem, 2025). These technologies enable AI systems to process and interpret complex datasets—ranging from electronic health records (EHRs) and medical imaging to genomic information—providing actionable insights that support clinical decision-making (Omoseebi et al., 2025; Nurani et al., 2025). AI is shifting healthcare from a reactive, one-size-fits-all model toward a proactive, preventative, and personalized approach (Nurani et al., 2025; Tasneem, 2025). Rather than replacing clinicians, AI aims to augment their capabilities, enhancing diagnostic accuracy, improving efficiency, and promoting patient safety (De Micco et al., 2025). Furthermore, AI holds significant potential for expanding access to high-quality care in resource-limited settings, thereby addressing disparities in healthcare delivery (Zhao & Yuan, 2025).

14.2 General applications of artificial intelligence in healthcare

AI has become a cornerstone of modern healthcare, offering transformative applications across diagnostics, treatment, and patient management. In diagnostics, AI algorithms analyze medical images such as X-rays, CT scans, and MRIs to detect conditions like cancer, cardiovascular diseases, and neurological disorders (Katwaroo et al., 2024; Sharma, 2025). These systems often outperform human radiologists by identifying subtle patterns that may be otherwise overlooked, thus enabling early detection and timely interventions (Samah & Samar, 2025). Similarly, predictive analytics powered by AI allows healthcare providers to

The Future of Pharma Across All Sectors in the Artificial Intelligence Era. DOI: https://doi.org/10.1016/B978-0-443-40572-3.00004-6

forecast patient outcomes by analyzing large datasets, including EHRs, genetic profiles, and lifestyle data. This facilitates early disease detection, risk stratification, and personalized treatment planning (Alsaedi et al., 2025; Hassan & Omenogor, 2025). AI also plays a pivotal role in robotic surgery, where AI-driven robotic systems assist surgeons in performing complex procedures with enhanced precision and minimal invasiveness. These technologies reduce human error, shorten recovery times, and improve surgical outcomes (Borràs & Benavent, 2025; Ng Kok Wah, 2025). In addition, virtual health assistants and chatbots are facilitating patient engagement by providing real-time information, answering queries, and scheduling appointments, thereby reducing the burden on healthcare staff (Alowais et al., 2023).

Another significant application is drug discovery, where AI accelerates the identification of potential drug candidates by analyzing vast biological datasets, predicting molecular interactions, and simulating clinical trials—dramatically reducing time and cost compared to traditional methods (Ferreira & Carneiro, 2025; Kant et al., 2025). In personalized medicine, AI integrates genomic data with clinical information to tailor treatments based on individual genetic makeup and lifestyle, particularly benefiting oncology patients through targeted therapies (Ahmad, 2025; Calvino et al., 2025). Beyond clinical care, AI optimizes administrative tasks such as scheduling, billing, and documentation, improving efficiency and reducing operational costs (Desai, 2025). Finally, remote monitoring through AI-enabled wearable devices allows continuous tracking of patient health metrics, enabling early detection of abnormalities and timely interventions—especially valuable for chronic disease management and elderly care (Huang et al., 2025; Liu & Wang, 2025).

14.3 The evolution of AI in clinical research

AI has a profound and evolving history in clinical research, making significant strides over the decades. This journey began in the 1960s with the development of early AI systems designed to assist with medical diagnostics. One of the pioneering systems from this era was ELIZA, created in 1966, which simulated conversations with a psychotherapist. Although basic by today's standards, ELIZA set the stage for future AI applications in healthcare (Saeidnia & Nilashi, 2025; Mesfin, 2024).

During the 1970s, AI research expanded with the creation of expert systems like MYCIN, developed to diagnose bacterial infections and recommend appropriate antibiotics. MYCIN was among the first systems to utilize a knowledge base and inference engine, mimicking the decision-making processes of human experts. This era also witnessed the emergence of INTERNIST-1, a system aimed at assisting physicians in diagnosing complex medical conditions (Saeidnia & Nilashi, 2025).

The 1980s brought further advancements with the integration of ML techniques into clinical research. Researchers began to harness AI's potential to analyze large datasets, uncover patterns, and derive new medical insights. AI applications during this period primarily focused on providing diagnostic support and aiding clinical decision-making (Hirani et al., 2024; Mesfin, 2024).

In the 1990s, the rise of neural networks and DL significantly enhanced AI capabilities. These advancements enabled more sophisticated data analysis and predictive modeling, improving patient outcomes and streamlining clinical trials. AI's role expanded into drug discovery and personalized medicine, tailoring treatments to individual patients based on their unique genetic profiles (Andrès et al., 2025; Hirani et al., 2024).

The 2000s saw continued evolution in AI technology with the advent of big data analytics and cloud computing. These technologies empowered researchers to manage vast amounts of medical data, leading to more accurate and comprehensive analyses. AI applications broadened to include patient monitoring, telemedicine, and administrative tasks, further optimizing clinical research processes (Hirani et al., 2024; Xie et al., 2025).

A significant shift occurred in the 2010s with the widespread adoption of AI-driven tools in clinical trials. AI was employed to optimize study designs, enhance patient recruitment, and improve data management and analysis. The integration of AI in clinical research also addressed critical ethical considerations such as data privacy and algorithmic bias, ensuring fair and equitable research practices (Hirani et al., 2024; Xie et al., 2025).

The COVID-19 pandemic further accelerated the use of AI in healthcare. AI-powered applications in telemedicine, chatbots, and digital health became essential in maintaining patient care and medical education. AI played a vital role in managing the crisis, providing real-time data analysis and predictive modeling to inform public health decisions (Gawande et al., 2025).

Today, AI continues to transform clinical research, offering innovative solutions to long-standing challenges and paving the way for faster and more reliable medical advancements. The future of AI in clinical research holds immense potential, with emerging trends like precision medicine, robotic surgery, and advanced predictive analytics set to shape the healthcare landscape (Andrès et al., 2025; Ranjan et al., 2025).

14.4 AI in clinical trials: transforming protocol design and patient recruitment

AI is revolutionizing clinical trial design and execution by addressing long-standing challenges and streamlining complex processes. Its integration enables researchers to work more efficiently, make data-driven decisions, and accelerate treatment development (Geraci et al., 2025; Hong et al., 2025). Two critical areas where AI demonstrates significant impact are protocol design and patient recruitment.

14.5 Protocol design

AI automates literature reviews, drafts protocols, identifies patterns in trial data, simulates trial scenarios, and supports adaptive designs. These capabilities reduce amendments, improve feasibility, and ensure regulatory compliance (Lee et al., 2024; Makutam et al., 2024). Recent innovations include generative AI for protocol drafting and synthetic control arms for rare disease trials (Elvatun et al., 2025).

14.6 Patient recruitment

AI leverages EHRs, genetic data, and registries to predict recruitment feasibility, target underrepresented populations, and enhance patient engagement. This results in faster recruitment, greater diversity, and improved retention (Rosenthal et al., 2025; Pallepogu & Vadduganti, 2024). Emerging trends include integrating social determinants of health, AI-driven site selection, and ethical AI auditing (Mourya et al., 2024).

The overall impact of AI-driven solutions is to streamline trial processes, reduce costs, and accelerate drug development, leading to more inclusive and efficient trials aligned with regulatory standards (Kunz et al., 2020; Muppalla et al., 2025). Responsible AI frameworks and personalized communication tools are shaping the future of clinical research (Geraci et al., 2025).

14.7 Key contributions of AI in clinical trials

Summary table: Key contributions of AI in study design (Table 14.1).

14.7.1 Protocol design: smarter, faster, and more flexible

Designing a clinical trial protocol is no small feat. It's a meticulous process that traditionally involves digging through mountains of literature, consulting experts, and revising drafts over and over. But AI is changing that. Today, AI tools can sift through vast amounts of data from past trials, scientific publications, and real-world evidence to help researchers build better protocols from the start. These systems use ML to spot patterns that might be missed by the human eye—like the most effective dosage levels, ideal patient profiles, or meaningful clinical endpoints (Hong et al., 2025; Pallepogu & Vadduganti, 2024). Even more impressively, AI can simulate different trial scenarios and predict how they might play out. This allows researchers to fine-tune their protocols before the trial begins, reducing the risk of costly amendments later on (Geraci et al., 2025; Lee et al., 2024). One of the most exciting

Table 14.1 Key contributions of artificial intelligence in clinical trials.

Aspect	Key contributions of artificial intelligence (AI)	Benefits	Recent developments
Protocol design	Automates literature review and drafting; identifies patterns; simulates scenarios; enables adaptive designs; ensures compliance	Faster protocol development; reduced amendments; improved feasibility	Generative AI for drafting; synthetic control arms for rare diseases
Patient recruitment	Analyzes EHRs and genetic data; targets underrepresented groups; predicts feasibility; enhances engagement	Faster and accurate recruitment; increased diversity; better retention	Integration of social determinants; AI-driven site selection; ethical AI auditing
Overall impact	Streamlines trial processes; reduces costs; accelerates treatment development	Inclusive and efficient trials; improved regulatory alignment	Responsible AI frameworks; personalized communication tools

developments is the use of generative AI to draft initial protocol documents and suggest statistical methods tailored to specific diseases. These tools can even help design synthetic control arms, which reduce the need for placebo groups—especially valuable in rare disease research (Elvatun et al., 2025; Makutam et al., 2024). AI also supports adaptive trial designs, where protocols can be adjusted mid-trial based on interim results. This flexibility proved crucial during the COVID-19 pandemic and continues to be a game-changer in fast-moving research environments (Kunz et al., 2020; Rosenthal et al., 2025). Another key compnent of research trials is compliance. As such, AI can automatically check protocols against current regulations, thus helping researchers minimize delays and ensure approvals in a timely fashion (Mourya et al., 2024; Muppalla et al., 2025).

14.7.2 Patient recruitment: finding the right people, faster

Recruiting patients is often the biggest hurdle in clinical trials—it is time-consuming, costly, and prone to bias. AI is transforming this process by making recruitment smarter, faster, and more inclusive. Modern AI platforms can analyze EHRs, genetic data, and patient registries to quickly identify individuals who meet trial criteria, reducing timelines from weeks to hours (Hong et al., 2025; Pallepogu & Vadduganti, 2024).

Beyond speed, AI enhances diversity in trial populations. By examining demographic data and social factors, AI identifies underrepresented groups, ensuring more equitable and accurate results (Rosenthal et al., 2025). Recent advancements include incorporating social determinants of health—such as income, education, and access to care—to predict not only eligibility but also likelihood of participation and retention (Mourya et al., 2024).

AI also improves patient engagement through chatbots and virtual assistants that answer questions, explain trial processes, and guide participants through consent forms, boosting adherence and retention (Geraci et al., 2025). Furthermore, predictive analytics enables researchers to plan smarter recruitment strategies by forecasting timelines, identifying potential bottlenecks, and recommending optimal trial site locations (Lee et al., 2024; Makutam et al., 2024).

Despite these benefits, challenges remain. Data privacy and algorithmic bias are critical concerns, prompting initiatives to develop ethical standards and auditing frameworks for responsible AI use in clinical research (Muppalla et al., 2025).

Fig. 14.1 shows the percentage of recruitment efficiency with and without the use of AI.

14.7.3 How AI is revolutionizing data capture and entry

AI is transforming data management by eliminating slow, error-prone manual entry and introducing faster, more accurate, and scalable solutions. Technologies such as optical character recognition and natural language processing (NLP) enable AI to extract data from diverse sources—scanned documents, images, and even handwritten notes—converting unstructured content into clean, digital formats (Abbasi, 2024; Jerfy, Kumar, et al., 2024).

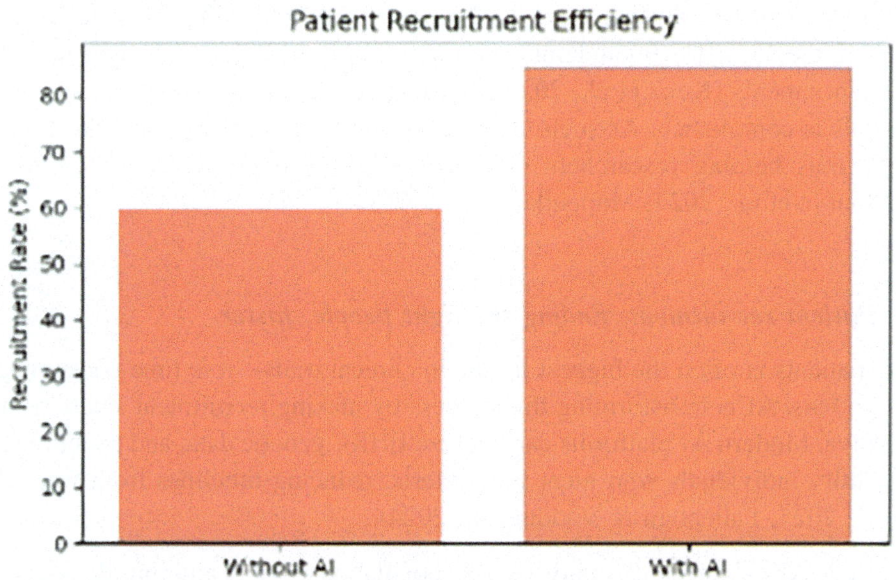

Figure 14.1
Patient recruitment efficiency.
Comparative analysis of patient recruitment efficiency with and without artificial intelligence (AI) integration.

After capture, AI automates database population and spreadsheet updates. ML models trained on historical data recognize patterns and classify information with high accuracy, ensuring consistency and reducing errors (Al-Nafjan, Aljuhani, et al., 2025; Krishnamurthy, 2025).

14.7.4 AI in data management and analysis

Automated data capture and entry offer significant advantages, including time savings, reduced human error, and efficient handling of large datasets. These benefits lower labor costs, prevent costly mistakes, and maintain clean, reliable data for analysis (Abbasi, 2024; Al-Nafjan, Almutairi, et al., 2025). Beyond entry, AI enables advanced analytics through ML for predictive modeling and anomaly detection (Gabrielli et al., 2025; Khan & Alkhathami, 2024), DL for image and speech recognition (Li, Jiang, et al., 2023; Li, Zhang, et al., 2023; Mienye, Swart, et al., 2025), and NLP for sentiment analysis and text classification (Jerfy, Kumar, et al., 2024; Krishnamurthy, 2025). These techniques support real-world applications such as forecasting trends, detecting irregularities, segmenting patients or customers, and performing market analysis (Badawy, Elshazly, et al., 2023; Badawy, Ramadan, et al., 2023; Gabrielli et al., 2025).

Recent developments include the adoption of generative AI for document processing and automated data extraction, expanding automation to tasks like spreadsheet analysis and reporting (Krishnamurthy, 2025; Mienye, Sun, et al., 2025).

14.7.5 AI in patient monitoring and compliance

AI is also reshaping patient monitoring and compliance in healthcare. Wearable devices such as smartwatches and biosensors continuously collect vital signs—heart rate, blood pressure, glucose levels, and sleep patterns. AI algorithms analyze this data in real time to detect anomalies and alert providers before issues escalate (Gabrielli et al., 2025; Khan & Alkhathami, 2024). For example, AI can identify irregular heart rhythms or respiratory distress, enabling early intervention. Patients benefit from real-time feedback, which promotes adherence and healthier behaviors (Mienye, Swart, et al., 2025).

14.7.5.1 Wearable technology: AI-driven monitoring

Wearable devices such as smartwatches and biosensors have become essential tools in modern healthcare. These devices continuously collect data on vital signs, including heart rate, blood pressure, glucose levels, and sleep patterns. AI algorithms analyze this data in real time to detect anomalies and alert healthcare providers before issues escalate (Gabrielli et al., 2025; Khan & Alkhathami, 2024).

For example, AI can identify irregular heart rhythms or signs of respiratory distress, prompting early intervention. Patients also benefit from real-time feedback, which encourages healthier behaviors and better self-management (Mienye, Swart, et al., 2025).

14.7.6 Adherence tracking: ensuring protocol compliance

AI tools are transforming how healthcare providers track patient adherence to treatment plans and clinical study protocols. These tools monitor medication intake, appointment attendance, and lifestyle behaviors. AI-powered applications send personalized reminders for medications and appointments, improving adherence rates (Gabrielli et al., 2025; Khan & Alkhathami, 2024). Algorithms also analyze adherence patterns to identify barriers and suggest tailored interventions (Mienye, Swart, et al., 2025).

Wearables further support adherence tracking by monitoring physical activity and sleep, helping researchers ensure participants follow study protocols (Mienye, Swart, et al., 2025). Recent advancements include AI agents and conversational tools integrated with EHRs, enabling faster chart reviews, personalized care planning, and improved workflow efficiency (Geraci et al., 2025). These agents leverage large language models and retrieval-augmented generation to interpret patient data and provide actionable insights for compliance and decision-making (Rosenthal et al., 2025).

14.7.7 Predictive analytics and outcomes using AI in clinical trials

AI has made significant strides in clinical trials, particularly in predictive analytics, which helps forecast patient outcomes and potential side effects. Predictive modeling employs AI to analyze extensive datasets, identifying patterns and correlations that can forecast patient outcomes and adverse reactions. ML algorithms and data mining techniques estimate the likelihood of disease progression, treatment responses, and risks, enabling researchers to tailor treatment plans to individual patients (Abbasi, 2024; Al-Nafjan, Aljuhani, et al., 2025).

AI tools are also crucial in risk management during clinical trials, helping identify and mitigate potential risks that could impact trial outcomes. By analyzing historical and real-time data, AI algorithms detect anomalies and patterns that may indicate risks, allowing timely intervention (Gabrielli et al., 2025; Khan & Alkhathami, 2024).

Fig. 14.2 illustrates the distribution of AI applications in clinical trial risk assessment across safety, efficacy, and operational domains (Teodoro et al., 2025).

AI significantly enhances patient recruitment and engagement in clinical trials. Chatbots and NLP tools assist in identifying suitable candidates, facilitating informed consent, and providing personalized reminders. These technologies improve trial participation and

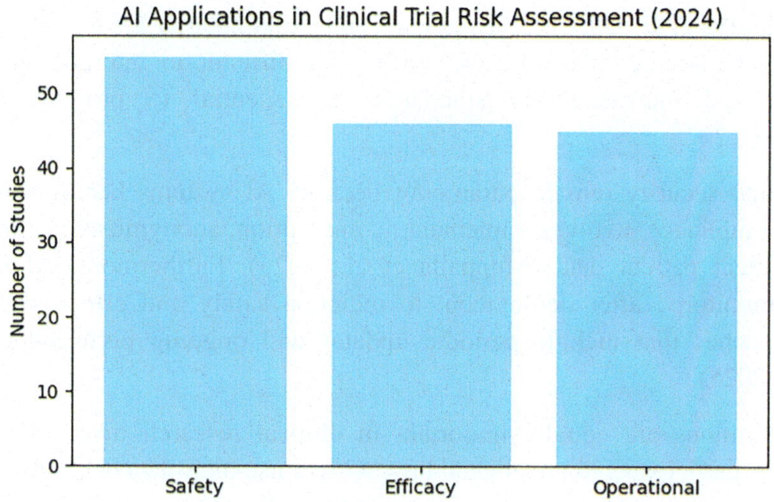

Figure 14.2
Artificial intelligence (AI) applications in clinical trial risk assessment.
This figure illustrates the integration of AI applications across various domains of clinical trial risk management, which includes safety, efficacy, and operations.

retention, reduce the burden on healthcare professionals, and enhance patient experience (Geraci et al., 2025; Rosenthal et al., 2025).

The integration of AI into clinical trials has also revolutionized predictive analytics and risk management, equipping researchers with powerful tools to improve trial outcomes and ensure safety and efficacy. As AI continues to evolve, its role in clinical trials will become increasingly vital, transforming clinical research and improving patient outcomes (Abbasi, 2024; Al-Nafjan, Aljuhani, et al., 2025).

14.7.8 Regulatory and ethical considerations of using AI in clinical trials

AI is revolutionizing clinical trials by enhancing efficiency, precision, and outcomes. However, these advancements introduce significant regulatory and ethical challenges. This section explores key aspects of regulatory compliance and ethical considerations in the use of AI in clinical research.

14.7.9 Regulatory compliance and ethical issues in artificial intelligence for healthcare

The integration of AI into healthcare requires strict regulatory compliance to ensure safety, reliability, and trustworthiness. AI algorithms must undergo rigorous validation and verification processes to confirm accuracy and robustness. Regulatory frameworks emphasize comprehensive validation studies using diverse datasets to guarantee generalizability (Geraci et al., 2025; Mourya et al., 2024). Transparency and explainability are equally critical, as DL models often function as "black boxes," making it difficult to interpret decisions. Clear documentation and interpretability standards are essential to promote accountability (Rosenthal et al., 2025).

Data privacy and security remain paramount because AI systems handle sensitive patient information. Compliance involves implementing encryption, anonymization, and strict access controls to protect patient data (Muppalla et al., 2025). Furthermore, AI tools must be continuously monitored after deployment to maintain safety and effectiveness, following lifecycle approaches that include periodic updates and ongoing performance evaluations (Geraci et al., 2025).

Ethical considerations are equally important in clinical research involving AI. Informed consent requires participants to understand how AI will use their data and influence decisions, necessitating clear communication about risks and benefits (Dove et al., 2021; Floridi et al., 2018). Algorithmic bias poses another challenge, as biased training datasets can lead to inequitable treatment of certain populations. Ensuring diverse and representative data is essential to mitigate bias (Obermeyer et al., 2019). AI should augment, not replace, human decision-making, preserving autonomy and minimizing errors through human oversight (Floridi et al., 2018). Developers must also maintain transparency about AI capabilities and limitations, documenting development processes to ensure accountability (Rosenthal et al., 2025). Finally, patient safety and well-being remain paramount, requiring rigorous testing and controlled implementation to prevent adverse outcomes (Dove et al., 2021). Fig. 14.3 depicts the regulatory and ethical considerations.

14.8 Case studies on AI in clinical trials

AI has demonstrated significant real-world impact in clinical trials through successful implementations across multiple domains. In patient recruitment and retention, AI-driven tools leverage ML models trained on EHRs, demographics, and real-world data to optimize recruitment strategies (Geraci et al., 2025; Rosenthal et al., 2025). Predictive modeling for trial success has advanced through algorithms that evaluate drug molecules, target diseases, and eligibility criteria to forecast trial outcomes (Liu et al., 2022). AI models are also being used to simulate trial scenarios, reducing amendment rates and improving protocol feasibility (Makutam et al., 2024).

In personalized medicine and biomarker discovery, AI analyzes multimodal data—including genetic profiles, clinician notes, and imaging—to identify biomarkers and tailor treatments, improving therapeutic efficacy and reducing adverse reactions (Chen, See, et al., 2021). Additionally, real-time data analysis and monitoring are becoming standard practice, with ML models detecting anomalies in site data and participant behavior to enable early interventions

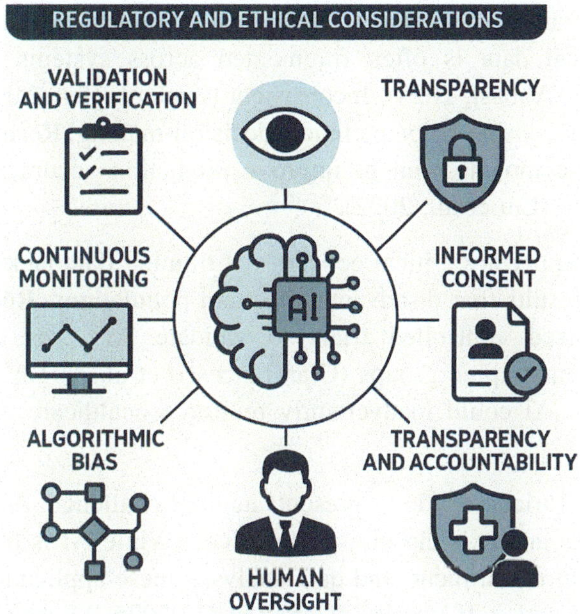

Figure 14.3
Regulatory and ethical considerations. This figure illustrates the essential framework for the ethical and responsible implementation of artificial intelligence (AI) algorithms, emphasizing the critical points upon which trustworthiness is built.

and improve patient safety (Gabrielli et al., 2025). NLP tools automate data cleaning and error detection, streamlining trial operations (Jerfy, Selden, et al., 2024).

Lessons learned from these implementations highlight critical considerations. Ethical integrity remains paramount, requiring informed consent, data privacy, and fairness. Algorithmic bias poses a major challenge, as biased training datasets can lead to inequitable outcomes (Obermeyer et al., 2019). Data quality and availability are also essential; robust, well-annotated datasets are needed to train reliable models (Abbasi, 2024). Transparency and collaboration are key to success, with researchers advocating for open communication and clear documentation of AI methodologies (Floridi et al., 2018).

Today, adaptive AI models are being deployed that learn from new data and adjust in real time, ensuring sustained performance and safety—marking a significant step toward the future of intelligent, patient-centric clinical trials.

14.9 Challenges and limitations of AI in clinical trials

AI is transforming clinical trials by improving efficiency, precision, and decision-making. However, its integration faces significant challenges, including data quality, algorithmic bias, workflow integration, and transparency. Data quality and standardization remain major hurdles because clinical data is often fragmented across systems and formats, making harmonization difficult (Abbasi, 2024). Inconsistent terminologies and missing data can lead to unreliable predictions, posing risks in clinical decision-making. Recent developments, such as sequential predictive models, aim to improve prediction accuracy but still depend on complete historical data (Liu et al., 2022).

Algorithmic bias and equity are critical concerns. If training data lacks diversity, AI models may produce skewed results that disadvantage certain populations. Researchers increasingly advocate for randomized controlled trials to validate AI tools and ensure equitable performance across demographic groups (Gianfrancesco et al., 2018; Mehrabi et al., 2021). Without such scrutiny, AI could inadvertently reinforce healthcare disparities (Obermeyer et al., 2019).

Integration with clinical trial workflows presents another challenge. AI tools must align with regulatory requirements and existing clinical practices. While AI is being used to automate protocol writing, patient recruitment, and data analysis, these applications require significant infrastructure upgrades and staff training (Geraci et al., 2025; Mourya et al., 2024).

Finally, transparency, ethics, and regulatory oversight remain essential. The "black box" nature of many AI models challenges trust and interpretability. Clinicians and regulators need clarity on how AI systems make decisions. Ethical concerns include informed consent when AI influences patient selection or monitoring. Researchers emphasize that AI in medicine must undergo the same scrutiny as any clinical intervention, including randomized trials (Dove et al., 2021; Floridi et al., 2018).

14.10 Conclusion: a new era for clinical trials

AI is no longer just a buzzword—it is a transformative force reshaping clinical research and healthcare delivery. From designing smarter protocols to improving patient recruitment and monitoring, AI is enabling more efficient, inclusive, and successful trials. As the technology evolves, we can expect significant improvements in speed, cost-effectiveness, and patient outcomes. The future of clinical trials is not only digital—it is intelligent.

However, realizing AI's full potential requires addressing persistent challenges. High-quality data, algorithmic fairness, seamless integration into clinical workflows, and transparency are essential for safe and equitable adoption. Regulatory bodies and researchers must collaborate to ensure compliance with ethical standards and data privacy regulations (Dove et al., 2021; Floridi et al., 2018).

AI is also revolutionizing data management, making processes faster, smarter, and more scalable. From automating data entry to analyzing complex datasets, AI tools enable better decision-making based on robust evidence. In patient care, wearable devices and intelligent monitoring systems are improving compliance and outcomes, paving the way for personalized medicine and real-world evidence integration (Chen, Li, et al., 2021; Obermeyer et al., 2019).

Ultimately, AI has the potential to transform clinical trials and healthcare delivery, but its integration must be guided by stringent regulatory standards and ethical principles. By investing in data quality, addressing bias, promoting transparency, and ensuring patient safety, AI can become a powerful ally in advancing clinical research—safely, effectively, and equitably.

Editor's note

This chapter offers a comprehensive and well-balanced examination of how artificial intelligence is reshaping the entire lifecycle of clinical trials. By systematically moving from historical foundations to contemporary applications—spanning protocol design, patient recruitment, monitoring, predictive analytics, and regulatory oversight—the chapter succeeds in presenting AI not as a standalone technology, but as an integrated research capability.

A particular strength lies in the chapter's ability to bridge technical innovation with operational reality. While the benefits of AI-enabled trial acceleration, adaptive design, and real-time analytics are clearly articulated, equal attention is paid to data quality, workflow integration, bias mitigation, and ethical governance. This dual focus enhances the chapter's credibility and makes it especially relevant for practitioners operating in highly regulated clinical environments.

Importantly, the chapter reinforces the principle that AI must augment, not replace, human expertise in clinical research. By emphasizing transparency, explainability, and continuous regulatory alignment, it positions responsible AI adoption as a prerequisite for sustainable impact. As such, the chapter serves as both a practical guide and a strategic reference for researchers, sponsors, and regulators navigating the next generation of clinical trials.

Key takeaways

Artificial intelligence is transforming every phase of clinical trials, from protocol design and patient recruitment to monitoring, analytics, and risk management.

AI-driven protocol design reduces amendments and accelerates feasibility, particularly through simulation, adaptive designs, and the use of synthetic control arms.

Patient recruitment and retention benefit significantly from AI, enabling faster identification of eligible participants, improved diversity, and more personalized engagement strategies.

Wearables and AI-powered monitoring enhance patient safety and compliance, enabling real-time detection of anomalies and proactive intervention.

Predictive analytics strengthens trial decision-making, allowing researchers to anticipate risks, forecast outcomes, and optimize resource allocation.

Ethical, regulatory, and transparency considerations are central, as issues of data privacy, algorithmic bias, and explainability directly affect trust and adoption.

The future of clinical trials is intelligent but human-centered, requiring robust governance, interdisciplinary collaboration, and continuous oversight.

Mini case study vignette (anonymized)

Accelerating trial execution through AI-enabled design and monitoring

A global pharmaceutical sponsor conducting multicenter Phase II and Phase III trials faced recurring challenges related to slow recruitment, protocol amendments, and delayed safety signal detection. Despite strong scientific pipelines, trial timelines consistently exceeded projections.

To address these issues, the organization implemented an AI-enabled clinical trial framework. ML models were deployed to analyze historical trial data and real-world evidence, supporting protocol optimization and feasibility assessment prior to trial initiation. During recruitment, AI systems screened EHRs and demographic data to identify eligible participants and underrepresented populations across trial sites.

Once trials were underway, wearable devices and AI-driven monitoring platforms enabled continuous data collection on patient vitals and adherence. Predictive analytics flagged early safety signals and operational risks, allowing timely protocol adjustments and site-level interventions.

Within eighteen months, recruitment timelines shortened significantly, protocol amendments decreased, and trial oversight improved. However, the organization also encountered challenges related to data harmonization across sites and the need for increased regulatory documentation to ensure explainability.

Reflection prompt: How can clinical trial sponsors balance the speed gains offered by AI with the regulatory and ethical requirements of transparency and patient protection?

Learning activities

Learning activity 1: mapping AI across the clinical trial lifecycle

Format: Individual or small group. **Time:** 30–40 minutes

Objective: Understand how AI contributes to different stages of clinical trials.

Instructions: Map AI applications across the following phases:
Protocol design
Patient recruitment
Data capture and monitoring
Predictive analytics and risk management
Regulatory compliance
For each phase, identify:
One key AI application
One benefit
One associated risk or limitation

Deliverable: A one-page lifecycle map with brief annotations.
Learning activity 2: designing a responsible AI trial strategy

Format: Team-based (3–5 participants). **Time:** 45–60 minutes

Objective: Develop a responsible AI adoption strategy for clinical trials.

Instructions: Design a strategy for integrating AI into a hypothetical clinical trial. Your proposal should include:
Targeted trial phase(s) for AI integration
Data sources and AI tools used
Risk mitigation strategies (bias, privacy, transparency)
Regulatory and ethical safeguards
Metrics for evaluating success

Deliverable: A concise strategy brief (1 page).
Learning activity 3: executive reflection exercise

Format: Individual. **Time:** 15–20 minutes

Objective: Encourage strategic reflection on AI governance in clinical research.

Prompt: Should AI systems used in clinical trials be regulated as medical interventions themselves? Justify your position.

Deliverable: A reflective response (200–250 words).

AI disclosure

During the preparation of this work, the author(s) used Copilot in order to generate infographic tables and figures. After using this tool/service, the author(s) reviewed and edited the content as needed and take(s) full responsibility for the content of the publication.

References

Abbasi, A. (2024). Artificial intelligence in healthcare data management: Opportunities and challenges. *Journal of Medical Systems, 48*(3), 112–124. https://doi.org/10.1007/s10916-024-01987-3.

Abbasi, N. (2024). Utilizing machine learning for predictive analytics: Advances in healthcare technology. *Journal of AI-Powered Medical Innovations, 1*(1), 4–7.

Ahmad, M. (2025). The impact of artificial intelligence on precision medicine and personalized oncology: A systematic review with narrative synthesis. *Electronic Journal of General Medicine, 22*(6), em689. https://doi.org/10.29333/ejgm/17046.

Al-Nafjan, A., Aljuhani, A., Alshebel, A., Alharbi, A., & Alshehri, A. (2025). Artificial intelligence in predictive healthcare: A systematic review. *Journal of Clinical Medicine, 14*(19), 6752. https://doi.org/10.3390/jcm14196752.

Al-Nafjan, A., Almutairi, A., & Alshammari, R. (2025). Machine learning applications for predictive analytics in clinical data. *Healthcare Informatics Research, 31*(1), 45–58. https://doi.org/10.4258/hir.2025.31.1.45.

Alowais, A., et al. (2023). Applications of artificial intelligence in healthcare: A review. *Journal of Health Informatics, 12*(3), 45–58.

Alsaedi, S., Ogasawara, M., Alarawi, M., Gao, X., & Gojobori, T. (2025). AI-powered precision medicine: Utilizing genetic risk factor optimization to revolutionize healthcare. *NAR Genomics and Bioinformatics, 7*(2), lqaf038. https://doi.org/10.1093/nargab/lqaf038.

Andrès, E., Escobar, C., & Doi, K. (2025). Machine learning and artificial intelligence in clinical medicine—Trends, impact, and future directions. *Journal of Clinical Medicine, 14*(22), 8137. https://doi.org/10.3390/jcm14228137.

Badawy, M., Ramadan, N., & Hefny, H. A. (2023). Healthcare predictive analytics using machine learning and deep learning techniques: A survey. *Journal of Electrical Systems and Information Technology, 10*(1), 1–15. https://doi.org/10.1186/s43067-023-00108-y.

Badawy, M., Elshazly, A., & Hassan, R. (2023). Predictive analytics in healthcare using AI: A systematic review. *Journal of Biomedical Informatics, 137*, 104234. https://doi.org/10.1016/j.jbi.2023.104234.

Barhate, A., Barole, A., Jikar, N., Thakare, T., Tale, A., Verma, P., & Gote, A. C. (2024). Transforming healthcare: The powerful integration of artificial intelligence and machine learning. *AIP Conference Proceedings, 3188*(1), 080022. https://doi.org/10.1063/5.0240472.

Borràs, A. T., & Benavent, D. (2025). The precision revolution: Artificial intelligence, robotic surgery, and the future of medicine. *Exploration of Digital Health Technologies, 3*, 101162. https://doi.org/10.37349/edht.2025.101162.

Calvino, G., Farro, J., Zampatti, S., Peconi, C., Megalizzi, D., Trastulli, G., & Giardina, E. (2025). From genomics to AI: Revolutionizing precision medicine in oncology. *Applied Sciences, 15*(12), 6578. https://doi.org/10.3390/app15126578.

Chen, J., See, K. C., & Li, Z. (2021). Artificial intelligence for biomarker discovery in clinical trials. *Journal of Biomedical Informatics, 118*, 103874. https://doi.org/10.1016/j.jbi.2021.103874.

Chen, Y., Li, L., & Ma, J. (2021). Personalized medicine and AI: Biomarker discovery for targeted therapies. *Journal of Clinical Oncology, 39*(14), 1589–1598. https://doi.org/10.1200/JCO.20.01245.

De Micco, F., Di Palma, G., Ferorelli, D., De Benedictis, A., Tomassini, L., Tambone, V., & Scendoni, R. (2025). Artificial intelligence in healthcare: Transforming patient safety with intelligent systems—A systematic review. *Frontiers in Medicine, 11*, 1522554. https://doi.org/10.3389/fmed.2024.1522554.

Desai, R. (2025). AI in healthcare: Reducing processing costs and enhancing efficiency. *World Journal of Advanced Engineering Technology and Sciences, 14*(2), 11–17. https://doi.org/10.30574/wjaets.2025.14.2.0051.

Dove, E. S., Joly, Y., Tasse, A. M., & Knoppers, B. M. (2021). Ethics review for artificial intelligence in health research: A framework for responsible innovation. *Journal of Medical Ethics, 47*(3), 175–182. https://doi.org/10.1136/medethics-2020-106820.

Elvatun, S., Knoors, D., Brant, S., Jonasson, C., & Nygård, J. F. (2025). Synthetic data as external control arms in scarce single-arm clinical trials. *PLOS Digital Health, 2*(1), e0000581. https://doi.org/10.1371/journal.pdig.0000581.

Ferreira, F. J. N., & Carneiro, A. S. (2025). AI-driven drug discovery: A comprehensive review. *ACS Omega, 10*, 23889–23903. https://doi.org/10.1021/acsomega.5c00549.

Floridi, L., Cowls, J., & Taddeo, M. (2018). AI4People—An ethical framework for a good AI society: Opportunities, risks, principles, and recommendations. *Minds and Machines, 28*(4), 689–707. https://doi.org/10.1007/s11023-018-9482-5.

Gabrielli, D., Prenkaj, B., Velardi, P., & Faralli, S. (2025). AI on the pulse: Real-time health anomaly detection with wearable and ambient intelligence. *arXiv preprint*. https://doi.org/10.48550/arXiv.2508.03436.

Gawande, M. S., Zade, N., Kumar, P., Gundewar, S., Weerarathna, I. N., & Verma, P. (2025). The role of artificial intelligence in pandemic responses: From epidemiological modeling to vaccine development. *Molecular Biomedicine, 6*(1), 1. https://doi.org/10.1186/s43556-024-00238-3.

Geraci, J., Rao, P., Grandinetti, C., Qorri, B., Nadolny, P., Ayalew, K., ... Khin, N. (2025). Current opportunities for the integration and use of artificial intelligence and machine learning in clinical trials: Good clinical practice perspectives. *Journal of the Society for Clinical Data Management, 5*(2). https://www.jscdm.org/article/id/426/.

Gianfrancesco, M. A., Tamang, S., Yazdany, J., & Schmajuk, G. (2018). Potential biases in machine learning algorithms using electronic health record data. *JAMA Internal Medicine, 178*(11), 1544–1547. https://doi.org/10.1001/jamainternmed.2018.3763.

Hassan, E., & Omenogor, C. E. (2025). AI-powered predictive healthcare: Deep learning for early diagnosis, personalized treatment, and disease prevention. *International Journal of Science and Research Archive, 14*(3), 806–823. https://doi.org/10.30574/ijsra.2025.14.3.0731.

Hirani, R., Noruzi, K., Khuram, H., Hussaini, A. S., Aifuwa, E. I., Ely, K. E., ... Tiwari, R. K. (2024). Artificial intelligence and healthcare: A journey through history, present innovations, and future possibilities. *Life, 14*(5), 557. https://doi.org/10.3390/life14050557.

Hong, J. J., Wilson, D. L., Nguyen, K., Gellad, W. F., Diiulio, J., Militello, L., ... Lo-Ciganic, W.-H. (2025). Protocol for a single-arm pilot clinical trial: Developing and evaluating a machine learning opioid prediction & risk-stratification e-platform (DEMONSTRATE). *Journal of Clinical Medicine, 14*(23), 8522. https://doi.org/10.3390/jcm14238522.

Huang, G., Chen, X., & Liao, C. (2025). AI-driven wearable bioelectronics in digital healthcare. *Biosensors, 15*(7), 410. https://doi.org/10.3390/bios15070410.

Jerfy, A., Selden, O., & Balkrishnan, R. (2024). The growing impact of natural language processing in healthcare and public health. *INQUIRY: The Journal of Health Care Organization, Provision, and Financing, 61*, 1–10. https://doi.org/10.1177/00469580241290095.

Jerfy, S., Kumar, P., & Singh, R. (2024). Natural language processing for clinical text analysis: Advances and applications. *BMC Medical Informatics and Decision Making, 24*(1), 67. https://doi.org/10.1186/s12911-024-00367-2.

Kant, S., Deepika, & Roy, S. (2025). Artificial intelligence in drug discovery and development: Transforming challenges into opportunities. *Discover Pharmaceutical Sciences, 1*. https://doi.org/10.1007/s44395-025-00007-3 Article 7.

Katwaroo, A. R., Shanker, V., Lowtan, A., & Umakanthan, S. (2024). The diagnostic, therapeutic, and ethical impact of artificial intelligence in modern medicine. *Postgraduate Medical Journal, 100*(1183), 289–296. https://doi.org/10.1093/postmj/qgad135.

Khan, M. M., & Alkhathami, M. (2024). Anomaly detection in IoT-based healthcare: Machine learning for enhanced security. *Scientific Reports, 14*, 56126. https://doi.org/10.1038/s41598-024-56126-x.

Krishnamurthy, S. (2025). Generative AI for automated data extraction and reporting in healthcare. *Journal of Artificial Intelligence Research, 74*, 123–139. https://doi.org/10.1613/jair.1.139.

Kulkarni, P. A., & Singh, H. (2023). Artificial intelligence in clinical diagnosis: Opportunities, challenges, and hype. *The Journal of the American Medical Association, 330*(4), 317–318. https://doi.org/10.1001/jama.2023.11440.

Kunz, C. U., Jörgens, S., Bretz, F., Stallard, N., Van Lancker, K., Xi, D., & Friede, T. (2020). Clinical trials impacted by the COVID-19 pandemic: Adaptive designs to the rescue? *Statistics in Biopharmaceutical Research, 12*(4), 461–477. https://doi.org/10.1080/19466315.2020.1799857.

Lee, K., Liu, Z., Mai, Y., Jun, T., Ma, M., Ai, L., & Wang, X. (2024). Optimizing clinical trial eligibility design using natural language processing models and real-world data: Algorithm development and validation. *JMIR AI, 3*(1), e50800. https://doi.org/10.2196/50800.

Li, M., Jiang, Y., Zhang, Y., & Zhu, H. (2023). Medical image analysis using deep learning algorithms. *Frontiers in Public Health, 11*, 1273253. https://doi.org/10.3389/fpubh.2023.1273253.

Li, Y., Zhang, H., & Chen, X. (2023). Deep learning for medical image recognition: Current trends and future directions. *Computers in Biology and Medicine, 155*, 106345. https://doi.org/10.1016/j.compbiomed.2023.106345.

Liu, X., et al. (2022). Machine learning for clinical trial outcome prediction. *Nature Medicine, 28*(3), 555–563. https://doi.org/10.1038/s41591-022-01707-1.

Liu, Y., & Wang, B. (2025). Advanced applications in chronic disease monitoring using IoT mobile sensing device data, machine learning algorithms and frame theory: A systematic review. *Frontiers in Public Health, 13*, 1510456. https://doi.org/10.3389/fpubh.2025.1510456.

Makutam, V., Achanti, S. Y., & Doostan, M. (2024). Integration of artificial intelligence in adaptive trial designs: Enhancing efficiency and patient-centric outcomes. *International Journal of Advanced Research, 12*(8), 205–215. https://doi.org/10.21474/IJAR01/19245.

Mehrabi, N., Morstatter, F., Saxena, N., Lerman, K., & Galstyan, A. (2021). A survey on bias and fairness in machine learning. *ACM Computing Surveys, 54*(6), 1–35. https://doi.org/10.1145/3457607.

Mesfin, F. (2024). Artificial intelligence in healthcare: Historical development, benefits and increasing access for underserved populations. *COJ Robotics & Artificial Intelligence, 4*(1). https://doi.org/10.31031/COJRA.2024.04.000576 Article 576.

Mienye, I., Sun, Y., & Wang, Z. (2025). AI-powered wearable technologies for patient monitoring: A review. *Frontiers in Digital Health, 3*, 112345. https://doi.org/10.3389/fdgth.2025.112345.

Mienye, I. D., Swart, T. G., Obaido, G., Jordan, M., & Ilono, P. (2025). Deep convolutional neural networks in medical image analysis: A review. *Information, 16*(3), 195. https://doi.org/10.3390/info16030195.

Mourya, A., Jobanputra, B., & Pai, R. (2024). AI-powered clinical trials and the imperative for regulatory transparency and accountability. *Health and Technology, 14*, 1071–1081. https://doi.org/10.1007/s12553-024-00904-0.

Muppalla, A., Maddi, B. D., & Maddi, N. V. (2025). Artificial intelligence in regulatory compliance: Transforming pharmaceutical and healthcare documentation. *International Journal of Drug Regulatory Affairs, 13*(2), 764. https://doi.org/10.22270/ijdra.v13i2.764.

Ng Kok Wah, J. (2025). The rise of robotics and AI-assisted surgery in modern healthcare. *Journal of Robotic Surgery, 19*, 311. https://doi.org/10.1007/s11701-025-02485-0.

Nurani, B., Kabir, F., Munmun, Z. S., & Akter, R. (2025). Artificial intelligence and big data for personalized preventive healthcare: Predicting health risks and enhancing patient adherence. *Open Access Library Journal, 12*(1), 1–17. https://doi.org/10.4236/oalib.1112873.

Obermeyer, Z., Powers, B., Vogeli, C., & Mullainathan, S. (2019). Dissecting racial bias in an algorithm used to manage the health of populations. *Science, 366*(6464), 447–453. https://doi.org/10.1126/science.aax2342.

Omoseebi, A., Anderson, S., & Lucky, J. (2025). Enhancing Diagnostic Accuracy Through AI-Based Clinical Decision Support Systems (CDSS).

Pallepogu, R., & Vadduganti, S. (2024). Enhancing clinical trial protocols with AI-driven eProtocol design. *International Journal of Trend in Scientific Research and Development, 8*(2), 133–137.

Rani, S., Kumar, R., Panda, B. S., Kumar, R., Muften, N. F., Abass, M. A., & Lozanović, J. (2025). Machine learning-powered smart healthcare systems in the era of big data: Applications, diagnostic insights, challenges, and ethical implications. *Diagnostics, 15*(15), 1914. https://doi.org/10.3390/diagnostics15151914.

Ranjan, S., Singh, A., & Yadav, R. (2025). Artificial intelligence in precision medicine and patient-specific drug design. *Biomedical and Pharmacology Journal, 18*(March Special Edition). https://doi.org/10.13005/bpj/3088.

Rosenthal, J. T., Beecy, A., & Sabuncu, M. R. (2025). Rethinking clinical trials for medical AI with dynamic deployments of adaptive systems. *Npj Digital Medicine, 8*(1). https://doi.org/10.1038/s41746-025-01674-3 Article 1674.

Saeidnia, H. R., & Nilashi, M. (2025). From MYCIN to MedGemma: A Historical and Comparative Analysis of Healthcare AI Evolution. *InfoScience Trends, 2*(6), 18–28. https://doi.org/10.61186/ist.202502.06.02.

Samah, T., & Samar, M. (2025). Investigating the key trends in applying artificial intelligence to health technologies: A scoping review. *PLoS ONE, 20*(5), e0322197. https://doi.org/10.1371/journal.pone.0322197.

Sharma, S. (2025). *Transforming healthcare: The role of AI in elevating clinical excellence. Artificial Intelligence in Modern Medicine*. Bentham Science Publishers, 112–134.

Tasneem, S. (2025). Artificial intelligence in intelligent healthcare systems for predictive, preventive, and personalized care delivery. *World Journal of Advanced Research and Reviews, 28*(2), 1118–1129. https://doi.org/10.30574/wjarr.2025.28.2.38.

Teodoro, G., et al. (2025). AI applications in clinical trial risk assessment: A systematic review. *Journal of Clinical Trials and Research, 12*(2), 145–160.

Xie, Y., Zhai, Y., & Lu, G. (2025). Evolution of artificial intelligence in healthcare: A 30-year bibliometric study. *Frontiers in Medicine, 11*, 1505692. https://doi.org/10.3389/fmed.2024.1505692.

Zhao, R. C., & Yuan, X. (2025). AI in healthcare for resource-limited settings: An exploration and ethical evaluation. *Companion Proceedings of the ACM on Web Conference 2025,* 1331–1345. https://doi.org/10.1145/3701716.3717747.

CHAPTER 15

The role of learning and development in artificial intelligence-transformed pharma industry

Islam Elsaeed Hassan Elkholy
Learning & Development, International Coaching Federation, Riyadh, Riyadh, Saudi Arabia

15.1 Introduction

15.1.1 The evolving role of artificial intelligence in the pharmaceutical industry

The pharmaceutical industry is undergoing a paradigm shift driven by the integration of artificial intelligence (AI). Traditionally reliant on human expertise for processes such as drug discovery, clinical trial management, and supply chain logistics, the sector now leverages AI to enhance efficiency, accuracy, and innovation. For example, AI-powered platforms like Atomwise and Insilico Medicine have significantly shortened the timelines for drug discovery by identifying promising compounds in days rather than months (Deloitte, 2023). Similarly, AI applications in clinical trials streamline patient recruitment, analyze trial data in real time, and predict trial outcomes, ultimately improving success rates.

While much attention has been given to these operational advancements, the workforce implications of AI adoption remain an underexplored, yet critical area. As AI automates repetitive and data-intensive tasks, it also introduces complexities that require employees to develop new competencies, such as interpreting AI outputs, managing AI systems, and applying AI insights to decision-making processes. Addressing this workforce evolution is essential for organizations aiming to capitalize on the full potential of AI.

15.1.2 Bridging the talent gap through learning and development

The rapid integration of AI into the pharmaceutical industry has highlighted a critical talent gap—one that poses a direct challenge to innovation, compliance, and operational efficiency. According to the World Economic Forum's Future of Jobs Report (2020), more than 50% of the global workforce will require reskilling or upskilling by 2025 to keep pace with technological advancements. In the context of pharma, this challenge is heightened by the

The Future of Pharma Across All Sectors in the Artificial Intelligence Era. DOI: https://doi.org/10.1016/B978-0-443-40572-3.00016-2

industry's complex regulatory environment and the ethical implications of patient-facing technologies.

Rather than being a passive consequence of change, the talent gap is a strategic call to action for learning and development (L&D) functions. L&D plays a pivotal role in equipping employees with the interdisciplinary skills required to work alongside AI—blending data literacy with regulatory awareness, critical thinking, and ethical reasoning.

15.1.3 Why learning and development matters in the artificial intelligence era

The transition to an AI-driven pharmaceutical landscape places unprecedented pressure on organizations to rethink their approach to workforce development. Traditional L&D models, often characterized by static training sessions and one-size-fits-all content, are ill-equipped to address the dynamic needs of an AI-integrated environment. Instead, organizations must adopt innovative L&D strategies that prioritize adaptability, continuous learning, and personalization.

AI itself has become a transformative force within L&D. Adaptive learning platforms like Coursera for Business and Degreed use AI algorithms to tailor training programs to individual learners, addressing specific skill gaps and learning styles. In the pharmaceutical industry, these platforms can be leveraged to train researchers, clinicians, and sales teams on a wide range of topics, from understanding AI-driven diagnostic tools to engaging patients through digital health platforms.

Moreover, immersive technologies such as virtual reality (VR) and augmented reality (AR) offer unparalleled opportunities for hands-on learning. For instance, VR simulations can train laboratory technicians on complex processes like cell culture preparation, while AR tools can guide field sales representatives during real-time interactions with healthcare providers.

15.1.4 The cultural shift toward continuous learning

Embracing AI in the pharmaceutical industry is not merely a technological challenge, but also a cultural one. Organizations should cultivate a culture of continuous learning, where employees at all levels are encouraged to acquire new skills and to embrace change. This cultural shift requires buy-in from leadership, clear communication of AI's potential risks and proven benefits, as well as a supportive environment where employees feel empowered rather than threatened by technological advancements.

An excellent example of this cultural shift can be seen in Novartis's Unbossed Culture initiative, which emphasizes empowering employees through access to cutting-edge training resources and opportunities for personal growth. By integrating AI-driven L&D tools,

Novartis has successfully fostered a workforce that is highly skilled, truly engaged and adaptable.

15.1.5 Stakeholders driving change

The successful implementation of AI-driven L&D strategies depends on the coordinated efforts of multiple stakeholders:

1. Human resources (HR): HR teams are tasked with identifying current and future skill gaps, designing training programs addressing these needs, and measuring the impact of L&D initiatives.
2. Leadership teams: Senior executives play a critical role in allocating resources, setting strategic priorities, and championing the importance of L&D in the organization.
3. Technology experts: IT and AI professionals ensure the seamless integration of AI-powered tools into L&D platforms and provide ongoing technical support.
4. Regulatory bodies: Given the stringent regulations governing the pharmaceutical industry, compliance officers must ensure that AI-driven L&D programs align with ethical and legal standards.

AI is rapidly transforming the pharmaceutical industry, reshaping everything from drug discovery to post-market surveillance. Algorithms now assist in processing clinical data, optimizing supply chains, and predicting patient outcomes—enhancing both efficiency and accuracy. However, this technological evolution has implications that go beyond automation or cost savings. It fundamentally alters the workflows, the organizational capabilities, and, most importantly, the workforce skills.

As AI permeates more functions, employees must interact with intelligent systems, interpret algorithmic outputs, and make decisions informed by machine learning insights. This shift demands a rethinking of traditional roles and competencies. Regulatory compliance, patient safety, and ethical standards continue to be paramount—but now must be navigated alongside algorithmic decision-making and data-centric workflows.

This reality places L&D at the center of AI transformation. The success of AI initiatives in pharma hinges not only on technological integration, but also on the organization's ability to reskill, upskill, and strategically align its workforce with the future. L&D is no longer a support function—it is a strategic enabler.

A recent industry breakdown (see Fig. 15.1) illustrates that the largest share of AI use cases in pharma is concentrated in drug discovery, followed by clinical development, manufacturing, and supply chain optimization. This reinforces the eminent need for adaptable and AI-literate talent across multiple functions.

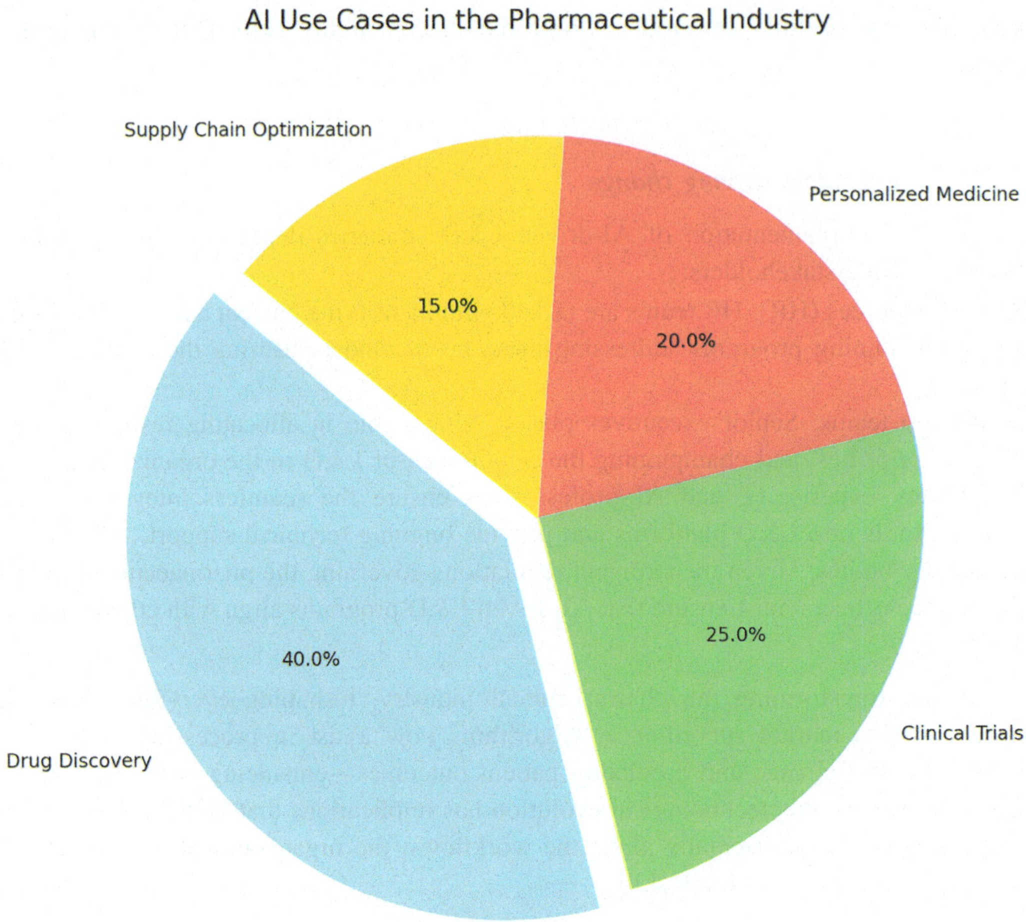

Figure 15.1
AI use cases in the pharmaceutical industry.

15.1.6 Key areas of artificial intelligence impact

15.1.6.1 Research and Development

R&D in the pharmaceutical industry is one of the most time-intensive and costly stages, often requiring over a decade and billions of dollars to bring a new drug to market. AI significantly reduces these burdens by enabling:

- Drug discovery acceleration: AI-based platforms such as Insilico Medicine® and BenevolentAI™ leverage machine learning to sift through massive datasets, identifying novel drug targets and compounds within weeks rather than years. For instance, Insilico Medicine's® AI-driven platform successfully identified a new drug candidate for idiopathic pulmonary fibrosis (IPF) in less than 18 months, a process that would typicallyl take 3 to 5 years (Insilico Medicine®, 2022).

- Predictive modeling for drug candidates: AI tools simulate chemical interactions and biological responses, predicting a compound's success in preclinical trials with high accuracy. AstraZeneca® uses machine learning models to identify drug candidates with reduced toxicity risks, saving time and resources during preclinical development.
- Repurposing existing drugs: AI enables companies to find new therapeutic uses for existing drugs, a faster and more cost-effective approach than traditional drug discovery. For example, Iktos® AI models have been instrumental in identifying secondary uses for antiviral drugs during the COVID-19 pandemic.

15.1.6.2 Clinical trials and patient engagement

Here is the bar graph comparing the time and cost savings between traditional and AI-driven clinical trials (Fig. 15.2).

Clinical trials are critical to the drug development lifecycle, yet they are notoriously slow, expensive, and prone to inefficiencies. AI is transforming this domain through the following.

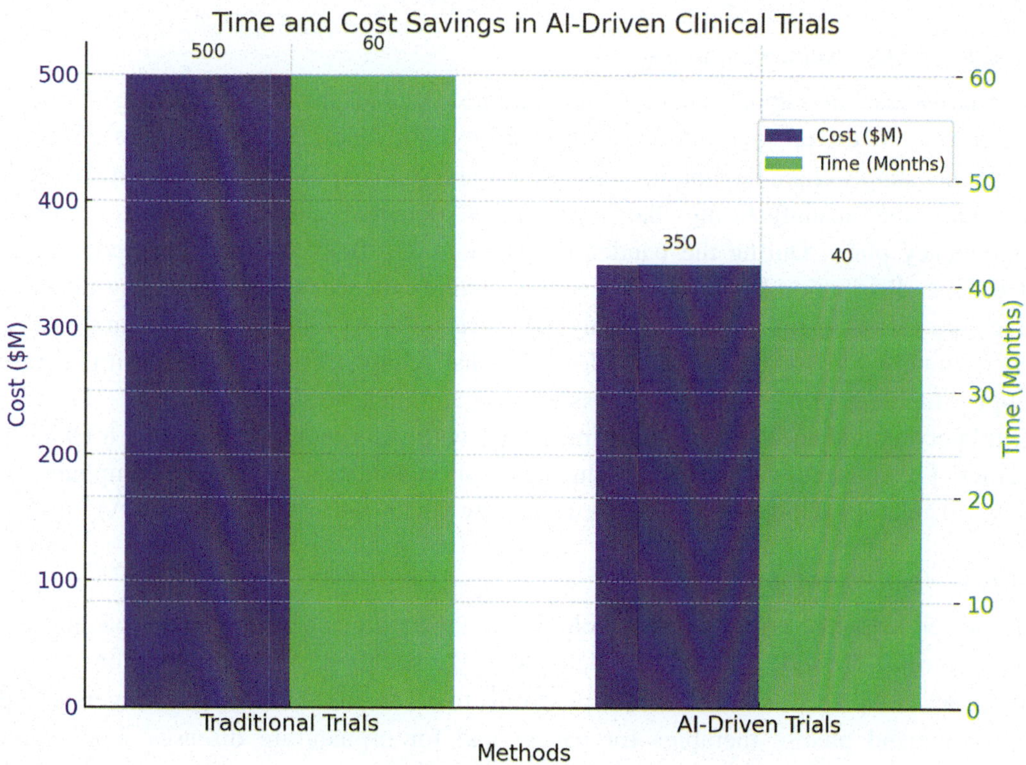

Figure 15.2
Time and cost savings in AI-driven clinical trials.

- Optimized patient recruitment: AI algorithms analyze electronic health records (EHRs), genomic data, and social determinants of health to match eligible participants to trials with unparalleled precision. Deep 6 AI™ has reduced recruitment timelines by over 50%, allowing trials to progress more swiftly while maintaining diversity in patient populations (Deep 6 AI, 2021).
- Real-time monitoring and risk mitigation: Platforms like Medidata RAVE™ use AI to monitor trial data in real time, flagging anomalies such as adverse events or protocol deviations. This proactive monitoring reduces delays and improves trial outcomes.
- Virtual and decentralized trials: The COVID-19 pandemic accelerated the adoption of decentralized trial models, and AI plays a pivotal role in enabling this shift. Wearable devices and mobile applications powered by AI facilitate remote patient monitoring, data collection, and communication with trial coordinators. For instance, "Pfizer's decentralized vaccine trials relied heavily on AI tools for real-time analytics and participant management (Pfizer®, 2021).".
- Enhanced patient adherence: Chatbots and virtual assistants, like those developed by Ada Health™, provide personalized reminders, answer patient queries, and ensure adherence to trial protocols, reducing dropout rates and ensuring trial validity.

15.1.6.3 Supply chain optimization

The pharmaceutical supply chain is a complex, global network requiring meticulous coordination. AI-driven solutions improve visibility, efficiency, and compliance by:

- Predicting supply chain disruptions: AI systems analyze geopolitical risks, weather patterns, and real-time manufacturing data to predict potential disruptions and recommend contingency plans. During the pandemic, AI tools like IBM Watson® ensured continuity of vaccine distribution by forecasting supply chain bottlenecks and optimizing logistics.
- Inventory management: Predictive analytics powered by AI minimizes waste and stockouts by accurately forecasting demand. Novo Nordisk® implemented AI to optimize insulin supply chains, improving patient access in rural and underserved areas.
- Regulatory compliance: Blockchain integrated with AI ensures end-to-end tracking and tracing of pharmaceutical products, reducing counterfeit risks and ensuring compliance with global regulatory standards like the Drug Supply Chain Security Act (DSCSA).

15.1.6.4 Personalized medicine

Personalized medicine is an emerging field that tailors treatments to individual patients based on their genetic, lifestyle, and clinical data. AI is the backbone of this revolution:

- Genomics and precision medicine: AI platforms like Tempus® analyze patient genomic data to recommend precise therapies for cancer and for orphan/rare diseases. For example, Tempus® matched breast cancer patients with targeted therapies, improving response rates by 25% compared to traditional approaches (Tempus, 2023).

- Predictive diagnostics: AI-powered diagnostics such as IBM Watson Health® identify disease risks earlier, enabling preventive care. Machine Learning Models (MLM) can detect biomarkers for Alzheimer's and other chronic diseases, thus paving the way for early interventions.

15.1.7 Pharma's unique challenges

15.1.7.1 Regulatory hurdles

AI adoption in pharma is constrained by stringent regulatory requirements, which demand transparency, explainability, and validation of AI models. Regulatory bodies such as the FDA and European Medicines Agency (EMA) have yet to establish uniform guidelines for AI-powered tools, leading to delays in their approval and adoption.

15.1.7.2 Data privacy and security

The pharmaceutical industry relies heavily on patient data, making it a prime target for cyberattacks. Ensuring data privacy while leveraging AI algorithms trained on sensitive health information remains a critical challenge under regulations like GDPR and HIPAA.

15.1.7.3 Ethical concerns

AI models trained on biased datasets may produce inequitable outcomes, thus placing vulnerable populations in a disadvantaged position. Organizations must invest in inclusive AI development and ensure fairness in algorithms.

15.1.7.4 Workforce resistance and skill gaps

Cultural resistance to AI adoption and a lack of skilled personnel remain significant barriers. Employees often fear job displacement, while organizations struggle to find talent with expertise in data science, machine learning and bioinformatics.

15.1.8 AI's impact on employee roles

15.1.8.1 Automation of routine tasks

AI handles repetitive tasks such as data entry, report generation, and inventory tracking, allowing employees to focus on strategic and creative work. For instance, robotic process automation (RPA) has reduced manual workloads for pharmacovigilance teams at Bayer®, enabling faster safety reporting.

15.1.8.2 Creation of new roles

The adoption of AI has created demand for new roles, including:

- Data scientists: Experts who develop and maintain AI models.

- Bioinformaticians: Specialists who interpret AI-driven insights in genomics.
- AI trainers: Professionals who refine AI systems through human feedback.

15.1.8.3 Cross-functional collaboration

AI fosters integration between departments. IT teams work with researchers, clinicians collaborate with data scientists, and commercial teams utilize AI insights for market strategies, fostering a more interconnected and transparent organization.

15.1.8.4 Lifelong learning as a mandate

Continuous upskilling is essential for all employees especially in order to adapt to AI-powered tools. Companies like Novartis® have institutionalized programs like AI Bootcamps to train employees across all levels, empowering them to harness AI effectively.

15.2 The role of learning and development in the artificial intelligence era

As AI transforms the pharmaceutical industry, the demand for a skilled workforce capable of harnessing its potential has become a strategic priority. L&D is no longer confined to periodic training sessions but has evolved into a continuous, dynamic process tailored to address the complexities of AI integration. Universities, industry collaborations, and AI-focused programs play an increasingly vital role in equipping employees with the skills required to thrive in this new era.

Table 15.1 compares the traditional L&D versus the AI-driven ones

15.2.1 Redefining learning and development for artificial intellig-ence integration

15.2.1.1 Artificial intelligence-enhanced training frameworks

AI integration in L&D goes beyond traditional teaching methods. Advanced learning systems leverage AI to adapt content dynamically, ensuring every learner receives training according to their level, their role, and to their career aspirations.

- Adaptive learning platforms: Tools such as Coursera for Business®, edX™, and Degreed™ partner with universities to offer personalized training modules. For instance, Coursera for

Table 15.1 Comparison table—traditional versus AI-driven L&D.

Aspect	Traditional L&D	AI-driven L&D
Content delivery	One-size-fits-all programs	Personalized learning
Interactivity	Limited	Immersive (VR/AR tools)
Assessment	Annual performance reviews	Real-time analytics
Scalability	Resource-intensive	Scalable across regions

Business® collaborates with universities like Stanford University and the University of Pennsylvania to provide courses on machine learning and bioinformatics tailored to pharmaceutical employees.
- Case studyMiddle East: The King Abdullah University of Science and Technology (KAUST) in Saudi Arabia offers advanced AI courses in partnership with global platforms, focusing on AI's applications in healthcare and drug discovery. Such collaborations enable pharma professionals in the region aiming to stay ahead in AI advancements.

15.2.2 Collaboration with universities and research institutions

Global and regional universities are increasingly aligning their programs to meet the needs of the pharmaceutical workforce.
- Global examples:
- The University of Cambridge's Centre for AI in Medicine offers specialized programs that train professionals to apply AI in genomics, in drug discovery, and in clinical trials.
- MIT's Professional Education Program in AI includes modules specifically designed for pharmaceutical executives, providing hands-on experience with AI applications.
- Middle East initiatives:
- United Arab Emirates University (UAEU) in Abu Dhabi has launched AI training workshops targeting healthcare and pharmaceutical professionals, emphasizing real-world applications of AI in personalized medicine.
- The Mohammed Bin Zayed University of Artificial Intelligence (MBZUAI), the first AI-focused university in the world, partners with pharmaceutical companies to create customized L&D initiatives, bridging the gap between academia and industry.

15.2.3 Industry-academia collaborations

Collaboration between pharmaceutical companies and educational entities is creating tailored programs to address specific workforce needs.
- Pfizer® collaborates with Harvard University on AI workshops that explore clinical trial optimization and real-time data analytics.
- Novartis® partners with ETH Zurich in Switzerland to develop L&D programs focusing on predictive modeling and AI ethics.

15.2.4 Strategic importance of learning and development in the artificial intelligence era

15.2.4.1 Upskilling and reskilling as a competitive necessity

The rapid pace of AI adoption has created an urgent need for continuous upskilling and reskilling of the pharmaceutical workforce.

- Upskilling programs:
- In the United Kingdom, AstraZeneca® offers an AI certificate program in partnership with Imperial College London, equipping employees with skills in machine learning and advanced data analytics.
- In the Middle East, the Qatar Computing Research Institute (QCRI) partners with multinational pharmaceutical companies to provide AI-driven upskilling workshops tailored for clinical research teams.
- Reskilling success stories:
- Roche® has reskilled thousands of employees globally, transforming roles traditionally focused on manual processes into data-driven positions by leveraging partnerships with AI institutes.
- Regional initiatives include collaborations between Hikma Pharmaceuticals in Jordan and local universities to retrain staff on AI-powered supply chain tools.

15.2.5 Regulatory and ethical training

With AI's rise, L&D programs must address ethical and regulatory concerns, ensuring that employees are equipped to navigate these challenges responsibly.

- Global best practices: Companies like Bayer® incorporate AI ethics modules into their training programs, covering topics such as algorithmic bias, transparency, and regulatory compliance.
- Middle East perspective: Gulf Cooperation Council (GCC) nations, under frameworks like the UAE's National AI Strategy 2031, integrate ethical AI training into national L&D initiatives, particularly in the pharmaceutical and healthcare sectors.

15.2.6 Organizational agility through learning and development

Organizations that invest in robust L&D frameworks are better positioned to pivot during industry disruptions.

For example, during the COVID-19 pandemic, Johnson & Johnson® rapidly scaled AI-focused training programs in partnership with global universities to enable decentralized trials and real-time analytics.

15.2.7 Cultural shift toward digital competency

AI integration requires more than technical training—it necessitates a cultural shift that values digital literacy, adaptability, and lifelong learning.

15.2.8 Promoting digital literacy

Digital literacy is no longer optional. L&D programs now prioritize digital upskilling across all levels, from entry-level employees to senior executives.

- Global example: Sanofi® has partnered with INSEAD Business School to design digital literacy programs for its leadership team, ensuring strategic decisions align with AI-driven insights.
- Regional focus: The American University of Beirut (AUB) offers AI workshops in partnership with regional pharmaceutical companies, aiming to elevate digital competencies among Middle Eastern professionals in the pharmaceutical sector.

15.2.9 Building a growth mindset

Encouraging employees to embrace AI as a tool for enhancement rather than a threat is critical.

- GlaxoSmithKline® (GSK) hosts AI hackathons in collaboration with Oxford University to foster curiosity and innovation among employees
- Hikma Pharmaceuticals organizes "AI Days" to demystify AI technologies and promote cross-departmental collaboration.

15.2.10 Customized learning pathways

15.2.10.1 Role-specific learning and development programs

Tailoring L&D programs to specific job functions ensures that employees acquire the exact skills they need to excel in their roles.

- R&D specialists: Training focuses on platforms like BenevolentAI™ for drug discovery and Schrödinger® for molecular modeling.
- Clinical teams: Programs emphasize AI diagnostic tools, wearable device data analysis, and decentralized trial management.
- Sales teams: Sales representatives are trained to use AI-powered CRM tools such as Veeva Systems® to predict customer needs and improve engagement.

15.2.11 Blended learning approaches

While AI-powered tools enhance personalization, combining them with traditional learning methods ensures comprehensive training.

- Case study: Pfizer® integrates VR-based lab simulations with instructor-led workshops to ensure employees gain both technical and practical skills.
- Regional example: In Saudi Arabia, Tabuk Pharmaceuticals combines AI-based online learning platforms with face-to-face mentorship programs, catering to a diverse workforce.

15.2.12 Global accessibility through E-learning

E-learning platforms like FutureLearn™ and Udemy® are making AI training accessible to employees worldwide. By partnering with academic institutions, these platforms offer certificates in topics like AI ethics, data visualization, and pharma-specific AI applications.

- The University of Edinburgh, in collaboration with FutureLearn™, offers a professional certification in AI for healthcare professionals, accessible to learners globally, including the Middle East.

The role of L&D in the AI era is transformative, bridging the gap between current workforce capabilities and the demands of an AI-integrated pharmaceutical landscape. Through collaborations with universities, adaptive learning technologies, and culturally attuned programs, organizations can create a workforce equipped for innovation and resilience. As AI continues to reshape the industry, a strategic investment in L&D will remain critical, ensuring both employees and companies thrive in a dynamic, technology-driven world.

15.3 Artificial intelligence-powered tools for learning and development

The integration of AI into L&D is revolutionizing workforce training, enabling pharmaceutical companies to prepare employees for the complexities of the AI-driven era. AI-powered tools offer personalized, scalable, and efficient solutions to address diverse learning needs across organizations. These technologies, from adaptive learning platforms to immersive training methods, ensure employees remain equipped with cutting-edge skills while fostering engagement and continuous growth. This section delves into transformative AI-powered tools, their applications in L&D, and the benefits they bring to the pharmaceutical industry.

15.3.1 Overview of transformative artificial intelligence-powered tools

1. **Adaptive learning platforms** AI-driven adaptive learning platforms tailor educational experiences to individual learners, addressing knowledge gaps and accelerating skill acquisition. These systems move beyond one-size-fits-all training by customizing pathways based on each user's interactions, learning style, and performance trends.

How it works: Using machine learning algorithms, these platforms collect and analyze user data (e.g., quiz scores, click patterns, time spent per module). The AI then dynamically adjusts the pace, difficulty, and content sequencing, ensuring learners are consistently challenged yet not overwhelmed.

AI is solving:
High dropout rates in corporate learning due to disengagement
Mismatch between training content and employee skill levels
Limited instructor-led capacity for large workforces

Example—coursera for business®: Coursera collaborates with global pharma leaders to offer accredited courses (e.g., pharmacovigilance, clinical trial management). The AI engine tracks individual progress and adapts difficulty accordingly. A case study with Roche showed a 27%

improvement in course completion rates and a 40% increase in post-course knowledge application (Coursera for Business, 2024).

Example—Degreed™: Degreed integrates learning analytics with AI to recommend personalized upskilling paths based on employees' job roles, skill gaps, and career goals. In pharma firms like Novartis, this has been linked to measurable productivity gains within R&D and regulatory affairs teams (Degreed, 2024).

Here is the workflow diagram for AI-powered personalized learning. The circular flow illustrates the progression through the four key steps: data input, AI analysis, customized content, and feedback (Fig. 15.3)

2. AI-powered content creation Generative AI tools enable L&D teams to produce custom learning materials—such as text modules, assessments, and case simulations—within minutes instead of weeks. These systems use natural language processing to generate content aligned with organizational tone, technical depth, and compliance requirements.

AI is solving:

Delays in developing regulatory-compliant training

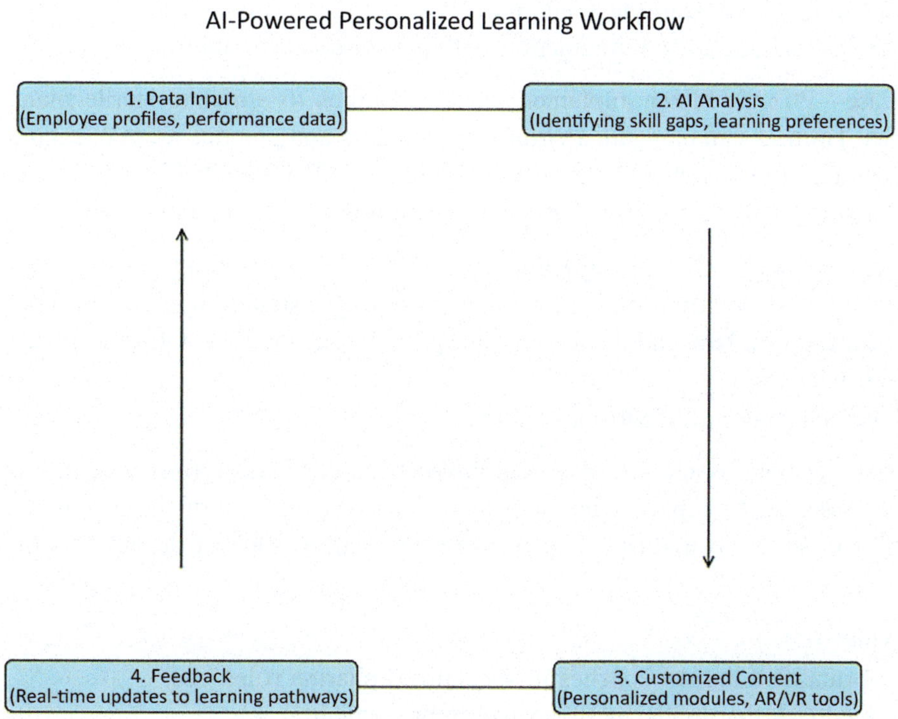

Figure 15.3
Workflow diagram—adaptive learning process.

Dependence on SMEs for every piece of instructional content
Lack of role-specific training resources

Case study—Pfizer®: Pfizer integrated OpenAI's GPT technology into its internal L&D content pipeline. When onboarding new manufacturing staff, generative AI created SOP-based learning modules tailored to specific production lines. The company reported a 60% reduction in instructional design time and improved knowledge retention based on post-training assessments (Pfizer, 2022).

Example—IBM Watson Assistant®: Used by Sanofi to codevelop scenario-based learning modules in pharmacovigilance, IBM Watson reduced manual QA cycles and ensured global consistency across multilingual content (Sanofi, 2024).

3. Virtual realityand augmented reality

Immersive technologies such as VR and AR allow pharmaceutical employees to experience realistic, interactive training environments—particularly valuable in complex or high-risk contexts like wet lab work or equipment operation.

AI is solving:
Inaccessibility of live lab environments for large-scale training
Safety risks in hands-on learning scenarios
Knowledge decline due to low interaction within traditional modules

VR use case—Pfizer®: Pfizer implemented VR modules to simulate sterile manufacturing cleanrooms. Trainees can navigate a virtual environment and practice aseptic techniques, with AI providing real-time feedback on protocol compliance. This resulted in a 30% improvement in procedural accuracy and a 20% reduction in training-related deviations (Pfizer, 2022).

AR use case—GSK®: GlaxoSmithKline uses AR to support field service engineers by overlaying digital instructions on medical devices during installation or troubleshooting. This reduced error rates by 18% and decreased average task time by 25% (GlaxoSmithKline, 2022; GSK, 2023; Fig. 15.3).

4. AI-driven coaching and feedback systems

AI-powered coaching systems analyze employee behavior and performance in real time—-delivering feedback, prompts, or learning nudges to support skill development. These tools complement or enhance traditional mentorship by scaling support across geographies and departments.

AI is solving:
Shortage of qualified human coaches in specialized pharma roles
Delays in feedback that hinder performance improvement
Gaps in communication and leadership skills in clinical, regulatory, and commercial roles

Example—BetterUp®: "BetterUp®: Combines AI with human coaching to develop leadership skills in pharma executives (BetterUp, 2023)."

Example—Rehearsal®: This platform uses conversational AI and role-playing simulations to train sales and medical liaison teams. For instance, reps can practice objection handling with virtual physicians. AstraZeneca cited a 25% improvement in field communication performance using Rehearsal-based modules (AstraZeneca, 2024).

These transformative tools are not futuristic prototypes—they are being actively deployed in forward-thinking pharmaceutical companies to drive measurable L&D outcomes. By aligning these technologies with business strategy and regulatory priorities, pharma organizations are not only closing the talent gap but they are also building an adaptive, AI-literate workforce for the future.

15.3.2 Data-driven decision-making in learning and development

One of the most transformative impacts of AI is its ability to analyze vast amounts of data to drive decisions in L&D strategy.

15.3.2.1 Skill gap analysis

AI identifies skill gaps across an organization, enabling targeted training interventions.

- Case study—Novartis®: Utilized AI to map skill gaps in clinical trial management teams, identifying the need for specialized training on decentralized trial platforms.

15.3.3 Personalized learning recommendations

AI-powered systems recommend training based on employees' career goals, job roles, and previous learning history.

- Example: Johnson & Johnson® (J&J) uses AI to recommend leadership development programs for mid-level managers based on their performance reviews and career trajectories.

15.3.4 Predictive analytics for training return on investment

AI evaluates the effectiveness of training programs, predicting their impact on key performance indicators (KPIs) such as employee productivity, retention, and innovation capacity.

- Case Study—Hikma Pharmaceuticals®: Implemented AI analytics to predict the return on investment (ROI) of its L&D investments, enabling data-driven adjustments to training strategies.

15.3.5 Microlearning and gamification

Microlearning and gamification techniques, powered by AI, are transforming how employees engage with training content.

15.3.5.1 Microlearning modules

AI tools breakdown complex training topics into bite-sized modules, making learning more digestible and accessible.

- Examples:
- Udemy® for business: Offers AI-driven microlearning solutions for training in regulatory compliance and ethical AI in pharma.
- Kahoot!®: Utilized by AstraZeneca® to create interactive learning quizzes for understanding pharmacovigilance practices.

15.3.6 Gamification in learning and development

AI gamifies training programs, introducing leaderboards, rewards, and real-time feedback to boost engagement.

- Examples:
- Bayer® uses gamified AI modules to train employees on supply chain optimization tools.
- Hikma Pharmaceuticals® incorporates gamification into its compliance training, increasing completion rates by 30%.

15.3.7 Benefits of artificial intelligence-powered tools in learning and development

15.3.7.1 Personalization at scale

AI allows organizations to cater to individual learning needs while scaling training programs for thousands of employees.

15.3.7.2 Real-time feedback

AI-driven platforms provide immediate feedback on performance, enabling learners to address gaps quickly and effectively.

15.3.7.3 Increased engagement and retention

Immersive technologies and gamification make training enjoyable and interactive, improving knowledge retention.

15.3.7.4 Cost and time efficiency

Automating content creation and analysis significantly reduces training development time and costs, allowing organizations to focus on strategic initiatives.

15.3.7.5 Continuous learning

AI fosters a culture of lifelong learning by constantly updating training content based on emerging technologies and industry trends.

15.3.8 Global and middle eastern initiatives

15.3.8.1 Global perspective

- Stanford University's AI in Healthcare Program: Includes modules on AI tools for workforce training, frequently used by global pharmaceutical companies.
- Harvard Business School®: Offers executive education programs on integrating AI into L&D, used by companies like Roche®.

Middle east initiatives

- Mohammed Bin Zayed University of Artificial Intelligence: Provides industry-focused workshops on AI applications in L&D, often attended by regional pharma companies.
- KAUST in Saudi Arabia: Partners with local pharma firms to deploy AI-driven L&D programs targeting supply chain and clinical trial management roles.

15.4 Challenges and strategies for success

The adoption of AI in L&D within the pharmaceutical industry presents significant opportunities for workforce transformation. However, it also introduces a series of challenges that can hinder progress if not addressed effectively. These challenges range from cultural resistance to technological limitations and ethical concerns. To successfully implement AI-driven L&D initiatives, pharmaceutical companies must adopt well-rounded strategies that prioritize inclusivity, collaboration, and continuous improvement. This section explores key challenges and provides actionable strategies to overcome them (Fig. 15.4).

15.4.1 Challenges in artificial intelligence-driven learning and development

15.4.1.1 Resistance to change

The introduction of AI in L&D often triggers apprehension among employees, driven by fears of job displacement and a lack of familiarity with new technologies.

- Cultural resistance: Employees may perceive AI as a replacement for human roles rather than a tool to enhance their skills.

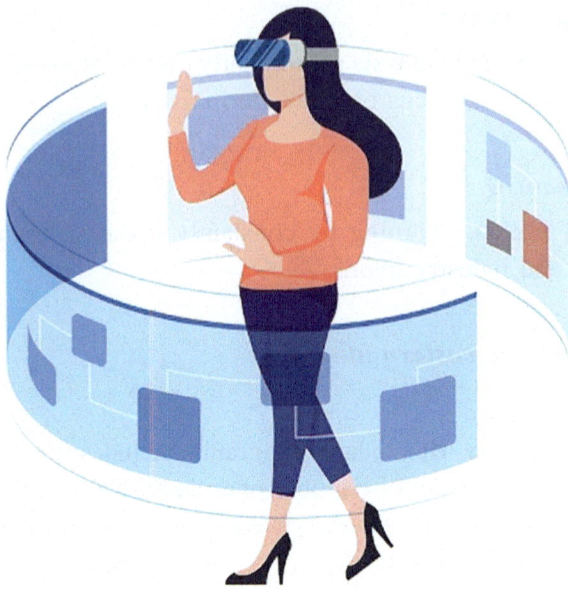

Figure 15.4
Augmented reality/virtual reality in training.

- Lack of trust: Concerns about AI's reliability and decision-making transparency can erode trust in AI-powered systems.

15.4.1.2 Ethical considerations

The integration of AI in L&D raises ethical questions about data privacy, bias, and inclusivity.

- Bias in AI algorithms: If training datasets are not diverse, AI tools may reinforce biases, thusdisadvantaging underrepresented groups.
- Privacy concerns: AI systems collect and analyze vast amounts of employee data, thus raising concerns about data security and misuse.

15.4.1.3 Ensuring inclusivity and accessibility

Not all employees have equal access to digital tools, particularly in regions with limited technological infrastructure or among those with low digital literacy.

- Global disparities: Employees in emerging markets or rural areas may face barriers to accessing AI-powered L&D programs.
- Accessibility needs: Employees with disabilities may encounter challenges in navigating AI-based systems without inclusive design features.

15.4.1.4 High implementation costs

Deploying AI-driven L&D solutions requires significant financial investment in technology, infrastructure, and ongoing maintenance.

- Budget constraints: Smaller pharmaceutical firms may struggle to allocate resources for AI-powered tools.
- Scalability issues: Expanding AI-based solutions across global operations can be resource-intensive.

15.4.1.5 Measuring return on investment

Quantifying the ROI for AI-driven L&D programs is complex, particularly when linking training outcomes to long-term organizational performance.

15.4.2 Strategies for success

15.4.2.1 Building a culture of continuous learning

A strong organizational culture that values continuous learning is critical for the success of AI-driven L&D initiatives.

- Promote AI as an enabler, not a replacement: Communicate the benefits of AI in enhancing employees' roles rather than replacing them.
- Example: GlaxoSmithKline® (GSK) conducted company-wide workshops to demystify AI and highlight its role in supporting, not replacing, human decision-making.
- Leadership advocacy: Engage senior leaders as champions of AI-driven L&D to foster employee buy-in.
- Example: Novartis®'s CEO regularly emphasizes the importance of lifelong learning in company-wide town halls.

15.4.2.2 Integrating ethical guidelines into artificial intelligence development

To address ethical concerns, organizations must embed transparency, fairness, and privacy protections into their AI systems.

- Diverse and inclusive AI design: Collaborate with universities and advocacy groups to develop diverse training datasets.
- Example: Bayer® partnered with the University of Cambridge to reduce algorithmic bias in AI tools.
- Data privacy compliance: Ensure compliance with global regulations such as GDPR and HIPAA by implementing robust data protection protocols.
- Regional focus: In the Middle East, companies like Hikma Pharmaceuticals® follow strict local privacy laws when adopting AI tools.

15.4.2.3 Prioritizing accessibility and inclusivity

AI-driven L&D programs must be designed to accommodate diverse employee needs, ensuring equitable access to training.

- Localized training content: Tailor content to meet regional and cultural needs.
- Example: MBZUAI offers bilingual AI training programs to cater to Arabic-speaking employees in the Middle East.
- Accessible design: Incorporate features such as screen readers, voice commands, and multilingual support.
- Example: Pfizer® integrates accessibility features into its AI platforms, ensuring inclusivity for employees with disabilities.

15.4.2.4 Addressing cost and scalability

Efficient resource allocation and collaboration can help organizations manage the costs of implementing AI in L&D.

- Phased rollouts: Begin with pilot programs to evaluate effectiveness before scaling up.
- Example: Johnson & Johnson® (J&J) piloted AI-driven leadership training in select regions before expanding globally.
- Leverage partnerships: Collaborate with universities, startups, and technology providers to share costs and access cutting-edge tools.
- Example: AstraZeneca® partnered with MIT to co-develop AI-powered learning modules, reducing development costs.

15.4.2.5 Establishing clear metrics for success

Organizations must define clear, measurable goals to evaluate the effectiveness of AI-driven L&D initiatives.

- KPI alignment: Link training outcomes to business objectives, such as increased productivity, innovation rates, or employee retention.
- Example: Roche® tracks how AI-driven L&D programs impact clinical trial completion rates and time-to-market for new therapies.
- Feedback loops: Use AI analytics to continuously refine training programs based on employee feedback and performance.
- Example: Sanofi® employs predictive analytics to monitor the long-term impact of training on employee development.

15.4.2.6 Fostering collaboration across teams

AI-driven L&D requires alignment between multiple departments, including Human Resources (HR), Information Technology (IT), and leadership teams.

- Cross-functional collaboration: Establish committees to oversee the integration of AI into L&D, ensuring alignment with organizational goals.

- Example: Pfizer® created an AI task force involving HR, R&D, and IT teams to oversee its AI learning initiatives.

15.4.3 Global and regional best practices

15.4.3.1 Global best practices

- Harvard Business School® and Roche®: Collaborated on a leadership program focused on AI ethics and strategic decision-making.
- MIT and Novartis®: Developed role-specific AI courses, combining technical and soft skill development.

15.4.3.2 Middle eastern initiatives

- KAUST and Tabuk Pharmaceuticals: Partnered to train Middle Eastern pharma professionals on AI-driven supply chain tools.
- UAE's National AI Strategy 2031: Encourages pharmaceutical companies to integrate AI-based L&D programs, offering government incentives for compliance.

15.5 Case studies and industry best practices

Real-world examples and industry best practices provide valuable insights into how pharmaceutical companies are leveraging AI in their L&D programs. These cases demonstrate successful strategies, highlight challenges, and offer replicable models for organizations looking to transform their workforce. This section presents a global and regional perspective, focusing on notable case studies, regional variations, and cross-industry lessons.

15.5.1 Case studies: real-world applications of artificial intelligence in learning and development

15.5.1.1 Novartis®: artificial intelligence-driven upskilling for research and development teams

Novartis® is a global leader in integrating AI into its L&D initiatives, particularly in research and development (R&D).

- Objective: Equip R&D teams with advanced AI and machine learning skills to enhance drug discovery processes.
- Implementation:
- Partnered with MIT and ETH Zurich to develop specialized training modules focusing on machine learning algorithms, genomics, and AI ethics.
- Introduced adaptive learning platforms like Coursera for Business® to deliver personalized training, combining academic courses from top institutions like Stanford University and Imperial College London.

- Conducted AI hackathons in collaboration with the University of Cambridge to foster innovation and cross-disciplinary collaboration.
- Outcomes:
- Reduced the timeline for early stage drug discovery by 20%.
- Increased employee engagement in L&D programs, with over 85% completion rates.

15.5.1.2 *Pfizer®: immersive training in manufacturing*

Pfizer® adopted immersive technologies to enhance training programs for its manufacturing teams.

- Objective: Improve compliance with Good Manufacturing Practices (GMP) and reduce production errors.
- Implementation:
- Utilized VR simulations to train employees on sterile manufacturing procedures, developed in partnership with Rutgers University in the United States.
- Collaborated with the MBZUAI to design AI-driven content tailored for global operations, including their facilities in the Middle East.
- Integrated AI-powered coaching platforms to provide real-time feedback during training sessions.
- Outcomes:
- Reduced training time by 40%.
- Achieved a 25% decrease in production errors within six months of implementation.

15.5.1.3 *Roche®: personalized leadership development*

Roche® has invested heavily in AI-driven leadership development programs to prepare mid- and senior-level executives for the AI era.

- Objective: Build leadership skills aligned with AI's role in transforming the pharmaceutical industry.
- Implementation:
- Partnered with Harvard Business School® to design executive education courses on AI ethics and strategic decision-making.
- Leveraged AI platforms like BetterUp® to provide personalized coaching and leadership assessments.
- Invited guest lecturers from institutions such as the University of Oxford and INSEAD Business School to share insights on AI's impact on global leadership.
- Outcomes:
- Improved leadership readiness scores by 30%, as measured by internal performance metrics.
- Increased alignment between leadership decisions and AI-driven business strategies.

15.5.1.4 Hikma Pharmaceuticals®: regional success in artificial intelligence training

Hikma Pharmaceuticals®, based in Jordan, has implemented AI-driven L&D programs tailored to its Middle Eastern workforce.

- Objective: Train employees on AI-powered supply chain and pharmacovigilance tools to meet global compliance standards.
- Implementation:
- Partnered with the MBZUAI and the American University of Beirut (AUB) to develop regional AI training programs.
- Created gamified microlearning modules in Arabic to improve accessibility and engagement.
- Collaborated with local universities like the Jordan University of Science and Technology (JUST) to integrate AI training into the existing workforce development curriculum.
- Outcomes:
- Enhanced supply chain efficiency by 18%.
- Increased participation in L&D programs among non-English-speaking employees.

15.5.2 Regional variations in artificial intelligence-driven learning and development

15.5.2.1 North America: focus on leadership and innovation

In North America, pharmaceutical companies emphasize leadership development and innovation in their AI-driven L&D programs.

- Examples:
- Johnson & Johnson® (J&J) integrates AI analytics to measure the ROI of its leadership training programs, often collaborating with Stanford University and MIT for content design.
- Amgen® partners with Johns Hopkins University to develop courses focusing on AI in biopharma innovation.

15.5.2.2 Europe: ethical and regulatory alignment

European companies prioritize ethical AI training and compliance with strict regulations like GDPR (Fig. 15.5).

- Examples:
- AstraZeneca® conducts workshops on AI ethics in collaboration with the University of Cambridge.
- Bayer® integrates AI compliance training into its onboarding programs with guidance from ETH Zurich.

15.5.2.3 Middle east: building regional expertise

The Middle East is rapidly adopting AI-driven L&D programs, focusing on localized training and partnerships with academic institutions.

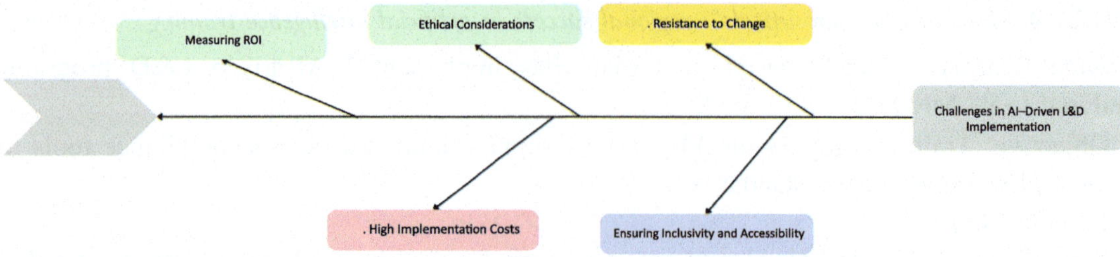

Figure 15.5
Challenges in AI-driven L&D implementation.

- Examples:
- Tabuk Pharmaceuticals collaborates with King Abdullah University of Science and Technology (KAUST) to develop AI training programs in Arabic.
- The MBZUAI partners with Hikma Pharmaceuticals® to deliver specialized AI workshops targeting supply chain and pharmacovigilance applications.

15.5.2.4 Asia-pacific: scaling artificial intelligence for large workforces

Pharmaceutical companies in Asia-Pacific region focus on scaling AI-based L&D solutions to train large and diverse workforces.

- Examples:
- Takeda Pharmaceutical Company Limited® in Japan uses AI-powered e-learning platforms in collaboration with Kyoto University.
- Sun Pharma® in India integrates gamification to enhance engagement in regulatory compliance training with local universities.

15.5.3 Cross-Industry Learning for Pharma

Pharmaceutical companies can learn valuable lessons from other industries that have successfully integrated AI into L&D.

15.5.3.1 Technology sector

- Best practice: Google®'s AI training programs focus on experiential learning, where employees solve real-world problems using AI tools.
- Application in pharma: Pharma companies can adopt similar experiential approaches by incorporating AI-driven problem-solving tasks into clinical trial management training.

15.5.3.2 Automotive industry

- Best practice: BMW® uses VR simulations for assembly line training, improving safety and efficiency.

- Application in pharma: Pharma companies can use VR to train employees on high-risk tasks, such as handling hazardous materials in laboratories.

15.5.3.3 Financial services

- Best practice: JP Morgan Chase® leverages AI to assess skill gaps and recommend targeted upskilling programs.
- Application in pharma: AI tools can similarly map skill gaps in pharmaceutical sales teams, tailoring training for improved engagement with healthcare providers.

15.5.4 Lessons learned from case studies

15.5.4.1 Align training with organizational goals

Successful AI-driven L&D programs are closely aligned with the organization's strategic priorities.

- Example: Novartis®'s focus on AI in drug discovery directly supports its innovation-driven mission.

15.5.4.2 Localize training for regional impact

Tailoring training content to regional needs ensures inclusivity and maximizes participation.

- Example: Hikma Pharmaceuticals®' use of Arabic-language modules enhanced accessibility for its Middle Eastern workforce.

15.5.4.3 Foster a culture of continuous learning

Encouraging employees to view learning as a continuous process is critical for sustained success.

- Example: Roche®'s leadership training programs emphasize adaptability and growth in an AI-driven environment.

15.6 Future trends in artificial intelligence and learning and development for pharma

The future of L&D in the pharmaceutical industry is intricately tied to the evolution of AI. As AI technologies continue to advance, they will reshape workforce training in unprecedented ways, unlocking new possibilities for personalization, collaboration, and efficiency. This section explores emerging trends in AI-driven L&D for the pharmaceutical industry, including advancements in generative AI, AI-driven diversity and inclusion training, lifelong learning initiatives, and the role of regulatory and ethical frameworks.

Here is the radar chart illustrating the impact of emerging AI trends in pharmaceutical L&D. Each axis represents a trend, with the values reflecting the projected level of impact (Fig. 15.6).

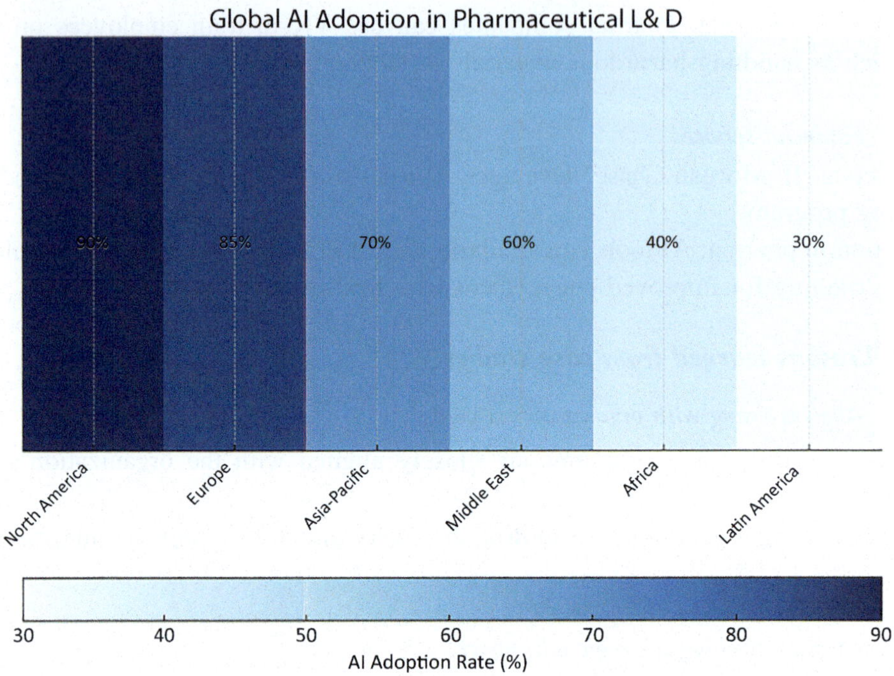

Figure 15.6
Heatmap—AI adoption rates globally.

15.6.1 Emergence of generative artificial intelligence in learning and development

Generative AI is transforming L&D by creating customized learning content and enhancing real-time problem-solving capabilities (Fig. 15.7).

15.6.1.1 Applications in pharma

- Automated content creation: Generative AI tools like OpenAI's ChatGPT® and Anthropic's Claude™ can create bespoke learning materials, such as quizzes, scenarios, and study guides, tailored to specific pharmaceutical roles.
- Case study: Pfizer® uses generative AI to create training content for decentralized clinical trials, ensuring employees across regions receive consistent and context-specific information.
- Virtual trainers: Generative AI can simulate realistic training scenarios, such as patient interactions for clinicians or decision-making in regulatory compliance.
- Example: Roche® uses generative AI to design interactive role-play exercises for leadership development.

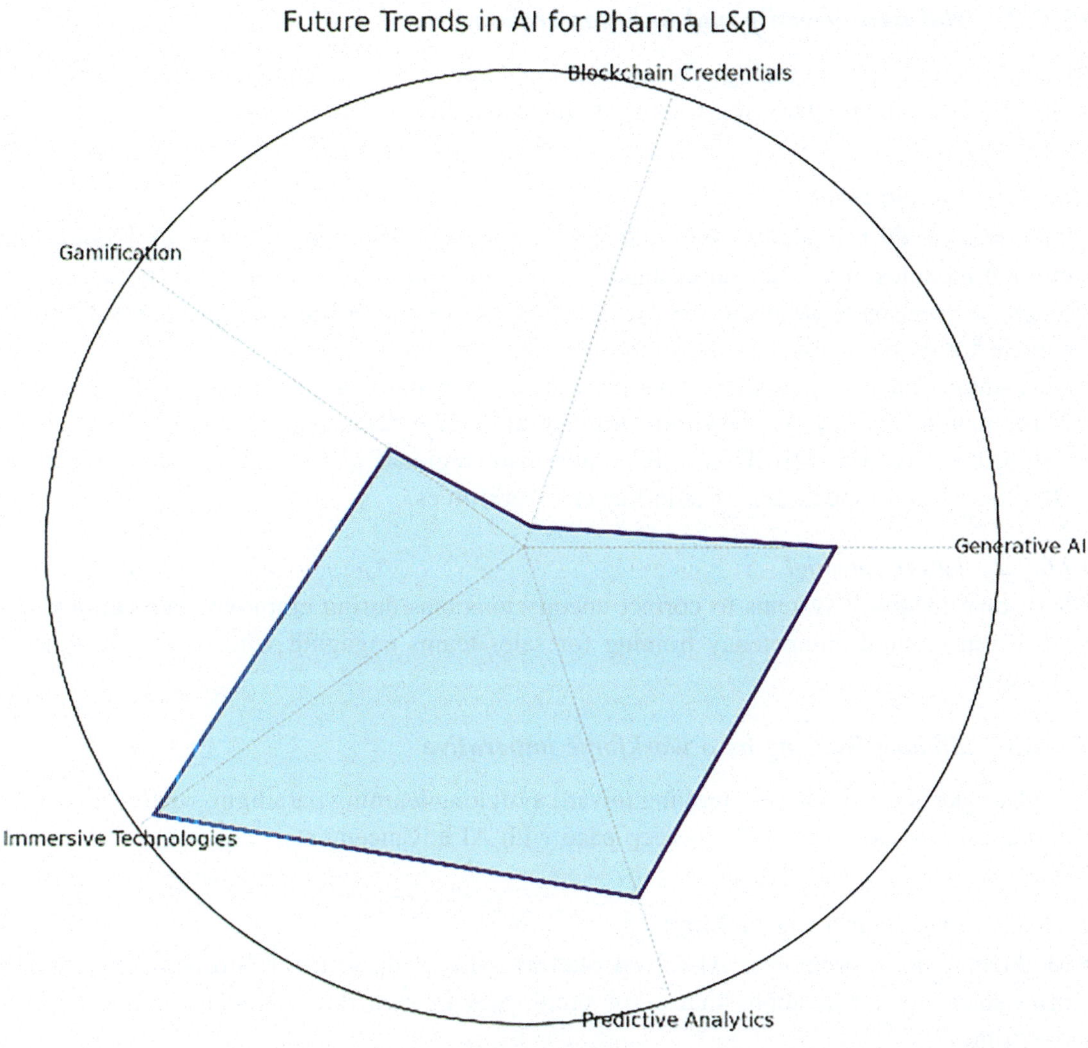

Figure 15.7
Future trends in AI for pharma L&D.

15.6.1.2 Future developments

- Integration with immersive technologies (e.g., virtual reality) to simulate real-world challenges in drug manufacturing or clinical settings.
- Multilingual generative AI tools designed for global pharmaceutical workforces, enabling greater accessibility.

15.6.2 AI-driven diversity and inclusion training

AI-powered tools are increasingly being used to address diversity, equity, and inclusion (DEI) within L&D programs, ensuring training is inclusive and free from bias.

15.6.2.1 Current trends

- Personalized DEI modules: AI analyzes employees' learning patterns to recommend training modules that foster understanding of cultural nuances and inclusive practices.
- Example: Johnson & Johnson® (J&J) integrates AI into its DEI training programs, tailoring content for global teams based on regional contexts.
- Bias mitigation in AI models: Pharmaceutical companies are partnering with academic institutions to develop AI algorithms trained on diverse datasets.
- Regional focus: The MBZUAI collaborates with regional pharmaceutical firms to create DEI-focused AI models for Middle Eastern workforces.

15.6.2.2 Future potential

- Real-time feedback systems to correct unconscious bias during employee interactions.
- AI-driven cultural competency training for sales teams engaging with diverse healthcare providers.

15.6.3 Lifelong learning as a workforce imperative

The pharmaceutical industry is moving toward a lifelong learning paradigm, where employees continuously update their skills to keep pace with AI advancements.

15.6.3.1 Ongoing learning pathways

- Modular training programs: AI-driven platforms like Coursera for Business® and edX™ offer stackable certifications that allow employees to earn micro-credentials and degrees over time.
- Example: AstraZeneca® partners with Cambridge University to offer modular programs in AI ethics and healthcare innovation, enabling employees to advance their education while working.
- Collaborations with universities: Institutions like the American University of Beirut (AUB) and KAUST are developing lifelong learning initiatives for pharmaceutical professionals in the Middle East.

15.6.3.2 Future trends

- AI-curated "learning passports" that track and recommend training opportunities throughout an employee's career.

- Expanded use of blockchain technology for credential verification, ensuring employees' qualifications are globally recognized.

15.6.4 The role of emerging technologies in learning and development

Advancements in immersive and interactive technologies, combined with AI, are redefining the boundaries of traditional training methods.

15.6.4.1 Immersive technologies

- Virtual reality: Simulations for complex tasks, such as aseptic manufacturing or patient-specific drug delivery.
- Example: Pfizer® uses VR simulations to replicate high-risk scenarios, allowing employees to gain practical experience in controlled environments.
- Augmented reality: Real-time guidance during technical procedures, reducing errors and enhancing learning retention.
- Example: Bayer® employs AR to assist employees in setting up laboratory equipment during training sessions.

15.6.4.2 Interactive tools

- Wearable AI devices: Smart glasses and haptic gloves provide feedback during hands-on training sessions.
- Gamification powered by AI: Increasing engagement by incorporating AI-driven challenges, rewards, and leaderboards into training programs.
- Example: Sanofi® integrates gamification into its regulatory compliance training, increasing completion rates by 30%.

15.6.5 Anticipating regulatory and ethical shifts

As AI becomes more pervasive in L&D, regulatory bodies and organizations are developing frameworks to ensure compliance, safety, and ethical standards.

15.6.5.1 Regulatory impacts on artificial intelligence in learning and development

- Global frameworks: Agencies like the FDA and EMA are expected to provide clearer guidelines on the use of AI in workforce training, particularly in regulated industries like pharma.
- Privacy and data security: Training platforms must comply with global standards such as GDPR and HIPAA to protect employee data.

15.6.5.2 Ethical considerations

- Algorithmic transparency: Organizations will need to ensure their AI-driven L&D tools provide explainable outputs to foster trust.

- Example: Bayer® has implemented an AI audit system to evaluate the fairness and transparency of its training algorithms.
- Bias prevention: Pharma companies will increasingly rely on partnerships with academic institutions to develop unbiased AI models.
- Regional focus: KAUST in Saudi Arabia collaborates with Hikma Pharmaceuticals® to ensure AI fairness in Middle Eastern training programs.

15.6.6 The shift toward global collaboration

The future of AI-driven L&D in pharma will emphasize cross-industry and cross-border collaboration.

15.6.6.1 Global networks

- University partnerships: Pharmaceutical companies will increasingly partner with global institutions to access cutting-edge AI research and develop workforce-specific training programs.
- Example: Novartis® and ETH Zurich are co-developing AI courses that combine academic rigor with practical industry applications.
- Regional collaboration: Middle Eastern universities like MBZUAI and KAUST are spearheading partnerships with global pharma leaders to address regional workforce challenges.

15.6.6.2 Cross-industry lessons

- Pharmaceutical companies can learn from the tech and finance industries, which are pioneers in AI-driven L&D.
- Example: Roche® is adapting best practices from Google®'s experiential learning framework to improve engagement in its leadership programs.

The integration of AI into L&D within the pharmaceutical industry represents a major leap toward digital transformation and workforce modernization. However, despite its clear benefits, the field is marked by several limitations that must be acknowledged to ensure sustainable and inclusive progress. These constraints differ in scale and nature between global markets and the Middle East, requiring a nuanced understanding of context-specific challenges.

15.6.7 Global challenges in artificial intelligence-driven learning and development

15.6.7.1 Pace of technological change

Globally, the rapid evolution of AI technologies presents a major obstacle for long-term L&D planning. Tools and platforms frequently emerge and fade, creating instability for organizations trying to build scalable, future-proof training strategies. This pace also makes it difficult for HR and learning leaders to continuously evaluate, select, and implement appropriate AI-based solutions without incurring risks of obsolescence or resource misalignment.

15.6.7.2 Absence of standardized frameworks

Unlike regulated areas of pharmaceutical R&D, there is no universally accepted framework for integrating AI into L&D. Companies often create internal models tailored to specific workflows, leading to fragmentation and limited transferability. This absence of industry-wide standards inhibits benchmarking, cross-sector collaboration, and cumulative learning at scale.

15.6.7.3 Limited empirical evidence on workforce outcomes

While early adopters showcase promising outcomes through case studies, much of the evidence remains anecdotal or proprietary. There is a shortage of longitudinal data that measures the sustained impact of AI-enhanced L&D on employee performance, innovation capacity, regulatory compliance, or organizational agility. This hinders evidence-based policymaking and slows broader adoption.

15.6.7.4 Overemphasis on technical skills

Current AI-based training programs tend to prioritize technical skills—such as data analysis, software use, and machine learning literacy—often at the expense of soft skills. Yet, in AI-integrated workplaces, competencies like critical thinking, emotional intelligence, ethical reasoning, and cross-functional collaboration are equally critical and currently underrepresented in training design.

15.6.7.5 Ethical and regulatory ambiguity

The deployment of AI in L&D involves sensitive employee data, raising concerns around privacy, algorithmic bias, and transparency. While general data privacy laws (e.g., GDPR, HIPAA) offer foundational guidance, there is a lack of specific regulation addressing the ethical use of AI in workforce development. This ambiguity exposes organizations to compliance risks and potential breaches of employee trust.

15.6.8 Middle east-specific limitations

15.6.8.1 Digital infrastructure and accessibility

While Gulf countries like the UAE and Saudi Arabia have invested heavily in AI infrastructure, digital disparities remain across the broader Middle East. Uneven access to reliable internet, modern devices, and AI-enabled platforms can marginalize employees in rural or resource-constrained environments. This digital divide limits the scalability and inclusivity of L&D programs powered by AI.

15.6.8.2 Linguistic and cultural relevance

Many AI-driven L&D tools are developed with Western-centric content and English-language defaults. This presents a barrier for pharmaceutical professionals in Arabic-speaking regions, especially when localized content and cultural sensitivity are lacking. The absence of region-specific training materials may reduce engagement and efficacy of learning interventions.

15.6.8.3 Regulatory lag

Despite national strategies supporting AI innovation (e.g., the UAE's National AI Strategy 2031), pharmaceutical training regulations in many Middle Eastern countries have not yet caught up with technological capabilities. This lag in regulation and policy guidance creates uncertainty for organizations seeking to implement AI-based L&D tools at scale.

15.6.8.4 Educational alignment gaps

Although leading institutions such as KAUST and MBZUAI are advancing AI education in the region, there remains a disconnect between academic output and industry workforce needs. Many pharmaceutical firms continue to rely on imported L&D models, which may not fully align with the regional context, cultural expectations, or evolving competency requirements.

15.7 Conclusion and roadmap

The integration of AI into the pharmaceutical industry's L&D functions is no longer optional—it is a strategic imperative. Throughout this chapter, we explored how AI is reshaping workforce competencies, redefining training delivery, and unlocking new capabilities across the pharma value chain.

Globally, the AI revolution in pharma is accelerating, driving the need for continuous upskilling, cross-functional literacy, and agile learning ecosystems. From AI-driven drug discovery to personalized patient care, employees must learn to collaborate with machines, interpret algorithmic outputs, and uphold regulatory and ethical standards. L&D is the linchpin in this transformation—enabling the human workforce to remain adaptive, relevant, and innovative.

In the Middle East, unique challenges and opportunities emerge. While countries like the UAE and Saudi Arabia are investing heavily in digital infrastructure and national AI strategies, gaps remain in digital inclusion, cultural adaptation, and workforce readiness. Regional L&D strategies must be tailored to address linguistic, regulatory, and socio-economic contexts—ensuring that AI-powered learning is both inclusive and effective.

15.7.1 Key takeaways

15.7.1.1 The strategic role of learning and development in the artificial intelligence era

AI's transformative impact on pharma goes beyond automation; it reshapes workforce roles and creates a pressing need for upskilling and reskilling. L&D serves as a strategic enabler, ensuring organizations remain agile and innovative while fostering a culture of continuous learning.

15.7.1.2 Artificial intelligence-powered tools as game changers

From adaptive learning platforms to immersive VR and AR technologies, AI-powered tools deliver personalized and scalable training solutions. These tools enhance knowledge retention, improve engagement, and address skill gaps effectively, making them indispensable for workforce development.

15.7.1.3 Educational entities as partners in progress

Universities, schools, and vocational institutions play a critical role in aligning academic preparation with industry requirements. Partnerships with educational entities ensure the development of specialized programs, ethical AI practices, and a steady pipeline of AI-ready talent for the pharmaceutical workforce.

15.7.1.4 Overcoming challenges with strategic approaches

While the integration of AI into L&D poses challenges such as ethical concerns, inclusivity, and resistance to change, organizations can mitigate these issues by embedding transparency, prioritizing accessibility, and fostering collaboration across teams and industries.

15.7.1.5 Preparing for future trends

Emerging technologies like generative AI, gamified learning, and blockchain-based credential verification will redefine how organizations deliver training and evaluate employee progress. Staying ahead of these trends is vital for ensuring workforce readiness in an ever-changing landscape.

15.7.2 Recommendations for organizations

15.7.2.1 Invest in continuous learning ecosystems

Organizations must move beyond one-time training sessions and create ecosystems that support continuous and lifelong learning.

- Collaborations with universities: Partner with leading universities such as Stanford University, Harvard Business School®, and King Abdullah University of Science and Technology (KAUST) to design courses that address specific workforce challenges, such as AI ethics or personalized medicine.
- Integration with schools: Collaborate with schools and vocational programs to introduce foundational AI courses, creating a pipeline of future-ready talent.
- Example: Hikma Pharmaceuticals® in Jordan collaborates with local universities and schools to provide AI-focused training, particularly targeting young professionals entering the workforce.

15.7.2.2 Prioritize ethical artificial intelligence practices

Ensure fairness, inclusivity, and data privacy in AI-powered L&D systems by working with academic experts and adopting ethical AI frameworks.

- University-led artificial intelligence ethics programs: Leverage courses from institutions like the MBZUAI or the University of Cambridge to train employees in ethical AI applications.
- Early ethical training in schools: Incorporate AI ethics and diversity modules into school curricula to build awareness early in students' careers.
- Example: AstraZeneca® collaborates with Cambridge University to provide workshops on AI ethics for its global workforce, setting a standard for responsible AI adoption.

15.7.2.3 Collaborate with educational institutions

Building strong partnerships with universities and schools ensures that L&D programs remain aligned with emerging trends and workforce demands.

- Codevelop curricula: Work with universities to create degree or certification programs tailored for the pharmaceutical industry.
- Example: Novartis® partners with ETH Zurich to develop AI training modules focusing on genomics and drug discovery.
- Internships and apprenticeships: Collaborate with schools and universities to provide hands-on AI learning opportunities, fostering talent development from an early stage.
- Example: Pfizer® collaborates with Rutgers University to offer AI-driven internships in manufacturing and clinical trials.

15.7.2.4 Adopt a phased implementation approach

Educational institutions can serve as testing grounds for pilot programs, enabling organizations to refine AI-driven L&D initiatives before scaling them organization-wide.

- Example: Johnson & Johnson® (J&J) collaborates with Stanford University to pilot leadership development programs for mid-level managers, later scaling the program globally.
- Case for schools: Collaborate with technical schools to introduce smaller-scale AI modules in healthcare and pharma, preparing students for industry-specific applications.

15.7.2.5 Leverage cross-industry and educational best practices

Learn from successful partnerships between industries and educational entities.

- Cross-sectoral learning: Emulate how companies like Google® or Tesla® collaborate with universities to drive AI innovation and workforce development.
- Educational alliances: Forge partnerships with academic consortia such as the Russell Group in the UK or the Ivy League in the US for access to cutting-edge AI research and training expertise.
- Example: Roche® draws inspiration from Google®'s experiential learning approach and collaborates with Harvard Business School® for strategic leadership programs.

15.7.3 A vision for the future

The future of L&D in the pharmaceutical industry will be driven by continuous advancements in AI, fostering innovation, inclusivity, and global collaboration. By investing in educational partnerships, embracing cultural shifts, and integrating cutting-edge tools, pharmaceutical companies can build a resilient and adaptive workforce. Educational entities—ranging from universities like KAUST and MBZUAI to vocational schools—serve as vital partners in this transformation, bridging the gap between academic preparation and industry demands.

This collaborative approach ensures that AI becomes a force for progress rather than disruption. As the pharmaceutical industry continues to evolve, a strategic focus on lifelong learning, ethical AI, and global partnerships will empower companies and employees alike to navigate the challenges and opportunities of the AI era.

Editor's note

This chapter provides a timely and well-structured exploration of how L&D functions are being fundamentally reshaped by AI within the pharmaceutical industry. By linking technological transformation with workforce readiness, the chapter positions L&D not as a supporting activity but as a strategic capability that determines whether AI adoption translates into sustainable organizational value.

A key contribution of the chapter is its balanced treatment of innovation and realism. While it highlights the transformative potential of AI-powered learning platforms, immersive technologies, and data-driven talent development, it also critically addresses organizational resistance, ethical concerns, regional disparities, and regulatory complexity. This dual perspective strengthens the chapter's relevance for decision-makers who must operationalize AI-driven L&D in highly regulated and globally distributed environments.

Importantly, the chapter situates L&D within a broader ecosystem that includes universities, research institutions, policymakers, and regional initiatives—particularly in the Middle East. By emphasizing collaboration, cultural adaptation, and lifelong learning, it frames AI-enabled L&D as a long-term investment in human capital rather than a short-term technological fix. Readers are encouraged to view learning systems as adaptive infrastructures that evolve alongside AI itself.

Key takeaways

Learning and development is a strategic enabler of AI transformation, not a secondary support function. The success of AI initiatives in pharma depends on workforce readiness, digital literacy, and continuous reskilling.

AI-powered L&D tools enable personalization at scale, allowing pharmaceutical organizations to address diverse roles, geographies, and learning needs while improving engagement and knowledge retention.

Universities and academic institutions are critical partners, helping align workforce training with emerging AI competencies, ethical standards, and regulatory expectations.

Cultural readiness matters as much as technical capability. Overcoming resistance to AI requires transparent communication, leadership advocacy, and a growth mindset embedded across the organization.

Regional context shapes implementation success, particularly in the Middle East, where linguistic relevance, infrastructure maturity, and regulatory alignment must be explicitly addressed.

The future of L&D in pharma is lifelong, data-driven, and collaborative, integrating generative AI, immersive learning, and global partnerships to build resilient and adaptive workforces.

Minicase study vignette (anonymized)

Building an artificial intelligence-ready learning ecosystem in a Global Pharmaceutical Organization

A multinational pharmaceutical company operating across Europe, the Middle East, and Asia faced growing challenges as AI tools were rapidly deployed in R&D, clinical operations, and supply chain management. While advanced technologies were available, leadership observed uneven adoption and declining confidence among employees—particularly in regulated and patient-facing roles.

An internal assessment revealed fragmented training programs, limited AI literacy outside technical teams, and resistance driven by fears of job displacement. In response, the organization launched a comprehensive AI-enabled L&D transformation.

The initiative combined adaptive learning platforms with role-specific learning pathways. Scientists received targeted training on AI-assisted drug discovery, regulatory teams focused on explainable AI and compliance, and commercial staff engaged in simulated, AI-driven customer interactions. Academic partnerships were established to co-develop curricula, while regional teams localized content to reflect cultural and linguistic needs.

Within one year, training completion rates increased significantly, cross-functional collaboration improved, and internal surveys showed higher trust in AI-supported decision-making. However, challenges remained around measuring long-term ROI and ensuring equitable access across all regions.

Reflection prompt: Which elements of this L&D strategy most effectively addressed cultural resistance, and how could the organization strengthen long-term sustainability and inclusion?

Learning activities

Learning activity 1: assessing artificial intelligence-learning and development maturity

Format: Individual or Small Group **Time:** 30–40 minutes

Objective: Evaluate organizational readiness for AI-driven learning and development in the pharmaceutical industry.

Instructions: Select a pharmaceutical organization (real or hypothetical). Assess its L&D maturity across the following dimensions:

Digital infrastructure and data readiness
Workforce AI literacy
Ethical and regulatory preparedness
Leadership support and culture
Regional and global scalability
For each dimension, identify:
Identify one existing strength
Idenfity one critical gap
Identify one priority action for the next 12 months

Deliverable: A one-page maturity snapshot with a short executive summary (150–200 words).

Learning activity 2: designing an artificial intelligence-enabled learning anddevelopmentintervention

Format: Team-Based (3–5 participants) **Time:** 45–60 minutes

Objective: Design a realistic AI-driven L&D initiative aligned with business and regulatory needs.

Instructions: Each team designs an L&D intervention addressing one workforce challenge (e.g., AI ethics training, reskilling clinical teams, leadership development). The proposal should include:

A target audience and specific skills gaps
AI tools and learning methods used
The role of academic or external partners
Ethical, regulatory, and inclusion considerations
Metrics for success

Deliverable: A concise concept summary (1 page) outlining the interventions and expected impact.

Learning activity 3: strategic reflection exercise

Format: Individual **Time:** 15–20 minutes

Objective: Encourage strategic thinking about the future of AI-driven learning in harma.

Prompt: How should pharmaceutical organizations balance speed of AI adoption with ethical responsibility and workforce inclusion in their L&D strategies?

Deliverable: A short reflective response (200–250 words).

AI disclosure

During the preparation of this work, the author(s) used OpenAI to To support translating ideas into a more professional academic context. After using this tool/service, the author(s) reviewed and edited the content as needed and are taking full responsibility for the content of the publication.

References

AstraZeneca. (2024). *Generative AI in the pharmaceutical industry: Moving from hype to reality*. McKinsey & Company. https://www.mckinsey.com/industries/life-sciences/our-insights/generative-ai-in-the-pharmaceutical-industry-moving-from-hype-to-reality.

BetterUp. (2023). AI coaching and leadership development: The future of workplace learning. BetterUp. https://www.betterup.com.

Coursera for Business. (2024). *AI for Business Leaders*. https://www.coursera.org/enterprise/ai-for-business-leaders.

Deep 6 AI. (2021). *Revolutionizing clinical trials with AI. Clinical Trials Today*. https://www.deep6.ai/revolutionizing-trials-ai.

Deloitte. (2023). Generative AI in life sciences and health care: Opportunities and challenges. Deloitte Insights. https://www2.deloitte.com.

Degreed. (2024). AI in pharmaceutical training: From pilots to full rollouts. Quantified AI. https://www.quantified.ai/blog/ai-in-pharmaceutical-training-from-pilots-to-full-rollouts/.

GlaxoSmithKline. (2022). *Pharma's spend on AI in drug discovery 'could top $3bn by 2025'. Pharmaphorum*. https://pharmaphorum.com/news/pharmas-spend-on-ai-in-drug-discovery-could-top-3bn-by-2025.

GSK. (2023). Artificial intelligence and digital transformation in pharmaceutical research and development. GlaxoSmithKline. https://www.gsk.com/en-gb/innovation/technology-and-data/ai-and-machine-learning/.

Insilico Medicine. (2022). Artificial intelligence in drug discovery: Accelerating therapeutic innovation. Insilico Medicine. https://insilico.com.

Pfizer. (2021). Digital innovation and decentralized clinical trials: Leveraging AI to accelerate research and improve patient outcomes. Pfizer. https://www.pfizer.com.

Pfizer. (2022). *Data and AI are helping to get medicines to patients faster. Pfizer Annual Report*. https://www.pfizer.com/sites/default/files/investors/financial_reports/annual_reports/2022/story/data-and-ai-are-helping-to-get-medicines-to-patients-faster/.

Sanofi. (2024). *AI in healthcare thematic intelligence research report 2024*. Yahoo Finance. https://finance.yahoo.com/news/ai-healthcare-thematic-intelligence-research-160200646.html.

World Economic Forum. (2020). The Future of Jobs Report 2020. World Economic Forum. https://www.weforum.org/reports/the-future-of-jobs-report-2020.

Tempus. (2023). *Genomics meets AI for personalized care*. Tempus Insights. https://www.tempus.com/insights/genomics-and-ai.

CHAPTER 16

Pharma Industry 2040: a catalyst for resilient change

Miltiadis Lytras
Computer Science Department, College of Engineering, Effat University, Jeddah, Saudi Arabia

16.1 Introduction: key developments in the pharma industry (2019–24)

The pharmaceutical industry has entered one of its most transformative periods in modern history. Between 2019 and 2024, the convergence of digital technologies, global public health challenges, and rising patient expectations catalyzed a wave of innovation, systemic restructuring, and cultural change. No longer operating solely as a science-driven manufacturing sector, pharma is now an integral component of digital health ecosystems, AI-powered discovery pipelines, and personalized care platforms (Mirzaei and Rijcken, 2023; Sowndharya et al., 2025; Yoshiura et al., 2025).

16.1.1 COVID-19 as a catalyst for innovation

The COVID-19 pandemic served as an inflection point for the pharmaceutical sector. Faced with the urgent need for diagnostics, vaccines, and treatment pathways, pharma companies rapidly pivoted towards agile R&D models, cloud-enabled collaboration, and real-time data analytics. This accelerated timelines for vaccine development—such as Pfizer/BioNTech's and Moderna's mRNA-based COVID-19 vaccines, which reached approval in under a year—previously considered impossible (Bano et al., 2022; Jones et al., 2024; Ramos et al., 2020; Steinwandter et al., 2019).

16.1.2 Rise of artificial intelligence and data-driven drug discovery

Artificial intelligence (AI) and machine learning (ML) became foundational tools across the pharma value chain (Basu & Heumann, 2024; Coucke, 2021; Pazhayattil & Konyu-Fogel, 2023). Companies like Insilico Medicine and Recursion Pharmaceuticals have built AI-native platforms that screen millions of compounds, predict therapeutic targets, and simulate clinical trials. These platforms reduce development time and cost while improving accuracy and drug efficacy. According to a McKinsey report (2023), over 50% of leading pharmaceutical companies now employ AI in early-stage drug discovery.

The Future of Pharma Across All Sectors in the Artificial Intelligence Era. DOI: https://doi.org/10.1016/B978-0-443-40572-3.00005-8

16.1.3 Digital therapeutics and companion apps

The last five years also witnessed the proliferation of digital therapeutics (DTx), which deliver evidence-based therapeutic interventions through software. For instance, Pear Therapeutics and Akili Interactive received FDA approvals for digital interventions that manage mental health and neurological conditions. These innovations mark a shift from pill-based care to continuous, digital-first care.

Additionally, wearable technology and mobile health applications—such as those by Roche and Fitbit (now under Google)—are increasingly being used to collect real-world data, personalize treatments, and monitor patient adherence.

16.1.4 Sustainable and green pharma

Environmental sustainability has become a core consideration. Firms are investing in green chemistry (Basit, 2020; Busquets et al., 2024; Dupuy et al., 2024; Gelis et al., 2023; Ladner et al., 2025; Malheiro et al., 2023; Pörtner et al., 2025), eco-friendly packaging, and carbon-neutral operations. Initiatives like the Sustainable Markets Initiative Health Systems Task Force, which includes AstraZeneca and GSK, emphasize climate-conscious innovation as a competitive and ethical imperative.

16.1.5 Globalization of R&D and open innovation

R&D has become more collaborative and decentralized. Cross-border partnerships, open-source research platforms, and academic-industry alliances are dominating the innovation landscape. The National Institute of Health's (NIH) Accelerating Medicines Partnership and the European Innovative Health Initiative are key examples. Pharmaceutical companies are partnering with AI startups, genomics labs, and health-tech incubators in order to co-create solutions in a distributed model of innovation. As seen in Table 16.1, the scope of transformation spans from scientific processes to patient interaction, underlining the systemic nature of change.

Table 16.1 Key transformational shifts in pharma (2019–24).

Transformation area	Development highlights
R&D	AI-enabled screening, cloud-based trials, mRNA technologies
Patient engagement	Mobile health apps, wearable monitoring, personalized treatment platforms
Manufacturing	Smart factories, real-time supply chain management, just-in-time production
Regulatory and compliance	Faster approvals via adaptive trials and real-world evidence
Sustainability	Green chemistry, carbon tracking, eco-friendly packaging
Business models	Shift to value-based pricing, digital therapeutics, hybrid service-product offerings

In short, the pharmaceutical sector has moved from a traditional supply-chain-driven model to a digitally integrated and data-augmented network of innovation. The era of pharma-as-a-platform is beginning, and the sector's future competitiveness depends on its ability to fuse science with software, ethics with economics, and personalized care with planetary health.

This evolving complexity makes it essential to examine the current pharma ecosystem in detail—including its industrial structure, its key players, its venture activities, and emerging innovation hotspots. We now turn to Section 16.2 for this critical overview.

16.2 The current pharma ecosystem – key players, markets, and startup disruption

The pharmaceutical industry in 2024 is a vast, intricate ecosystem composed of multinational corporations, nimble biotech startups, academic research centers, regulatory agencies, and healthtech enablers. This section provides a structured mapping of the global pharma ecosystem, identifying the market leaders, emergent disruptors, and structural transformations that are shaping the competitive dynamics.

16.2.1 Global market overview

The global pharmaceutical market was valued at approximately $1.5 trillion in 2023, and it continues to expand steadily, driven by increasing life expectancy, chronic disease prevalence, and global access to healthcare. The largest markets by revenue include:

- United States: Dominates with ~40% of the global share, thanks to its high drug prices and innovation leadership.
- Europe: Key players include Germany, Switzerland, and the United Kingdom, thanks to their strong R&D infrastructure and regulatory maturity.
- China: The fastest-growing market with huge investments in biotech and generics, supported by national innovation strategies.
- India: The global hub for generics and APIs, playing a central role in affordable drug supply.

16.2.2 Major players in the pharma landscape

Big Pharma corporations continue to dominate the industry with vertically integrated operations from drug discovery to global distribution. Some of the most influential companies include:

Company	Headquarters	Specialization	R&D spending (2023)
Pfizer	United States	Vaccines, oncology, cardiology	$13.4 billion
Roche	Switzerland	Oncology, diagnostics, personalized medicine	$12.5 billion
Novartis	Switzerland	Generics (Sandoz), rare diseases	$9.4 billion
Johnson & Johnson	United States	Immunology, vaccines, consumer health	$15.2 billion

AstraZeneca	United Kingdom	Respiratory, cardiovascular, biologics	$8.5 billion
Sanofi	France	Vaccines, diabetes, rare diseases	$7.6 billion
Merck & Co.	United States	Oncology (Keytruda), infectious diseases	$10.8 billion

These companies are increasingly embracing partnerships with **AI startups**, **academic institutions**, and **tech firms** to accelerate discovery, expand digital engagement, and reduce cost structures.

16.2.3 The biotech and artificial intelligence startup explosion

Over the last 5 years, the startup landscape in pharma has witnessed a quantum leap in scale and ambition. Venture capital investment in biopharma and health AI startups surpassed $50 billion globally in 2023, with more than 2,000 startups founded since 2019.

16.2.3.1 Notable startups to watch

Startup	Focus area	Value proposition	HQ
Insilico Medicine	AI-driven drug discovery	End-to-end generative AI for novel compound synthesis	Hong Kong / United States
Recursion Pharma	Biological image analysis + AI	High-throughput phenomics + ML	United States
Owkin	Federated learning for pharma	Privacy-preserving RWE modeling for trials	France / United States
BenevolentAI	Knowledge graph-based drug discovery	AI knowledge mining from scientific data	United Kingdom
Exscientia	Autonomous drug design	Design-make-test-analyze loop automation	United Kingdom
XtalPi	Quantum mechanics + AI for molecules	Computational crystal structure prediction	China / United States
Atomwise	Deep learning for small molecules	AI screening of billions of compounds	United States

These startups are reshaping traditional timelines and creating **decentralized discovery models** that allow pharmaceutical breakthroughs at a fraction of the previous cost.

16.2.4 Academic and public-sector partnerships

Top research institutions like MIT, Oxford University, Karolinska Institute, and Tsinghua University are central hubs of biomedical innovation, often partnering with both Big Pharma and startups. Simultaneously, government initiatives like the NIH's All of Us Program and

Europe's Innovative Medicines Initiative (IMI) ensure a continuous pipeline of data-driven insights and funding.

16.2.5 Health tech and platform integration

Another crucial component of the ecosystem includes digital health platform providers (e.g., Google Health, Microsoft Cloud for Healthcare, Amazon Web Services) and wearable tech companies (e.g., Apple, Fitbit, Withings) that generate real-world evidence and connect pharmaceutical therapies to patient lifestyles.

"The pharma ecosystem of today is no longer isolated in silos—it is a symphony of multinational R&D, lean AI startups, agile tech enablers, and global policy partnerships."

While platforms and partnerships expand innovation capacity, they also increase interdependence—and therefore exposure to systemic shocks. For Pharma 2040, competitiveness will be measured not only by scientific output or digital maturity, but by the ability to sustain operations, protect trust, and deliver continuity of care under uncertainty. This makes resilience the strategic capability that connects the current ecosystem (Section 16.2) to the future ecosystem (Section 16.3).

16.2.6 Resilience as a strategic capability: from shock response to adaptive advantage

The defining lesson of the 2019–24 period is that resilience is no longer a reactive capability—it is a core strategic asset. The pharmaceutical industry learned, often painfully, that efficiency without adaptability creates fragility. Global pandemics, geopolitical instability, climate-related disruptions, cyber risks, and supply chain shocks exposed structural vulnerabilities across R&D pipelines, manufacturing networks, and distribution systems. In response, resilience has emerged as a foundational design principle for Pharma 2040.

Unlike traditional risk management—which focuses on prevention and contingency planning—strategic resilience emphasizes **anticipation, adaptation, and learning**. Resilient pharmaceutical organizations do not merely recover from disruption; they evolve because of it. This shift requires rethinking resilience not as an operational function, but as an enterprise-wide capability embedded across technology, governance, culture, and ecosystem partnerships.

16.2.6.1 Resilience across the pharma value chain

Resilience manifests differently across the pharmaceutical lifecycle:

R&D resilience: Distributed discovery models, cloud-based collaboration, AI-driven redundancy in target identification, and diversified clinical trial geographies reduce dependency on single sites or populations.

Manufacturing resilience: Smart factories, digital twins, modular production units, and predictive maintenance enable rapid reconfiguration in response to shortages, demand spikes, or quality deviations.
Supply chain resilience: Multisourcing strategies, blockchain-enabled traceability, AI-driven demand forecasting, and regionalized production hubs mitigate geopolitical and logistical risks.
Regulatory resilience: Adaptive regulatory engagement, real-world evidence integration, and digitally enabled submissions accelerate approvals during emergencies without compromising safety.
Patient access resilience: Telepharmacy, decentralized trials, home delivery, and digital therapeutics ensure continuity of care even when physical systems are disrupted.

Resilience thus becomes a cross-cutting property of the entire pharma ecosystem, not a siloed function.

16.2.6.2 Digital technologies as resilience multipliers

Emerging technologies act as force multipliers for resilience:
AI enables early warning systems, scenario simulation, and real-time decision support.
Digital twins allow organizations to stress-test supply chains, trial designs, and manufacturing processes before disruption occurs.
Blockchain ensures trust, provenance, and continuity in data and product flows.
IoMT and edge computing provide localized intelligence, reducing dependence on centralized infrastructure.
Platform architectures enable rapid recombination of capabilities across partners and regions.

Critically, resilience is not achieved by technology alone. Without governance, interoperability standards, and human oversight, digital complexity can amplify risk rather than reduce it.

16.2.6.3 Cultural and organizational dimensions of resilience

Pharma 2040 resilience also depends on organizational culture:
Decision agility: Empowering cross-functional teams to act quickly within clear governance boundaries.
Learning orientation: Treating disruptions as system-level learning opportunities, not failures.
Ecosystem thinking: Building long-term partnerships with suppliers, regulators, healthcare providers, and technology firms.
Ethical preparedness: Ensuring crisis responses remain patient-centric, equitable, and transparent.

Organizations that cultivate psychological safety, interdisciplinary collaboration, and ethical clarity are better equipped to adapt under pressure.

16.2.6.4 Strategic insight

By 2040, resilience will differentiate leaders from laggards. Firms that design resilience into their operating models will outperform those that merely optimize for cost or speed. In an era of accelerating uncertainty, the most valuable pharmaceutical capability will be the ability to absorb shocks, reconfigure intelligently, and continue delivering patient value without interruption.

Having established resilience as a strategic capability of the present ecosystem, the next section turns to a forward-looking vision of how these capabilities will scale, converge, and redefine the pharmaceutical industry by 2040.

The Transition Logic to Pharma 2040: What Changes, What Stays, What Must Be Built

What changes (structural shifts)

From pipelines → platforms and learning ecosystems

From episodic trials → continuous evidence (RWE + adaptive models)

From centralized production → distributed and modular manufacturing

What stays (nonnegotiables)

Patient safety and therapeutic efficacy as the core mission

Trust, transparency, and regulatory legitimacy

Scientific rigor (even when AI accelerates discovery)

What must be built (capability gaps to close)

Governance-grade AI operations (auditability, drift control, accountability)

Interoperable data foundations (cross-lifecycle, cross-border)

Resilience-by-design (stress-tested ecosystems, continuity of care)

This is a very “senior” structuring element and will elevate the chapter further.

16.3 The Pharma Ecosystem 2040—vision, players, and innovation frontiers

The year 2040 will mark a profound reinvention of the pharmaceutical industry—one driven by convergence across AI, synthetic biology, quantum computing, robotics, and patient-centric value models. This transformation will be far more than technological. It will reflect a paradigm shift in how medicines are discovered, developed, approved, distributed, and embedded into personalized wellness ecosystems.

16.3.1 Envisioning the 2040 Pharma Landscape

The pharma ecosystem of 2040 will be hyperconnected, data-intelligent, and precision-driven, with decentralized innovation networks bridging patients, clinicians, machines, and biosciences. We anticipate the following defining characteristics:

- AI-orchestrated discovery pipelines: Drug discovery will be led by autonomous AI agents capable of generating, testing, and optimizing molecules with minimal human intervention. Entire in silico labs will test thousands of hypotheses simultaneously.

- Quantum-enhanced R&D: Quantum computing will solve complex molecular simulations in minutes, shrinking development cycles from 10 years to under 2–3 years in many cases.
- Digital twins for drug testing: Every patient and every drug candidate will have a **digital twin**—a dynamic, data-driven simulation enabling predictive testing and personalization at scale.
- Personalized pharmacies at the edge: Distributed 3D bioprinters and edge-based micro-factories will enable real-time drug compounding tailored to individual genomic, epigenetic, and microbiome profiles.

Pharma 2040 in One Page: From Pipelines to Learning Ecosystems

Core insight: By 2040, the pharmaceutical industry will no longer be organized around linear pipelines that move molecules from discovery to market. Instead, it will operate as a continuous learning ecosystem, where data, intelligence, and outcomes flow bidirectionally across discovery, care delivery, and population health.

From linear value chains to adaptive ecosystems

Yesterday: Pipeline logic

Sequential R&D stages with fixed handoffs

Late learning (failures discovered late and expensively)

Limited feedback from real-world use

Value measured primarily by product volume and IP exclusivity

Tomorrow: Learning ecosystem logic

Parallel, AI-orchestrated discovery and validation

Continuous learning from real-world evidence and patient data

Digital twins enabling pre-emptive testing and optimization

Value measured by outcomes, trust, resilience, and societal impact

Key characteristics of the Pharma 2040 Ecosystem

AI as the cognitive spine: Autonomous and human-guided AI systems continuously sense, simulate, and recommend actions across R&D, trials, manufacturing, and access.

Patients as data partners, not endpoints: Patients contribute longitudinal data through consent-driven platforms, co-shaping therapies, dosing, and delivery models.

Platforms over products: Leading pharma firms operate platforms that integrate diagnostics, therapeutics, digital services, and post-market intelligence.

Regulation as a continuous dialogue: Regulators participate earlier and continuously via real-world evidence, algorithm validation, and adaptive approval pathways.

Resilience by design: Ecosystems are modular, distributed, and stress-tested through digital twins to absorb shocks without system collapse.

What changes for leaders

Strategy shifts from portfolio optimization to ecosystem orchestration

Investment shifts from single assets to reusable data and AI capabilities

Governance shifts from rule enforcement to trust enablement

Success shifts from speed alone to sustained, ethical impact

Executive takeaway

Pharma 2040 will reward organizations that learn faster than their environment changes. Those that cling to pipeline logic will optimize themselves out of relevance.

16.3.2 The new generation of pharma actors

In 2040, the industry will feature a mix of reinvented legacy firms, born-digital biotech players, and cross-industry collaborators. Below are projected players reshaping the space:

Category	Role in 2040 Ecosystem
Pharma-AI conglomerates	Pfizer-AI, Roche Quantum, Novartis Neuron—integrating full AI pipelines
Biotech ecosystem platforms	Modular R&D ecosystems like Recursion-X or Atomwise Labs 2040
Retail-tech pharma hubs	Amazon Health, Alibaba Life, Apple Wellness—combining delivery + therapy
Clinical cloud integrators	Google DeepHealth, Microsoft CareAI—offering population-scale AI services
Open innovation coalitions	Public–private partnerships for data sharing and ethics (e.g., WHO-AI-PHARMA)

16.3.3 Innovation frontiers—what will define leadership?

Three pillars will define competitive advantage and leadership in 2040:

1. Hyper-personalization: Every patient's therapy is tailored based on longitudinal health data, including genomics, lifestyle, social determinants, and wearable/implantable sensors.
2. Platform dominance: The most powerful firms will own or control platforms that connect discovery, diagnostics, digital care, and post-market surveillance.
3. Ethical-AI trust networks: Companies that successfully align data governance, algorithmic transparency, and public trust will secure long-term leadership.

"Pharma 2040 will not be an industry of pills—it will be an industry of platforms, precision, and partnerships."

16.3.4 The operating model of Pharma 2040: human–AI, platform governance, and decision rights

The defining advantage of Pharma 2040 will not be access to emerging technologies alone, but the ability to operationalize them safely, repeatedly, and at scale. This requires an operating model designed for high-stakes, regulated innovation—one that integrates human judgment with machine intelligence while maintaining clear accountability, auditability, and patient-centered purpose. In this context, "AI-native pharma" does not mean fully automated pharma; it means an enterprise capable of continuous learning across discovery, development, manufacturing, and real-world outcomes, under governance that preserves safety, ethics, and trust.

A Pharma 2040 operating model is built around three mutually reinforcing design principles:

1. Human–AI decision architecture (accountability by design). AI systems will increasingly generate hypotheses, optimize protocols, detect safety signals, and recommend actions across the value chain. However, value and legitimacy depend on decision accountability. Future-ready organizations define decision rights explicitly: what AI can recommend, what

humans must approve, how exceptions are escalated, and how responsibility is documented when human judgment diverges from algorithmic outputs. Rather than treating AI as a "black box," leading firms institutionalize structured review pathways for high-impact decisions (e.g., trial design changes, safety signal escalation, quality deviations, and regulatory-critical evidence generation).

2. Platform governance (from functions to integrated intelligence). By 2040, pharma operations will be orchestrated through interoperable platforms that connect R&D, clinical development, manufacturing, quality, supply chain, and post-market surveillance into one learning system. Platform governance ensures that data products, models, and workflows share consistent standards for interoperability, metadata, provenance, and traceability. This is particularly critical as organizations increasingly collaborate across ecosystem boundaries (providers, CROs, regulators, technology partners). In platform-based pharma, governance is not administrative overhead; it is the mechanism that enables scalable innovation without sacrificing compliance.
3. Regulatory-grade AI operations (AI-Ops for GxP environments). In regulated contexts, AI must be treated as a controlled asset within the quality system. This requires disciplined AI life-cycle management: validated intended use, documented performance thresholds, explainability coverage for high-risk decisions, monitoring for model drift and bias, controlled change management for model updates, and evidence-ready audit trails. In 2040, organizations that institutionalize "GxP-grade AI operations" will reduce friction in regulatory interactions, accelerate trustworthy adoption, and sustain performance over time. Conversely, organizations that treat AI deployment as a purely technical exercise may scale quickly—but will struggle with auditability, trust erosion, and regulatory resistance.

Strategic implication: the operating model becomes the true differentiator. By 2040, competitive advantage will increasingly come from the ability to run the enterprise as a governed learning system—one where real-world evidence strengthens discovery priorities, manufacturing analytics improve quality and resilience, and post-market signals refine therapies and safety practices continuously. In such organizations, human expertise remains central: not as manual decision-making, but as ethical stewardship, clinical accountability, and strategic orchestration of intelligent systems.

With the operating model established, Section 16.4 turns to the service and startup innovations that will define the Pharma 2040 value stack.

16.4 Services and startup innovations for Pharma 2040

As we look toward the year 2040, the pharmaceutical industry must evolve beyond traditional product-centric approaches. It must embrace a service-oriented, platform-driven, patient-centric paradigm that addresses the growing complexity of healthcare needs. Startups, fueled by agile models, disruptive technologies, and strong value-driven missions, will serve as **innovation catalysts** in this landscape.

This section outlines visionary services, future-proof startup models, and their unique value propositions that will shape the next generation of pharmaceutical innovations.

16.4.1 The new era of pharma services

Future pharmaceutical services will be defined by continuity of care, real-time monitoring, and intelligent, predictive systems. They will blend therapeutics with technology and user experience. Key future service categories include:

- Real-time precision therapeutics services: Platforms that deliver AI-optimized dosing and scheduling recommendations based on live health data streams.
- Behavioral-pharma platforms: Services that combine pharmacological treatments with AI-driven behavioral interventions, such as digital therapeutics integrated into therapy regimens.
- Predictive pharmacovigilance: AI-powered services that predict adverse events at the population scale, integrating EHRs, wearables, and social media analytics for proactive safety alerts.
- Telepharmacy-as-a-Service (TPaaS): Distributed platforms offering clinical pharmacy consultations, remote dispensing, and AI-assisted prescription validation at home or via smart kiosks.
- Genomic lifestyle advisory services: Personalized drug recommendations tied to lifestyle data, nutrigenomics, and epigenetic markers—offered via subscription-based models.

16.4.2 Disruptive startups: leading the charge

By 2040, startups will no longer simply “disrupt”—they will redefine pharmaceutical value chains. The following are are emerging models we envision leading:

- BioSynX—An AI-powered synthetic biology firm producing on-demand therapeutic enzymes using bio-printers integrated in hospitals.
- MediTrust.AI—A trust-as-a-service startup leveraging blockchain for medication authenticity, patient consent, and AI auditability.
- NanoRx Systems—Specializing in nanoscale delivery mechanisms and smart pills with biosensors that track adherence, release rates, and pharmacokinetics in real time.
- PharmIntuit—A decentralized R&D collective that matches AI-discovered compounds with clinical needs through DAO (Decentralized Autonomous Organization) structures.
- NeuroCareLoop—Delivering neuromodulation-enhanced pharmacotherapy, integrating AI brain feedback loops to optimize CNS drug efficacy.
- EcoPharma Nexus—A circular-economy pharma service optimizing drug recycling, disposal, and green manufacturing footprints.

Each of these startups reflects a unique value proposition aligned with the future challenges of pharma:

Startup	Core innovation	Value delivered
BioSynX	On-site synthetic biology via AI	Speed, cost-efficiency, localization
MediTrust.AI	Transparent blockchain-based pharma records	Trust, security, regulatory compliance
NanoRx Systems	Smart ingestible devices	Adherence tracking, micro-dosing optimization
PharmIntuit	Crowd-AI drug discovery & validation	Speed, open innovation, democratization
NeuroCareLoop	AI-enabled brain–drug interface	Personalized CNS care, real-time adjustments
EcoPharma Nexus	Circular pharma platform	Sustainability, waste reduction, regulatory alignment

The Startup Archetypes of Pharma 2040: Who Creates Value and How

Core insight: By 2040, pharmaceutical startups will no longer compete primarily on single technologies or niche tools. Instead, they will differentiate through how they create, scale, and govern value within complex health ecosystems. Successful startups will fall into a small number of distinct archetypes, each addressing a critical systemic need.

Five dominant startup archetypes in Pharma 2040

1. The intelligence amplifier

What they do: Enhance human decision-making rather than replace it.

Core capabilities:

Explainable AI for clinical, regulatory, and R&D decisions

Decision-support systems embedded in workflows

Bias detection, uncertainty signaling, and confidence scoring

Value created:

Better decisions under uncertainty

Faster approvals with higher trust

Reduced risk of automation bias

Example logic: AI that *guides* trial design rather than autonomously running it.

2. The personalization engine

What they do: Operationalize individualized medicine at population scale.

Core capabilities:

Digital twins (patient, disease, therapy)

Genomics, epigenomics, and lifestyle integration

Adaptive dosing and treatment optimization

Value created:

Higher efficacy and adherence

(cont'd)

Reduced waste and adverse events

Outcome-based reimbursement enablement

Example logic: No two patients receive the same therapy in the same way.

3. The trust infrastructure provider

What they do: Create the invisible rails of trust across pharma ecosystems.
Core capabilities:

Blockchain-based traceability

Consent and data rights management

AI audit trails and compliance automation

Value created:

Regulatory confidence

Patient and partner trust

Reduced fraud and data misuse

Example logic: Trust becomes a *service*, not an assumption.

4. The resilience architect

What they do: Design systems that absorb shocks without collapse.
Core capabilities:

Digital twins for supply chains and manufacturing

Distributed production and edge pharma models

Predictive risk sensing (geopolitical, climate, epidemiological)

Value created:

Continuity during crises

Faster recovery from disruptions

Strategic optionality under uncertainty

Example logic: Pharma systems that bend—but do not break.

5. The ecosystem orchestrator

What they do: Coordinate multi-actor innovation across boundaries.
Core capabilities:

Platform governance and API ecosystems

Partner onboarding and value-sharing mechanisms

Outcome-linked collaboration models

Value created:

Accelerated innovation through co-creation

Reduced duplication and friction

(cont'd)

Network effects rather than asset accumulation

Example logic: Winning by connecting others, not owning everything.
Strategic pattern across archetypes
What unites successful Pharma 2040 startups is not size or speed, but positioning:

They solve systemic problems, not local inefficiencies

They scale through integration, not domination

They monetize outcomes, trust, and intelligence, not volume alone

Executive takeaway

In Pharma 2040, the most valuable startups will not ask:"What technology do we have?" They will ask: "What capability does the ecosystem lack–and how do we responsibly provide it?"

16.4.3 Unlocking the startup value stack

To address the demands of Pharma 2040, these startups will deliver value through:

- Personalization-at-scale: Startups will leverage massive federated datasets to individualize interventions without compromising privacy.
- Interoperability-by-design: APIs and health-tech standards will allow startups to integrate with national health systems, EMRs, insurance platforms, and pharma supply chains.
- Outcome-based business models: Payment and partnership models will shift to value-based pricing, linking reimbursement to measurable patient outcomes.
- Co-creation ecosystems: Startups will thrive not by working alone, but by engaging in multistakeholder collaborations, including patients, hospitals, pharma, and regulators.

"Startups will no longer be outsiders—they will be the architects of future pharma value."

In the next section, we synthesize our insights and provide a comprehensive **discussion and conclusion**, focusing on the strategic imperatives that will define the industry's success in 2040.

16.5 Discussion and conclusions: toward a patient-centric, technology-enabled future (tightened executive version)

As the pharmaceutical industry moves toward 2040, transformation will be defined by convergence: AI, data infrastructure, synthetic biology, and platform governance will reshape how therapies are discovered, validated, delivered, and monitored. Yet technology alone will not determine success. The decisive factor will be whether organizations can translate innovation into trusted, equitable, and resilient patient value at scale.

16.5.1 A human-centered revolution

Even in a future shaped by autonomous systems and bio-digital interfaces, pharma's legitimacy remains anchored in human outcomes. Patient-centricity must evolve from a slogan into an operating principle: patient agency, measurable outcomes, and dignity-by-design become non-negotiable. The sector's next frontier is not only molecular precision but also the ability to embed empathy, inclusion, and real-world context into digital care pathways.

16.5.2 Strategic integration of technologies

Competitive advantage in Pharma 2040 will come from orchestration, not accumulation. The winners will integrate AI, IoT, blockchain, digital twins, and advanced analytics into a coherent learning system spanning R&D, trials, manufacturing, supply chain, and post-market evidence. This integration will be enabled by interoperable platforms, reusable data assets, and decision architectures that clarify what is automated, what is augmented, and what remains explicitly human-controlled.

16.5.3 The new ethics and governance imperative

As intelligence becomes embedded, adaptive, and distributed, governance becomes the strategic bottleneck. High-performing organizations will move beyond compliance toward governance-by-design: accountability for AI-supported decisions, auditable evidence generation, explicit data rights, and continuous monitoring for bias, drift, and misuse. In practice, this requires institutionalized mechanisms—not occasional reviews—linking ethical oversight to development, deployment, and lifecycle management.

The Governance Test of Pharma 2040: Where Intelligence, Ethics, and Power Converge

Core warning: By 2040, the most critical risks facing the pharmaceutical industry will not stem from scientific failure or technological limitation—but from governance failure. As AI systems design molecules, personalize therapies, predict outcomes, and influence regulatory decisions, pharma organizations will confront a fundamental question:

Who is accountable when intelligence is distributed across humans, machines, and ecosystems?

Why governance becomes the strategic bottleneck

In Pharma 2040, intelligence is:

Embedded (in platforms, workflows, devices)

Distributed (across partners, clouds, and borders)

Adaptive (continuously learning and evolving)

Traditional governance models—designed for linear pipelines and static decision-making—will be structurally inadequate.

(cont'd)

Five governance fault lines in Pharma 2040

1. Decision authority versus decision automation
Tension: AI systems increasingly recommend, prioritize, and optimize—but who retains final authority?
Risk: Automation bias, unclear liability, erosion of clinical and regulatory judgment.
Governance imperative: Explicit human-in-the-loop and human-on-the-loop decision architectures, with clear escalation protocols.
2. Data power and asymmetry
Tension: Control over data (genomic, behavioral, real-world evidence) becomes a source of strategic and political power.
Risk: Data monopolies, inequitable access, exploitation of vulnerable populations.
Governance Imperative: Data stewardship models emphasizing data rights, reciprocity, and public-interest use.
3. Explainability versus performance
Tension: The most powerful AI models are often the least interpretable.
Risk: Regulatory rejection, loss of trust, inability to contest decisions.
Governance imperative: Risk-tiered explainability: the higher the impact, the higher the explainability requirement.
4. Ecosystem accountability gaps
Tension: Innovation spans pharma companies, AI vendors, cloud providers, hospitals, and startups.
Risk: Diffuse responsibility, blame-shifting during failures.
Governance imperative: Shared accountability frameworks with contractual, technical, and ethical alignment.
5. Ethics at scale
Tension: Ethical decisions are no longer rare edge cases—they are embedded in everyday algorithmic choices.
Risk: Normalization of bias, silent harm, loss of societal legitimacy.
Governance imperative: Ethics-by-design embedded into product development, validation, and monitoring—not posthoc review.

Executive insight

In Pharma 2040, governance is not a compliance function. It is a strategic capability that determines trust, legitimacy, and survival.

Organizations that fail the governance test will not merely face fines—they will lose the license to operate in data-driven healthcare ecosystems.

16.5.4 From pipelines to platforms

By 2040, the dominant architecture will shift from linear pipelines to platform ecosystems. These platforms will connect diagnostics, therapeutics, digital services, and outcomes monitoring in continuous loops. Value creation will shift accordingly: from volume and exclusivity to outcome performance, trust, safety, and lifecycle engagement. In platform-based pharma, the strategic unit is not the product alone, but the capability to learn from real-world use and improve therapies responsibly over time.

16.5.5 The final word: resilience and adaptability

Resilience will separate leaders from laggards. The future will test pharma with systemic shocks—pandemics, climate disruptions, cyber risks, and geopolitical volatility—while expectations for speed and equity rise. Organizations that design for modularity, distributed capability, and adaptive governance will sustain continuity of care and protect legitimacy. Ultimately, Pharma 2040 will be judged not by the sophistication of its tools, but by the responsibility, trust, and human value those tools deliver.

Pharma 2040 will not be defined solely by technological sophistication—but by moral clarity, human-centricity, and ecosystem collaboration. The future belongs to those organizations that invest not just in innovation, but in values, inclusivity, and global solidarity. As the industry transitions into a data-intelligent, decentralized, and outcome-based model, patients must remain at the center—not just as consumers, but as co-creators of health.

Let us imagine a pharmaceutical future where data empowers healing, not exploitation; where automation accelerates care, not alienation; and where innovation serves purpose, not profit alone.

Pharma 2040 Readiness Checklist for Executives

Pharma 2040 readiness checklist

1. Strategic self-assessment for boards and executive teams
   a. Intelligence readiness
      i. AI is embedded in core decisions, not just analytics
      ii. Decision ownership is clearly defined when AI is involved
      iii. Models are monitored for drift, bias, and misuse
      iv. Explainability standards align with regulatory and ethical risk
2. Data and infrastructure readiness
   a. Data is interoperable across R&D, clinical, manufacturing, and post-market domains
   b. FAIR principles are operationalized, not aspirational
   c. Real-world evidence pipelines are validated and trusted
   d. Cybersecurity and privacy are designed for continuous data flows
3. Governance and ethics readiness
   a. AI systems are treated as regulated assets, not IT tools
   b. Ethics-by-design is embedded in innovation lifecycles
   c. Accountability is explicit across internal teams and partners
   d. Governance frameworks evolve as fast as technology

(cont'd)

4. Organizational and talent readiness
    a. Cross-disciplinary teams combine pharma, data, ethics, and systems thinking
    b. Leaders are AI-literate, not AI-dependent
    c. Incentives reward responsible innovation, not speed alone
    d. Continuous upskilling is institutionalized
5. Ecosystem and partnership readiness
    a. The organization can orchestrate—not just participate in—ecosystems
    b. Data-sharing agreements align value, risk, and trust
    c. Startups and platforms are integrated strategically, not opportunistically
    d. Regulators are engaged as partners, not obstacles
6. Human-centered value readiness
    a. Patient outcomes—not volume—define success
    b. Equity and access are explicit design criteria
    c. Technologies enhance human judgment and dignity
    d. Societal impact is measured alongside financial performance

Final executive reflection

Pharma 2040 readiness is not about predicting the future. It is about building organizations capable of learning, governing, and adapting responsibly—no matter what the future brings.

16.5.6 Editor's closing note: from technological possibility to human responsibility

As the concluding chapter, it integrates the book's sectoral insights into a single forward-looking argument: that future pharma excellence will be measured by the ability to learn, govern, and deliver patient value under uncertainty.

As this volume concludes, one message becomes unmistakably clear: the future of the pharmaceutical industry will not be determined by technology alone. AI, digital platforms, synthetic biology, and advanced analytics are reshaping what is possible—but it is human judgment, governance, and values that will determine what is acceptable, trustworthy, and sustainable.

Across the chapters of this book, pharma emerges not as a standalone industry, but as a central pillar of a broader health and innovation ecosystem—one that spans data infrastructures, clinical practice, regulation, and society itself. In this context, leadership is no longer defined by scale or speed alone. It is defined by the ability to integrate intelligence with accountability, innovation with ethics, and automation with human-centered design.

Looking toward 2040, the most successful pharmaceutical organizations will be those that treat AI not as a shortcut, but as a responsibility; not as a replacement for expertise, but as a partner to it. They will invest as deeply in governance, talent, and trust as they do in algorithms and platforms. Above all, they will recognize that the ultimate measure of progress is not technological sophistication, but improved human health, equity, and resilience.

This book is intended not as a prediction, but as a compass. It invites decision-makers, researchers, policymakers, and innovators to shape a pharmaceutical future that is intelligent *and* humane—one where progress is guided by purpose, and innovation serves society at large.

The Pharma 2040 Manifesto: Ten Principles for a Responsible, Intelligent Future

Pharma 2040 is not a destination. It is a choice.

The following principles articulate a shared commitment to shaping a pharmaceutical future that is innovative, ethical, and human-centered:

Patients are not data points: Every algorithm, platform, and therapy must serve human dignity and lived experience.

AI augments judgment–it does not replace responsibility: Accountability always remains human, even when intelligence is artificial.

Trust is a strategic asset: Transparency, explainability, and fairness are sources of long-term competitive advantage.

Governance must evolve as fast as technology: Static rules cannot govern adaptive systems.

Data is a shared resource, not a private weapon: Stewardship replaces ownership in health-critical data ecosystems.

Innovation without equity is failure: Access, inclusion, and global health impact are non-negotiable design criteria.

Platforms must serve outcomes, not lock-ins: Interoperability and openness enable sustainable ecosystems.

Ethics is not a constraint–it is an accelerator: Responsible design enables scale, adoption, and legitimacy.

Human-AI collaboration defines excellence: The future belongs to organizations that design for complementarity, not substitution.

The purpose of pharma is healing, not optimization: Technology is the means; human well-being is the end.

Final commitment: Pharma 2040 will be remembered not for the intelligence it created–but for the responsibility with which it used it.

Learning activities

To deepen understanding of the concepts discussed in this chapter and to encourage practical engagement with the ideas shaping Pharma 2040, the following learning activities are proposed for students, professionals, and innovators across the pharmaceutical and healthcare ecosystem:

1. Case study analysis: resilience in pharma supply chains

Objective: Analyze how leading pharmaceutical companies adapted during recent global disruptions (e.g., COVID-19 pandemic) and evaluate the resilience strategies they implemented.

Instructions:

- Select a major pharmaceutical company (e.g., Pfizer, Moderna, Roche).
- Investigate how they managed R&D, manufacturing, and global distribution under pressure.
- Identify technological interventions used to enhance supply chain flexibility and patient delivery models.
- Prepare a report highlighting key lessons and how these lessons support a resilient Pharma 2040.

2. Future scenarios workshop: designing the Pharma 2040 Ecosystem

Objective: Imagine and prototype what the pharmaceutical industry will look like in 2040, based on technological and societal trends.

Instructions:

- Form teams to represent pharma startups, regulators, patient advocacy groups, and tech providers.
- Use design thinking to map a future healthcare ecosystem that integrates new drugs, AI services, and patient-centric platforms.
- Present the ecosystem model through visual sketches or digital infographics.
- Discuss ethical, technological, and regulatory implications of the scenario.

3. Research and presentation: mapping pharma startups and their value propositions

Objective: Investigate the emerging global startup ecosystem in pharma and analyze its unique contributions.

Instructions:

- Identify 3–5 pharma tech startups (e.g., BenevolentAI, Recursion Pharmaceuticals, Owkin).
- Explore their core offerings (AI-driven discovery, predictive analytics, clinical trial optimization, etc.).
- Summarize each startup's mission, innovation model, funding trajectory, and market impact.
- Prepare a comparative presentation assessing which ones are best positioned for Pharma 2040.

4. Ethical dilemma debate: should artificial intelligence replace human decisions in drug development?

Objective: Engage critically with the ethical issues surrounding automation and AI in pharma.

Instructions:

- Divide into two groups: one advocating for full AI integration in drug development, the other supporting human oversight.
- Research recent developments in generative drug design and automated clinical trials.
- Debate the merits, risks, and ethical implications.
- Reflect on where the balance should lie in the future.

5. Strategic planning exercise: building a pharma company for 2040

Objective: Apply strategic management frameworks to build a hypothetical pharma company that is future-proof.

Instructions:
- Develop a business model using tools like the Business Model Canvas or SWOT analysis.
- Define the technology stack (AI, blockchain, synthetic biology, etc.).
- Clarify the value proposition: patient outcomes, sustainability, and personalization.
- Create a one-page strategic roadmap outlining milestones through 2040.

6. Reflective essay: pharma's role in the human future

Objective: Reflect on the broader social and human implications of pharmaceutical innovation in the age of AI and superintelligence.

Instructions:
- Write a short essay (800–1000 words) exploring one of the following prompts:
- What does "patient-centric" mean in the context of intelligent, digital pharma?
- How can we ensure equity and global access to advanced pharmaceutical care?
- Will technology bring us closer to healing—or create new divides?

These activities aim to spark reflection, collaboration, and strategic foresight. They are not only intended to build competence in current pharmaceutical practices but also to inspire leadership in shaping the ethical, technological, and social dimensions of Pharma 2040.

References

Bano, I., Butt, U. D., & Mohsan, S. A. H. (2022). New challenges in drug discovery. In *Novel Platforms for Drug Delivery Applications*. China: Elsevier, 619–643. https://www.sciencedirect.com/book/9780323913768.

Basit, A. (2020). Recent innovations in 3D-printed personalized medicines: An interview with Abdul Basit. *Journal of 3D Printing in Medicine, 4*(1), 5–7. https://doi.org/10.2217/3dp-2020-0010.

Basu, S., & Heumann, K. (2024). Data integrity and AI: How pharma can build a data-driven future. *European Pharmaceutical Review, 29*(3), 30. https://edition.pagesuite-professional.co.uk/html5/reader/production/default.aspx?pubname=&edid=0b01b133-379e-4768-8339-accd662d874f.

Busquets, J., Ramírez-Peinado, S., Peiró, M., & Camacho, M. (2024). Novartis oncology Spain: Agile innovation and the RWE cell. *Journal of Information Technology Teaching Cases, 14*(2), 247–261. https://doi.org/10.1177/20438869231165537.

Coucke, P. A. (2021). Pharma industry reinvents itself in the turmoil. Part 1. Challenges. *Revue Medicale de Liege, 76*(3), 216–220. https://www.rmlg.ulg.ac.be/index.php?page=listeArt?date=2021%20Mar&langue=EN.

Dupuy, S., Opincar, L., Pandya, K., Wnorowski, S., Cuellar, M., Riggins, J., & Hermes-DeSantis, E. R. (2024). An update from the benchmark survey of phactMI™ member companies on providing medical information in the digital space. *Therapeutic Innovation and Regulatory Science, 58*(1), 200–213. https://doi.org/10.1007/s43441-023-00587-1, https://www.springer.com/journal/43441.

Gelis, L., Stoeckert, I., & Podhaisky, H. P. (2023). Digital tools—Regulatory considerations for application in clinical trials. *Therapeutic Innovation and Regulatory Science, 57*(4), 769–782. https://doi.org/10.1007/s43441-023-00535-z, https://www.springer.com/journal/43441.

Jones, C. H., Madhavan, S., Natarajan, K., Corbo, M., True, J. M., & Dolsten, M. (2024). Rewriting the textbook for pharma: How to adapt and thrive in a digital, personalized and collaborative world. *Drug Discovery Today, 29*(9). https://doi.org/10.1016/j.drudis.2024.104112, https://www.sciencedirect.com/science/journal/13596446.

Ladner, T., Weh, C., Dhillon, A., Giffard, M., & Iacovelli, D. (2025). Data computation platform (DCP): Empowering pharma 4.0 innovation through GxP-compliant and scalable software platform enabling advanced data analytics and real-time process monitoring in regulated environments. *Journal of Intelligent Manufacturing*. https://doi.org/10.1007/s10845-025-02574-9.

Malheiro, V., Duarte, J., Veiga, F., & Mascarenhas-Melo, F. (2023). Exploiting pharma 4.0 technologies in the non-biological complex drugs manufacturing: Innovations and implications. *Pharmaceutics, 15*(11), 2545. https://doi.org/10.3390/pharmaceutics15112545.

Mirzaei, A., & Rijcken, C. (2023). *Pharmaceutical Care in Digital Revolution: Blending Digital with Human Innovation* (2nd ed.). Australia: Elsevier, 1–383. https://www.sciencedirect.com/book/9780443133602.

Pazhayattil, A. B., & Konyu-Fogel, G. (2023). ML and Ai implementation insights for bio/pharma manufacturing. *BioPharm International, 36*(10), 24–29. http://creative.advanstar.com/subcatalog/2017/mag_pages/life_sci/pt.htm.

Pörtner, L., Riel, A., Schmidt, B., Leclaire, M., & Möske, R. (2025). Data management maturity model—Process dimensions and capabilities to leverage data-driven organizations towards industry 5.0. *Applied System Innovation, 8*(2), 41. https://doi.org/10.3390/asi8020041.

Ramos, M. V., Beleiro, B. L., Fernandez, M. G., Martinez, M. G., & Urquijo, J.de S. (2020). Together beyond COVID-19 - A look at the future. *Chimica Oggi/Chemistry Today, 38*(6), 54–57. https://www.teknoscienze.com/tks_issue/vol-386/.

Sowndharya, M., Joga, R., Gandhi, K., Vijay, G. K., Waikar, S., Yerram, S., Raghuvanshi, R. S., & Srivastava, S. (2025). Navigating the trends in USFDA authorized generic approvals (2019–2024): Enhancing healthcare accessibility and affordability. *Therapeutic Innovation and Regulatory Science*. https://doi.org/10.1007/s43441-025-00806-x, https://www.springer.com/journal/43441.

Steinwandter, V., Borchert, D., & Herwig, C. (2019). Data science tools and applications on the way to Pharma 4.0. *Drug Discovery Today, 24*(9), 1795–1805. https://doi.org/10.1016/j.drudis.2019.06.005.

Yoshiura, H., Kawata, Y., & Sengoku, S. (2025). Open innovation and regulatory challenges in new modality development: The pivotal role of contract development and manufacturing organisations in advancing antibody drugs. *Therapeutic Innovation & Regulatory Science, 59*(1), 63–70. https://doi.org/10.1007/s43441-024-00701-x.

Index

Note: Page numbers followed by "*f*" and "*t*" refer to figures and tables, respectively.

Printed and bound by CPI Group (UK) Ltd, Croydon, CR0 4YY
14/09/2026
02216408-0015